Updates on Endoscopic Submucosal Dissection and Third Space Endoscopy

Editor

AMRITA SETHI

GASTROINTESTINAL ENDOSCOPY CLINICS OF NORTH AMERICA

www.giendo.theclinics.com

Consulting Editor
CHARLES J. LIGHTDALE

January 2023 • Volume 33 • Number 1

ELSEVIER

1600 John F. Kennedy Boulevard • Suite 1800 • Philadelphia, Pennsylvania, 19103-2899

http://www.theclinics.com

GASTROINTESTINAL ENDOSCOPY CLINICS OF NORTH AMERICA Volume 33, Number 1
January 2023 ISSN 1052-5157, ISBN-13: 978-0-323-96085-4

Editor: Kerry Holland
Developmental Editor: Jessica Cañaberal

Photocopying

Single photocopies of single articles may be made for personal use as allowed by national copyright laws. Permission of the Publisher and payment of a fee is required for all other photocopying, including multiple or systematic copying, copying for advertising or promotional purposes, resale, and all forms of document delivery. Special rates are available for educational institutions that wish to make photocopies for non-profit educational classroom use. For information on how to seek permission visit www.elsevier.com/permissions or call: (+44) 1865 843830 (UK)/(+1) 215 239 3804 (USA).

Derivative Works

Subscribers may reproduce tables of contents or prepare lists of articles including abstracts for internal circulation within their institutions. Permission of the Publisher is required for resale or distribution outside the institution. Permission of the Publisher is required for all other derivative works, including compilations and translations (please consult www.elsevier.com/permissions).

Electronic Storage or Usage

Permission of the Publisher is required to store or use electronically any material contained in this periodical, including any article or part of an article (please consult www.elsevier.com/permissions). Except as outlined above, no part of this publication may be reproduced, stored in a retrieval system or transmitted in any form or by any means, electronic, mechanical, photocopying, recording or otherwise, without prior written permission of the Publisher.

Notice

No responsibility is assumed by the Publisher for any injury and/or damage to persons or property as a matter of products liability, negligence or otherwise, or from any use or operation of any methods, products, instructions or ideas contained in the material herein. Because of rapid advances in the medical sciences, in particular, independent verification of diagnoses and drug dosages should be made.

Although all advertising material is expected to conform to ethical (medical) standards, inclusion in this publication does not constitute a guarantee or endorsement of the quality or value of such product or of the claims made of it by its manufacturer.

Gastrointestinal Endoscopy Clinics of North America (ISSN 1052-5157) is published quarterly by Elsevier Inc., 360 Park Avenue South, New York, NY 10010-1710. Months of issue are January, April, July, and October. Business and Editorial Offices: 1600 John F. Kennedy Blvd., Suite 1800, Philadelphia, PA, 19103-2899. Periodicals postage paid at New York, NY and additional mailing offices. Subscription prices are $381.00 per year for US individuals, $703.00 per year for US institutions, $100.00 per year for US and Canadian students/residents, $419.00 per year for Canadian individuals, $830.00 per year for Canadian institutions, $501.00 per year for international individuals, $830.00 per year for international institutions, and $245.00 per year for international students/residents. To receive student/resident rate, orders must be accompanied by name of affiliated institution, date of term, and the signature of program/residency coordinator on institution letterhead. Orders will be billed at individual rate until proof of status is received. Foreign air speed delivery is included in all Clinics subscription prices. All prices are subject to change without notice. POSTMASTER: Send address change to Gastrointestinal Endoscopy Clinics of North America, Elsevier Health Sciences Division, Subscription Customer Service, 3251 Riverport Lane, Maryland Heights, MO 63043. Customer Service: 1-800-654-2452 (US). From outside the United States, call 1-314-447-8871. Fax: 1-314-447-8029. E-mail: JournalsCustomerService-usa@elsevier.com (for print support) or JournalsOnlineSupport-usa@elsevier.com (for online support).

Reprints. For copies of 100 or more, of articles in this publication, please contact the Commercial Reprints Department, Elsevier Inc., 360 Park Avenue South, New York, NY 10010-1710. Tel. 212-633-3874; Fax: 212-633-3820; E-mail: reprints@elsevier.com.

Gastrointestinal Endoscopy Clinics of North America is covered in Excerpta Medica, MEDLINE/PubMed (Index Medicus), and MEDLINE/MEDLARS.

Contributors

CONSULTING EDITOR

CHARLES J. LIGHTDALE, MD
Professor of Medicine, Division of Digestive and Liver Diseases, Columbia University Medical Center, New York, New York, USA

EDITOR

AMRITA SETHI, MD, MASGE, NYSGEF
Professor of Medicine, Director of Interventional Endoscopy, Program Director, Advanced Endoscopy Fellowship, Division of Digestive and Liver Disease, Columbia University Irving Medical Center-NYP, New York, New York, USA

AUTHORS

HIROYUKI AIHARA, MD, PhD
Division of Gastroenterology, Hepatology, and Endoscopy, Brigham and Women's Hospital, Harvard Medical School, Boston, Massachusetts, USA

SARAH S. AL GHAMDI, MBBS, FRCPC
Division of Gastroenterology and Hepatology, Department of Medicine, King Abdulaziz University, Jeddah, Saudi Arabia

SUNIL AMIN, MD
Division of Digestive Health and Liver Diseases, Department of Medicine, University of Miami, Miller School of Medicine at the University of Miami, Miami, Florida, USA

AMOL BAPAYE, MD, (MS), FASGE, FJGES, FISG, FSGEI
Shivanand Desai Center for Digestive Disorders, Deenanath Mangeshkar Hospital and Research Center, Pune, India

JAY BAPAYE, MD
Department of Internal Medicine, Rochester General Hospital, Rochester, New York, USA

MING-YAN CAI, MD, PhD, FASGE
Endoscopy Center and Endoscopy Research Institute, Zhongshan Hospital, Fudan University, Shanghai Collaborative Innovation Center of Endoscopy, Shanghai, China

PHILIP WAI-YAN CHIU, MD, FRCSED
Division of Upper GI and Metabolic Surgery, Department of Surgery, Institute of Digestive Disease, Faculty of Medicine, The Chinese University of Hong Kong, Hong Kong; Multi-Scale Medical Robotics Center, Hong Kong, China

ZHIWEI DONG, MSURG
Division of Upper GI and Metabolic Surgery, Department of Surgery, Institute of Digestive Disease, Faculty of Medicine, The Chinese University of Hong Kong, Hong Kong; Multi-Scale Medical Robotics Center, Hong Kong, China

PETER V. DRAGANOV, MD
Professor of Medicine, Director of Advanced Therapeutic Endoscopy, University of Florida, Gainesville, Florida, USA

NORIO FUKAMI, MD, AGAF, FACG, MASGE, FJGES
Professor of Medicine, Mayo Clinic College of Medicine and Science, Mayo Clinic Arizona, Scottsdale, Arizona, USA

ASHISH GANDHI, MD, DNB
Shivanand Desai Center for Digestive Disorders, Deenanath Mangeshkar Hospital and Research Center, Pune, India

ZI-HAN GENG, MD
Endoscopy Center and Endoscopy Research Institute, Zhongshan Hospital, Fudan University, Shanghai Collaborative Innovation Center of Endoscopy, Shanghai, China

AMYN HAJI, MA, MBBCHIR, MSC, MD, FRCS
Consultant, Laparoscopic Colorectal Surgeon and Interventional Endoscopist, Director of Surgery, King's College Hospital, London, United Kingdom

MUHAMMAD K. HASAN, MD
Center for Interventional Endoscopy, AdventHealth, Orlando, Florida, USA

JOO HA HWANG, MD, PhD
Division of Gastroenterology and Hepatology, Department of Medicine, Stanford University School of Medicine, Stanford, California, USA

HARUHIRO INOUE, MD
Professor and Chair, Digestive Diseases Center, Showa University Koto Toyosu Hospital, Tokyo, Japan

PICHAMOL JIRAPINYO, MD, MPH
Division of Gastroenterology, Hepatology, and Endoscopy, Brigham and Women's Hospital, Harvard Medical School, Boston, Massachusetts, USA

GRACE E. KIM, MD
Section of Gastroenterology, Hepatology, and Nutrition, Gastroenterology Fellow, University of Chicago, Chicago, Illinois, USA

SHIVANGI KOTHARI, MD
Division of Gastroenterology/Hepatology, Associate Professor of Medicine, Associate Director of Endoscopy, University of Rochester Medical Center & Strong Memorial Hospital, Rochester, New York, USA

ANDREW A. LI, MD
Division of Gastroenterology and Hepatology, Department of Medicine, Stanford University School of Medicine, Stanford, California, USA

ROBERTA MASELLI, MD, PhD
Department of Biomedical Sciences, Pieve Emanuele, Humanitas University, Rozzano, Italy; Humanitas Clinical and Research Center -IRCCS-, Endoscopy Unit, Rozzano, Italy

THOMAS R. MCCARTY, MD, MPH
Division of Gastroenterology, Hepatology, and Endoscopy, Brigham and Women's Hospital, Harvard Medical School, Boston, Massachusetts, USA

MARC JULIUS H. NAVARRO
Clinical fellow, Digestive Diseases Center, Showa University Koto Toyosu Hospital, Tokyo, Japan

SAOWANEE NGAMRUENGPHONG, MD
Division of Gastroenterology and Hepatology, Johns Hopkins Hospital, Baltimore, Maryland, USA

GAIA PELLEGATTA, MD
Humanitas Clinical and Research Center -IRCCS-, Endoscopy Unit, Rozzano, Italy

ALESSANDRO REPICI, MD
Professor, Department of Biomedical Sciences, Pieve Emanuele, Humanitas University, Rozzano, Italy; Humanitas Clinical and Research Center -IRCCS-, Endoscopy Unit, Rozzano, Italy

RAHIL H. SHAH, MD
Department of Medicine, University of Miami/Jackson Memorial Hospital, Miami, Florida, USA

YUTO SHIMAMURA
Assistant Professor, Digestive Diseases Center, Showa University Koto Toyosu Hospital, Tokyo, Japan

UZMA D. SIDDIQUI, MD
Section of Gastroenterology, Hepatology, and Nutrition, Professor of Medicine, Director of Director, Center for Endoscopic Research and Therapeutics (CERT) and Advanced Endoscopy Training, University of Chicago, Chicago, Illinois, USA

CEM SIMSEK, MD
Division of Gastroenterology, Hepatology, and Endoscopy, Brigham and Women's Hospital, Harvard Medical School, Boston, Massachusetts, USA

MARCO SPADACCINI, MD
Department of Biomedical Sciences, Pieve Emanuele, Humanitas University, Rozzano, Italy; Humanitas Clinical and Research Center -IRCCS-, Endoscopy Unit, Rozzano, Italy

MAYO TANABE
Assistant Professor, Digestive Diseases Center, Showa University Koto Toyosu Hospital, Tokyo, Japan

AKIKO TOSHIMORI
Assistant Professor, Digestive Diseases Center, Showa University Koto Toyosu Hospital, Tokyo, Japan

MANU VENKAT, MD
Instructor in Medicine, Department of Medicine, Columbia University Irving Medical Center, New York Presbyterian Hospital, New York, New York, USA

KAVEL VISRODIA, MD
Assistant Professor, Division of Digestive and Liver Diseases, Columbia University Irving Medical Center, New York Presbyterian Hospital, Herbert Irving Pavilion, New York, New York, USA

DENNIS YANG, MD
Center for Interventional Endoscopy, AdventHealth, Orlando, Florida, USA

MARGARET J. ZHOU, MD
Division of Gastroenterology and Hepatology, Department of Medicine, Stanford University School of Medicine, Stanford, California, USA

PING-HONG ZHOU, MD, PhD, FASGE
Endoscopy Center and Endoscopy Research Institute, Zhongshan Hospital, Fudan University, Shanghai Collaborative Innovation Center of Endoscopy, Shanghai, China

SIRAN ZHOU, MMED
Division of Upper GI and Metabolic Surgery, Department of Surgery, Institute of Digestive Disease, Faculty of Medicine, The Chinese University of Hong Kong, Hong Kong; Multi-Scale Medical Robotics Center, Hong Kong, China

Contents

> With the advent of endoscopic submucosal dissection, a variety of endoscopic devices including knives and high-frequency electrosurgical unit have become available. In addition, the concept of natural orifice transluminal endoscopic surgery pushed flexible endoscopic surgery ahead. In this review, the birth of peroral endoscopic myotomy and its expansion into the field of submucosal endoscopy are reviewed.

> Endoscopic submucosal dissection (ESD) is the preferred strategy for the resection of large superficial neoplasia throughout the gastrointestinal tract in Asian countries. The transition of ESD to the West has been slower because of various regional and training differences. Nonetheless, over the past couple of decades, the steady growth of ESD mentors in the West and the introduction of viable training pathways and dedicated devices and accessories have led to the increasing adoption of ESD and other third space endoscopic procedures.

 A video of double-clip traction method used during rectal ESD accompanies this article at http://www.giendo.theclinics.com.

> Endoscopic submucosal dissection (ESD) is a technically complex and still evolving procedure. As a result, there are many advances in the technology and tools available to assist the endoscopist. This article delves into the various tools developed for ESD including electrosurgical knives, caps, injection agents, and traction devices. The authors discuss tools available as well as their respective pros, cons, and technical considerations for use. Overall, the choice of tools depends on a multitude of factors from availability, cost, lesion characteristics, and the endoscopist's familiarity and proficiency.

endoscopic resection of EGC are if patients are presumed to have a less than 1% risk of lymph node metasta endoscopic submucosal dissection-sis, and long-term outcomes are similar to those with surgical gastrec-tomy. Duodenal ESD is more technically difficult and requires expertise in ESD in other locations.

> The concept of third space endoscopy is based on the principle that the deeper layers of the gastrointestinal tract can be accessed by tunneling in the submucosal space. The mucosal flap safety valve enabled endoscopists to use submucosal space securely. The era of third space endoscopy has expanded to treat various gastrointestinal disorders, such as mucosal lesions, SMTs, extraluminal tumors, achalasia, and others. Third space endoscopy emerged as a minimally invasive alternative to conventional surgery. Our review focused on the indications, techniques, clinical management, and adverse events of submucosal tunneling techniques for tumor resection.

> Colorectal cancer is the third most common cancer worldwide and the fourth leading cause of cancer-related deaths in the world, second in the United States. Although most lesions are managed surgically especially when they have already invaded into the submucosal layer, endoscopic full-thickness resection (EFTR) has become an emerging technique that can serve as a safe and effective alternative management for locally invasive gastrointestinal cancers. This article discusses the indications and various techniques and limitations of nontunneled EFTRs of gastrointestinal cancer and reviews the current literature on the outcomes of EFTR.

> The rapid expansion of third space endoscopy has necessitated development of innovative endoscopic defect closure devices and techniques. This article discusses commonly used endoscopic closure devices and techniques, data on their safety and efficacy, and a description of the authors' own practice patterns.

> The risk–benefit profile of submucosal endoscopic procedures is generally favorable but there exist unique considerations regarding the recognition, treatment, and prevention of submucosal endoscopic complications. Bleeding during the procedure can be managed with knife electrocautery, tamponade by injection of additional submucosal agent, or hemostatic forceps, depending on the location and degree of bleeding. Delayed bleeding should be managed with repeat endoscopy. Potential means to reduce the risk of delayed bleeding include anticipatory coagulation of visible vessels in the dissection ulcer base, applied hemostatic chemicals, snares, clips, and sheets of cultured cells.

Philip Wai-yan Chiu, Siran Zhou, and Zhiwei Dong

 Video content accompanies this article at http://www.giendo. theclinics.com.

Endoscopic resection has been widely applied especially in endoscopic submucosal dissection and third space endoscopy (TSE). Flexible endoluminal robotics allow performance of endoscopic submucosal dissection with exposure of the submucosal plane for precise dissection using two robotic arms. The introduction of TSE revolutionized the horizon of therapeutic endoscopy to the submucosal space beneath and beyond the mucosa. Advantages of TSE include avoidance of full thickness incision in gastrointestinal tract through the submucosal tunneling for performance of peroral endoscopic myotomy and submucosal tunneling endoscopic resection. In future, robotic-driven devices should be developed to enhance performance of complex endoluminal procedures and TSE.

GASTROINTESTINAL ENDOSCOPY CLINICS OF NORTH AMERICA

FORTHCOMING ISSUES

April 2023
Pediatric Endoscopy
Catherine M. Walsh, *Editor*

July 2023
Advances in Diagnosis and Therapy of Pancreatic Cystic Neoplasms
Tamas A. Gonda, *Editor*

October 2023
Updates in Pancreatic Endotherapy
D. Nageshwar Reddy and Rupjyoti Talukdar, *Editors*

RECENT ISSUES

October 2022
Interventional Inflammatory Bowel Disease: Endoscopic Treatment of Complications
Bo Shen, *Editor*

July 2022
Advances in Biliary Endoscopy
Mouen Khashab, *Editor*

April 2022
Colorectal Polyps
Aasma Shaukat, *Editor*

SERIES OF RELATED INTEREST

Gastroenterology Clinics
(www.gastro.theclinics.com)
Clinics in Liver Disease
(www.liver.theclinics.com)

Foreword

Third Space Endoscopy: Expanding Therapeutic Power

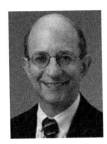

Charles J. Lightdale, MD
Consulting Editor

In an audacious and amazing progression, gastrointestinal (GI) endoscopists have opened a new vista where none seemed to exist–the submucosal space. A verb "to tunnel" has become central to the endoscopic method called third space endoscopy. Tunnelling through the mucosal lining of the GI tract into the submucosa with endoscopic instruments to create a space that can accommodate the scope itself was a truly disruptive achievement. Therapeutic applications of this technique have rapidly multiplied, adding tremendous new power to interventional endoscopy.

This is an extraordinary issue of the *Gastrointestinal Endoscopy Clinics of North America* devoted to the subject of third space endoscopy. The Editor for the issue is Dr Amrita Sethi, an internationally renowned interventional endoscopist, who is a central figure in guiding third space endoscopy into mainstream practice. Dr Sethi has provided a true state-of-the-art review of third space endoscopy topics with an over-the-top group of authors from around the world.

The issue begins with an authoritative history of the origins of the method in Asia, where the need for en bloc resection of early mucosal cancer in the stomach was a priority. The previous method, endoscopic mucosal resection, using cautery snares, often resulted in piecemeal removal associated with increased cancer recurrence. Japanese pioneers developed methods using needle-knife instruments based on those used for biliary endoscopy to tunnel around and under the lesions to be removed. I well remember when they came up with the name for this method: endoscopic submucosal dissection (ESD). The procedures, requiring skill and stamina, were first carried out in the stomach, and then with more difficulty in the esophagus, duodenum, colon, and rectum. As instruments and techniques improved, ESD spread from East to West and is performed widely throughout the world with accumulating results showing significant benefit. For removal of deeper tumors in submucosa and muscularis propria, the technique of endoscopic full-thickness resection (EFTR) has

Gastrointest Endoscopy Clin N Am 33 (2023) xiii–xiv
https://doi.org/10.1016/j.giec.2022.10.005
1052-5157/23/© 2022 Published by Elsevier Inc.

giendo.theclinics.com

been developed, with and without tunnelling. All the indications, techniques, and results so far are summarized in separate articles in this issue.

The next great leap came from extending the submucosal tunnel through long lengths of the esophagus to the esophagogastric junction, exposing the esophageal muscularis propria, which could then be excised (per-oral endoscopic myotomy or POEM) for treatment of achalasia and other esophageal motility disorders. Like ESD, POEM has been performed from the top to the bottom of the GI tract for a variety of smooth muscle disorders, with pyloric myotomy for selected cases of gastroparesis gaining traction. Again, articles describing indications, techniques, and results are included in this issue.

Training in third space endoscopy is the next big hurdle. In the West, these procedures are currently done mostly by top-gun interventionists in academic centers. Aside from training more GI Fellows, live case demonstrations in postgraduate courses can be helpful along with hands-on training models. Critical to third space endoscopy is the mastering of electrocautery instruments and techniques, selecting settings and devices for cutting and coagulating as needed. Separate articles in this issue cover devices and electrocautery principles in depth. Methods for closure of tunnel entrances and areas following EFTR are also provided in another article, as are avoidance and management of adverse events.

There is a final article on the future of third space endoscopy, including a discussion of incorporating robotics with the potential for increased safety and efficiency. When I read through the entire contents of this outstanding issue, I suspect that three decades ago I probably would have thought where we are today was science fiction. There has been fantastic progress for third space endoscopy, clearly a less-invasive method that will in many cases replace more costly and morbid operations for the benefit of our patients. This issue is a don't miss!

Charles J. Lightdale, MD
Department of Medicine
Columbia University Medical Center
161 Fort Washington Avenue
New York, NY 10032, USA

E-mail address:
CJL18@columbia.edu

Preface

Navigating a Path in Submucosal Endoscopy: Learning from the Past and Forging Ahead

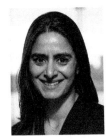

Amrita Sethi, MD, MASGE, NYSGEF
Editor

In this issue of *Gastrointestinal Endoscopy Clinics of North America*, we explore the field of submucosal endoscopy. Work in this space first started in Asia with descriptions of endoscopic submucosal dissection (ESD). The value of working in the submucosal space and the recognition that there can be controlled and safe access beyond not only the mucosal layer but also the entire gastrointestinal (GI) wall inspired the field of Third Space Endoscopy (TSE) and endoscopic full-thickness resection (EFTR). As the introduction, training, and adoption of this field moves from Eastern to Western countries, there is a need to reconsider classical training patterns that require lengthy apprenticeship and focused indications, and adopt changes more rapidly as advances are being made in device and technique innovation. Given the differences in disease prevalence (ie, gastric cancer), training models, and the structure of practice settings, there is a need to reframe and even redefine the way in which we consider this field and make it more accessible to Western endoscopists. In addition, there is a recognition that these techniques are not limited to one disease entity, such as GI cancers, but have applications throughout many GI disorders and sometimes even outside of the discipline.

In this issue, we are reminded of the origins of ESD as well as the considerations that must be made as we integrate the field into Western practice. We learn of indications and techniques of submucosal endoscopy for early neoplasms and submucosal lesions, in the esophagus, stomach, duodenum, colon, and rectum. Furthermore, we discuss resection of lesions not traditionally considered GI in nature but made possible by such techniques as TSE and EFTR. The expansive reach of the access created by the submucosal tunneling techniques in treating disorders that target muscular layers, such as achalasia, is thoroughly explored, including indications, outcomes, and techniques. For innovation to proceed, we must understand all aspects of submucosal endoscopy, including electrocautery principles, the tools currently available to perform these techniques, ways in which to manage adverse events, and how to consider training and measuring competency. It is equally important to see modifications and developing technology (ie, robotics) that will help guide growth in the field.

Given the rapid pace at which the field of ESD and TSE is moving, it is important to not only maintain perspectives from the pioneers in the field but also appreciate how emerging endoscopists are adopting and innovating techniques to make these procedures safe and more effective and develop novel indications. I am grateful to the authors for providing their excellent guidance to help navigate the path ahead. And, on behalf of myself and all of the authors, I thank the editor, Dr Lightdale, for this opportunity to share our passion for this field.

Amrita Sethi, MD, MASGE, NYSGEF
Division of Digestive and Liver Disease
Columbia University Irving Medical Center-NYP
New York, NY 10032, USA

E-mail address:
as3614@cumc.columbia.edu

The Journey from Endoscopic Submucosal Dissection to Third Space Endoscopy

Haruhiro Inoue, MD*, Marc Julius H. Navarro, Yuto Shimamura,
Mayo Tanabe, Akiko Toshimori

KEYWORDS

- Submucosal endoscopy • Third space endoscopy • POEM

KEY POINTS

- Endoscopic submucosal dissection pushed forward development of peroral endoscopic myotomy (POEM).
- POEM opened the door of submucosal endoscopy.
- Treatment with submucosal endoscopy covers various muscle layer–related diseases.

BACKGROUND

Until the development of endoscopic submucosal dissection (ESD),[1–4] therapeutic endoscopy of the gastrointestinal tract was referred to as endoscopic mucosal resection (EMR). EMR was an extension of polypectomy, in which a snare was used to strangle and remove mucosal lesions.[5] There are several methods, including direct strangulation of the mucosa with a snare and EMR using a cap.[6,7] EMR using a ligature device has been established as a simple and safe method of mucosal resection.[8] However, EMR using a snare device is limited to resecting a 1 to 2 cm specimen in a single strangulation. In practice, resection of large mucosal lesions is ultimately limited to piecemeal resection. Fragmented resection has the potential risk of leaving a small amount of epithelial component at the resection margin; this was thought to lead to a risk of recurrence if cancer developed. Therefore, pioneers attempted to resect extensive mucosal lesions in one piece.[9]

Endoscopic Submucosal Dissection

In ESD, the mucosa is incised circumferentially, and the submucosa is detached. Although ESD seems simple at first glance, it is actually a technically difficult and

Digestive Diseases Center, Showa University Koto Toyosu Hospital, Toyosu 5-1-3, Koto-Ku, Tokyo 135-8577, Japan
* Corresponding author.
E-mail address: haru.inoue@med.showa-u.ac.jp

Gastrointest Endoscopy Clin N Am 33 (2023) 1–6
https://doi.org/10.1016/j.giec.2022.09.004
1052-5157/23/© 2022 Elsevier Inc. All rights reserved.

time-consuming procedure. Reasons for the technical difficulty of ESD include the complex 3-dimensional structure and soft walls of the gastrointestinal tract, respiratory movement, heartbeat, peristalsis, and effect of insufflation and suction of the endoscope. In addition, the digestive endoscope has only 1 or 2 channels for instruments compared with laparoscopy that allows 4 to 5 trocars to be used. In the early days of ESD due to these constrained platforms, the following measures were naturally developed.

Knives

Initially, the only knife that existed was a simple needle scalpel. However, pushing the needle scalpel forward into the gastrointestinal wall often resulted in full-layer puncture. Therefore, the insulated tip knife (Olympus Medical, PA, USA) was designed, in which an insulator was attached to the tip of the needle scalpel to prevent puncture.[1] Many knives have since appeared, but the Dual Knife (Olympus Medical, PA, USA) is probably the most widely used today. It is an excellent knife because the outer sheath of the knife applies tension to the tissue to be incised.

Transparent hood

A transparent hood is an essential tool for ESD because it maintains a certain distance between the scope lens and the mucosa to prevent contact. Tapered hoods such as ST hoods (Fujifilm, Tokyo, Japan), short ST hoods (Fujifilm, Tokyo, Japan), and space adjusters (soft and flexible hood, Top) have been developed.[2,7,10]

Carbon dioxide insufflation system

Insufflation of air was originally used in gastrointestinal endoscopy. A carbon dioxide (CO_2) insufflation system was developed to relieve discomfort caused by large amounts of air accumulation after colonoscopy. This CO_2 insufflation system can prevent gas retention in the small intestine even after prolonged ESD. It is also critical in preventing disruptive pressures in the case of perforation or breach of the muscle layer and the resulting pneumoperitoneum.

Electrosurgical devices

Originally, hot biopsy forceps were used for hemostasis and now have been switched to coagulation forceps. The establishment of a soft coagulation mode on the high-frequency power supply enabled effective control of bleeding. Subsequently, the introduction of the spray coagulation mode effectively contributed to tissue dissection with adequate hemostasis.

Development of the clip

Clips were originally developed for hemostasis of peptic ulcers.[11] Today, the primary role of clips has shifted to closure of tissue defects. Clips are often used with end loops to close large defects. To make it simple, several methods including clip closure with a line or "loop (thin slip knot tying to fix clips on the edge of defect)" method were developed.[12,13] The over-the-scope clip (OTSC, Ovesco Endoscopic AG, Tubingen, Germany) was also used for tight closure of full-layer defect.[14]

Evolution of local injection

Initially, epinephrine was added to saline to reduce a risk of bleeding. However, the use of epinephrine has declined in order to avoid vasoconstriction of cardiac disease cases. On the other hand, the use of high-viscosity solution such as hyaluronic acid has made it possible to maintain the mucosal layer elevation for a longer period of time, which helps prevent muscle injury, especially in duodenal and colorectal

ESD.[2,15] Later, with the advent of knives with a water delivery function, the local injection solution again returned to simple saline solution.[16]

Traction method

The traction method was very effective in reducing ESD procedure time.[17] By retracting the specimen, the submucosal layer can be opened widely. Traction particularly makes the procedure easier when the specimen becomes floppy after mobilization of most of the lesion.

Control of pneumoperitoneum

Pneumoperitoneum (or capnoperitoneum) may happen during submucosal endoscopy. Abdominal decompression with a needle is a simple, effective way to control the high pressure caused by pneumoperitoneum.

Development to Submucosal Endoscopy (Third Space Endoscopy)

Submucosal endoscopy and third space endoscopy can be considered synonyms.[18] Submucosal endoscopy indicates the layers to be incised, whereas third space endoscopy is understood conceptually: the first space is the lumen of the digestive tract, second space is the abdominal cavity or thoracic cavity, and the third space is the artificially created submucosal space.

Development of peroral endoscopic myotomy

The natural orifice transluminal endoscopic surgery (NOTES) concept, as proposed by Dr A. Kalloo, attracted a great deal of attention as a minimally invasive procedure that would bridge the gap between gastrointestinal endoscopy and surgery.[19] As background for the development of POEM, the mucosal flap safety valve concept by Sumiyama K and colleagues[20,21] and the animal experiments of myotomy by Pasricha and colleagues were noted. In 2008, the first clinical case of POEM was performed.[22] At our institution alone, we have treated more than 2500 cases in last 14 years. Now it became the standard care of achalasia in place of laparoscopic Heller-Dor surgery.[23]

Peroral endoscopic tumor (submucosal tunnelling endoscopic reaction)

During POEM, we sometimes encountered small leiomyomas (originating from the muscularis propria). Removal of small leiomyomas through the submucosal tunnel was technically feasible,[24,25] and this has led to development of the submucosal tunnelling endoscopic reaction procedure where a submucosal tunnel is specifically created in order to remove submucosal tumors less than 4 cm.[26]

Diverticulum peroral endoscopic myotomy

Epiphrenic diverticulum sometimes appears in patients with achalasia. Originally, full-thickness septotomy (including the mucosa and the muscle layer) was performed to improve the symptom of dysphagia caused by the diverticulum. Diverticulum peroral endoscopic myotomy is when the POEM technique is used to perform muscular septotomy of the epiphrenic diverticulum.[27]

Gastric peroral endoscopic myotomy

A pyloric sphincterotomy via the POEM procedure can be performed for gastroparesis.[28] It is a safe and effective procedure in expert hands.[29]

From peroral endoscopic myotomy for Zenker diverticulum to peroral endoscopic septotomy

POEM for Zenker diverticulum has also been performed, and we now prefer to perform peroral endoscopic septotomy (POES), where the incision is performed along the edge of the septum.[30,31]

Peroral endoscopic fundoplication

Post-POEM gastroesophageal reflux disease (GERD) was discussed from the beginning of the development of POEM. It has been shown to be preventable by adjusting the length of the gastric myotomy and preserving the collar-sling muscle.[32,33] In order to reduce the risk of potential reflux disease, POEM with endoscopic fundoplication in a single session was successfully carried out.[34] Anti-reflux effect continues one year after POEM + F.[35] POEM + F is theoretically appropriate but it takes a longer procedure time. Now we perform POEF alone as a standard procedure. Just in case of refractory reflux POEF is independently performed.[36] In POEF, the transoral endoscope enters the abdominal cavity through the submucosal tunnel of the esophagus, thus providing a pure NOTES procedure.[19]

From Endoscopic Submucosal Dissection to Deeper Layer Dissection to Pure Natural Orifice Transluminal Endoscopic Surgery

From the early experience of perforation during ESD, it has been shown that even if perforation occurs in a clean gastrointestinal tract, there is no major problem if the gastrointestinal wall is closed tightly by clipping or other means. Therefore, we have developed the endoscopic muscle layer dissection, endoscopic subserosal dissection, endoscopic full-thickness resection, and pure NOTES.[37–39] Pure NOTES is represented by POEF.[36]

SUMMARY

With the advent of ESD, therapeutic endoscopy has greatly expanded from treatment using a snare to flexible endoscopic surgery and allowed endoscopists to potentially parallel laparoscopic surgery.

CLINICS CARE POINTS

- Check your endoscopy processor air insufflation is off even when CO_2 insufflator is on.

REFERENCES

1. Ono H. Endoscopic submucosal dissection for early gastric cancer. Chin J Dig Dis 2005;6:119–21.
2. Yamamoto H, Kawata H, Sunada K, et al. Success rate of curative endoscopic mucosal resection with circumferential mucosal incision assisted by submucosal injection of sodium hyaluronate. Gastrointest Endosc 2002;56:507–12.
3. Yahagi N, Kato M, Ochiai Y, et al. Outcomes of endoscopic resection for superficial duodenal epithelial neoplasia. Gastrointest Endosc 2018;88:676–82.
4. Oyama T. Esophageal ESD; technique and prevention of complications. Gastrointest Endosc Clin N Am 2014;24:201–12.
5. Deyhle P, Sauberhi H, Nuesch HJ, et al. Endoscopic "jumbo biopsy" in the stomach with a diathermy loop. Acta Hepatogastroenterol (Stuttg) 1974;21:228–32.
6. Suehendra N, Binmoeller KF, Bohnacker S, et al. Endoscopic snare mucosectomy in the esophagus without any additional equipment: a simple technique for resection of flat early cancer. Endoscopy 1997;29:380–3.
7. Inoue H, Endo M, Takeshita K, et al. A new simplified technique of endoscopic esophageal mucosal resection using a cap-fitted panendoscope (EMRC). Surg Endosc 1992;6:264–5.

8. Seewald S, Ang TL, Smar S, et al. Endoscopic mucosal resection of early esophageal squamous cell cancer using the Duette mucosectomy kit. Endoscopy 2006;38:1029–31.
9. Ono H, Yao K, Fujishiro M, et al. Guidelines for endoscopic submucosal dissection and endoscopic mucosal resection for early gastric cancer. Dig Endosc 2016;28:3–15.
10. Fujiyoshi Y, Shimamura Y, Inoue H. Usefulness of a newly developed distal attachment: super soft hood (Space adjuster) in therapeutic endoscopy. Dig Endosc 2020;32:e38–9.
11. Hachisu T, Miyazaki S, Hamaguchi K. Endoscopic clip-marking of lesions using the newly developed HX-3L clip. Surg Endosc 1989;3:142–7.
12. Soga K, Shimomura T, Suzuki T, et al. Usefulness of the modified clip-with-line method for endoscopic mucosal treatment procedure. J Gastrointestin Liver Dis 2018;27:317–20.
13. Inoue H, Tanabe M, Shimamura Y, et al. A novel endoscopic purse-string suture technique, "loop 9", for gastrointestinal defect closure: a pilot study. Endoscopy 2022;54:158–62.
14. Haito-Chavez Y, Law JK, Kratt T, et al. International multicenter experience with an over-the-scope clipping device for endoscopic management of GI defects. Gastrointest Endosc 2014;80:610–22.
15. Fujishiro M, Yahagi N, Nakamura M, et al. Successful outcomes of a novel endoscopic treatment for GI tumors: endoscopic submucosal dissection with a mixture of high-molecular-weight hyaluronic acid, glycerin, and sugar. Gastrointest Endosc 2006;63:243–9.
16. Takeuchi Y, Uedo N, Ishihara R, et al. Efficacy of an endo-knife with a water-jet function (Flushknife) for endoscopic submucosal dissection of superficial colorectal neoplasms. Am J Gastroenterol 2010;105:314–22.
17. Imaeda H, Hosoe N, Kashiwagi K, et al. Advanced endoscopic submucosal dissection with traction. World J Gastrointest Endosc 2014;6:186–95.
18. Maydeo A, Dhir V. Third-space endoscopy: stretching the limits. Gastrointest Endosc 2017;85:728–9.
19. Kalloo AN. Closing the gap: progress for NOTES. Endoscopy 2009;41:1080–1.
20. Sumiyama K, Gostout CJ, Rajan E, et al. Submucosal endoscopy with mucosal flap safety valve. Gastrointest Endosc 2007;65:688–94.
21. Pasricha PJ, Hawari R, Ahmed I, et al. Submucosal endoscopic esophageal myotomy: a novel experimental approach for the treatment of achalasia. Endoscopy 2007;39:761–4.
22. Inoue H, Minami H, Kobayashi Y, et al. Peroral endoscopic myotomy (POEM) for esophageal achalasia. Endoscopy 2010;42:265–71.
23. Akintoye E, Kumar N, Obaitan I, et al. Peroral endoscopic myotomy: a meta-analysis. Endoscopy 2016;48:1059–68.
24. Inoue H, Ikeda H, Hosoya T, et al. Submucosal endoscopic tumor resection for subepithelial tumors in the esophagus and cardia. Endoscopy 2012;44:225–30.
25. Xu MD, Cai MY, Zhou PH, et al. Submucosal tunneling endoscopic resection: a new technique for treating upper GI submucosal tumors originating from the muscularis propria layer. Gastrointest Endosc 2012;75:195–9.
26. Onimaru M, Inoue H, Bechara R, et al. Clinical outcomes of per-oral endoscopic tumor resection for submucosal tumors in the esophagus and gastric cardia. Dig Endosc 2020;32:328–36.

27. Yang J, Zeng X, Yuan X, et al. An international study on the use of POEM in the management of esophageal diverticula: the first multicenter D-POEM experience. Endoscopy 2019;51:346–9.

28. Khashab MA, Stein E, Clarke JO, et al. Gastric peroral endoscopic myotomy for refractory gastroparesis: first human endoscopic pyloromyotomy. Gastrointest Endosc 2013;78:764–8.

29. Kahaleh M, Gonzalez JM, Xu MM, et al. Gastric peroral endoscopic myotomy for the treatment of refractory gastroparesis: a multicenter international experience. Endoscopy 2018;50:1053–8.

30. Hernández Mondragón OV, Solórzano Pineda MO, Blancas Valencia JM. Zenker's diverticulum: Submucosal tunneling endoscopic septum division (Z-POEM). Dig Endosc 2018;30:124.

31. Repici A, Spadaccini M, Belletrutti PJ, et al. Peroral endoscopic septotomy for short-septum Zenker's diverticulum. Endoscopy 2020;52:563–8.

32. Shiwaku H, Inoue H, Sato H, et al. Peroral endoscopic myotomy for achalasia: a prospective multicenter study in Japan. Gastrointest Endosc 2020;91:1037–44.

33. Tanaka S, Toyonaga T, Kawara F, et al. Novel per-oral endoscopic myotomy method preserving oblique muscle using two penetrating vessels as anatomic landmarks reduces postoperative gastroesophageal reflux. J Gastroenterol Hepatol 2019;34:2158–63.

34. Inoue H, Ueno A, Shimamura Y, et al. Peroral endoscopic myotomy and fundoplication: a novel NOTES procedure. Endoscopy 2019;51:161–4.

35. Bapaye A, Dashatwar P, Dharamsi S, et al. Single-session endoscopic fundoplication after peroral endoscopic myotomy (POEM+F) for prevention of post gastroesophageal reflux - 1-year follow-up study. Endoscopy 2021;53:1114–21.

36. Toshimori A, Inoue H, Shimamura Y, et al. Peroral endoscopic fundoplication: a brand-new intervention for GERD. VideoGIE 2020;5:244–6.

37. Liu F, Zhang S, Ren W, et al. The fourth space surgery: endoscopic subserosal dissection for upper gastrointestinal subepithelial tumors originating from the muscularis propria layer. Surg Endosc 2018;32:2575–82.

38. Quarta Colosso BM, Abad MRA, Inoue H. Traction method for endoscopic subserosal dissection. VideoGIE 2020;5:148–50.

39. Stavropoulos SN, Modayil R, Friedel D, et al. Endoscopic full-thickness resection for GI stromal tumors. Gastrointest Endosc 2014;80:334–5.

East versus West
Comparisons and Implications in Adaptation to Practice

Dennis Yang, MD[a], Muhammad K. Hasan, MD[a],
Peter V. Draganov, MD[b],*

KEYWORDS

- Endoscopic submucosal dissection • Training • Per-oral endoscopic myotomy
- Endoscopic mucosal resection

KEY POINTS

- The traditional Japanese master-apprenticeship model cannot be directly applied for endoscopic submucosal dissection (ESD) training in the West.
- In recent years, the steady growth of available Western ESD mentors, suitable training pathways, and dedicated devices has significantly narrowed the gap of ESD practice between Asia and the West.
- Future efforts to reduce procedural technical demand and address the lack of proper reimbursement are necessary for ESD's widespread adoption.

BACKGROUND

Endoscopic submucosal dissection (ESD) is a specialized endoscopic resection technique initially developed in Japan in the 1990s as a treatment for early gastric cancer (EGC). As opposed to conventional snare-assisted endoscopic mucosal resection (EMR) approaches, ESD permits the en bloc resection of lesions irrespective of size. This in turn procures an ideal specimen for accurate histopathological assessment, translates into higher R0 resection rates, and decreases the risk of residual or recurrent neoplasia.[1] Furthermore, when compared with conventional surgery, ESD is less invasive and associated with a faster recovery.[2,3] As such, over the last few decades, ESD has been disseminated in Asian countries as not only the preferred strategy for EGC but also as the gold standard technique for the resection of large superficial neoplasias throughout the gastrointestinal (GI) tract. The transition of

[a] Center for Interventional Endoscopy, AdventHealth, Orlando, FL, USA; [b] Division of Gastroenterology, Hepatology and Nutrition, University of Florida, 1329 SW 16th Street, Room #5262, Gainesville, FL 32608, USA
* Corresponding author. University of Florida, 1329 SW 16th Street Room # 5251, Gainesville, FL 32608.
E-mail address: peter.draganov@medicine.ufl.edu

Gastrointest Endoscopy Clin N Am 33 (2023) 7–13
https://doi.org/10.1016/j.giec.2022.07.004
1052-5157/23/© 2022 Elsevier Inc. All rights reserved.

giendo.theclinics.com

ESD has been slower in the West, given the vastly regional and training differences between the East and the West. Nonetheless, over recent years, the authors have witnessed an increase in the clinical adoption of ESD and other third space endoscopic procedures catapulted by the steady growth of ESD mentors in the West, the introduction of viable training pathways, and new dedicated devices and accessories.

DISCUSSION

Endoscopic Submucosal Dissection Training in Asia: a Traditional Master-Apprenticeship Model

ESD is a technically demanding procedure associated with a steep learning curve that encompasses not only the acquisition of technical skills of endoscopic resection, but an in-depth knowledge on appropriate lesion assessment and selection. In Japan and other Asian countries, ESD training follows a traditional master-apprentice model, in which cognitive and technical proficiency are acquired through a stepwise introduction to the procedure.[4] The initial phases involve comprehensive knowledge-based self-training and a focus on establishing basic endoscopic skills. Subsequently, trainees are expected to undergo a short course of training with ex vivo animal models before assisting ESD cases and finally advancing to human ESD procedures under supervision.[4] Nearly all trainees begin by targeting smaller lesions in the gastric antrum, which carry the lowest degree of technical difficulty, before embarking on lesions in other parts of the stomach. Although the minimum case load necessary for ESD competency has not been defined, several studies suggest that at least 30 to 50 gastric ESDs are needed to achieve proficiency, a benchmark that is often regarded as a prerequisite in Japan before embarking on ESD in the esophagus and colon, because of its higher degree of technical complexity.[5,6]

This stepwise master-apprenticeship model has been successful in developing highly skilled ESD endoscopists in Asia. Yet, this model is not adaptable to training conditions in the West. For one, the incidence of EGC is substantially higher in Japan compared with the West, which allows Japanese trainees to have ample opportunities for hands-on introductory ESD before their gradual progression to more complex lesions in other parts of the GI tract. Even more importantly, the prior lack of qualified Western ESD endoscopists to serve as mentors is perhaps the most apparent barrier for trainees, who inevitably need to travel to Asia and take extended time off for training, a strategy that is neither pragmatic nor sustainable in the long run. These and other factors, including the lack of proper reimbursement for a long procedure associated with higher procedural risk, have significantly hindered the dissemination of ESD in the West.

Peroral Endoscopic Myotomy and Its Implications on Endoscopic Submucosal Dissection Training in the West

Peroral endoscopic myotomy (POEM) was a transcendental innovative technique initially introduced as a concept by Pasricha and colleagues[7] in 2007 and then clinically by Inoue and colleagues[8] for the treatment of achalasia. POEM involves the myotomy of the lower esophageal sphincter through a submucosal tunneling approach, a prime example of the concept of third space or submucosal endoscopy, which is founded on the principle that the deeper layers of the GI tract can be accessed by tunneling in the submucosal space without compromising the integrity of the overlying mucosa.

Shortly after the report by Inoue and colleagues,[9] POEM was quickly and simultaneously adopted by multiple centers across Asia, Europe, and the Americas, with more than 2400 cases documented within 5 years from the first human study of POEM. The authors speculate that several factors contributed to the rapid uptake of POEM and its incorporation into clinical practice in the rest of the world outside of Asia. On the surface, POEM appears to be similar to ESD, both offshoots of third space endoscopy. Yet, POEM is conceptually and technically easier to assimilate compared with ESD, because the procedure follows well-defined steps, with easy-to-identify tissue landmarks in an environment that provides relative stable scope position within the confines of the submucosal tunnel.[10] Furthermore, POEM is a technique with no endoscopic equivalent. Prior to its introduction into clinical practice, botulinum toxin injection and pneumatic balloon dilation were the main endoscopic alternatives to conventional surgical myotomy, which remained as the long-term standard of care for most patients with achalasia. POEM offered the benefit of surgical myotomy through a less invasive approach, an attractive and novel concept that received universal acceptance shortly after multiple specialized centers across the globe consistently reported similar favorable outcomes.[10–12] Soon thereafter, several consensus documents were introduced by various GI professional societies establishing the role of POEM for the treatment of esophageal motility disorders.[13–15] At the same time, with the assimilation of POEM worldwide, local experts across various centers began to emerge, which translated into a larger pool of trainers and thereby more accessible training opportunities. This in turn led to the development of different training pathways and rekindled the interest of ESD training in the West.[4]

The Current Status of Endoscopic Submucosal Dissection in the West

The dissemination and adoption of POEM into clinical practice helped change the landscape of ESD training in the West. As endoscopists became more comfortable with venturing into third space endoscopy with POEM, many of them realized that it shared a similar cognitive and technical skill set required for ESD. Importantly, in recent years there has been an increasing recognition of the need to broaden the endoscopic resection armamentarium, as unnecessary surgical referral over EMR for benign disease remains a common practice in the United States.[16,17] In response, the authors have witnessed an exponential growth in educational resources for individuals interested in training in POEM and ESD.[18] Although many Western endoscopists have continued to pursue training by visiting and observing Japanese ESD masters, there has been an increasing number of live and hands-on courses in third space endoscopy that have become readily available at national and international endoscopy conferences offered by institutions and professional societies.[18] This noticeable growth in local ESD expertise with the expanding pool of Western ESD endoscopists and educational resources has been the foundation of ESD training in the West.

One of the ongoing criticisms toward the dissemination of ESD in the West has been that the superb results achieved by Japanese endoscopists have not being duplicated in the West. In a prior systematic review and meta-analysis, Fuccio and colleagues reported lower resection rates among Western ESD endoscopists compared with their Eastern counterparts.[19] However, in more recent years, improvements in ESD technique and training opportunities have translated into better clinical outcomes through many Western tertiary referral centers. The authors recently conducted and published the largest multicenter prospective study on ESD in North America with nearly 700 cases.[20] Notably, the technical resection outcomes achieved in this study (92% en bloc, 84% R0, 78% curative resection) were in line with the current established consensus quality parameters supporting the feasibility and efficacy of ESD for the treatment of select GI neoplasia when performed at highly specialized centers.[20]

Shortly thereafter, Fleischmann and colleagues presented the results of a multicenter cohort study of ESD in 1000 patients from Germany.[21] Similarly, ESD achieved en bloc, R0 and curation resection of 92%, 79%, and 72% respectively. Notably, in both studies, these favorable outcomes were attained despite submucosal fibrosis being commonly identified, a less frequent issue among Asian studies as tattooing, partial snare resections, and biopsies are seldom performed. In aggregate, these studies have added to the body of evidence that ESD can be performed safely and effectively in the West at tertiary referral centers.

FUTURE DIRECTIONS

Over the past 2 decades, it has been learned that the traditional Japanese master-apprenticeship model cannot be directly applied for training in the West. Although the number of POEM/ESD mentors continues to steadily increase in the West, the pool is still limited to tertiary referral centers. As such, hands-on practice on animal models should remain an integral component of training, particularly in the initial phases.[22] Yet, animal laboratories are costly and not widely available. Further research should focus on the role of endoscopy simulators, as these may represent a viable alternative to accelerate skill acquisition in a low-risk environment and implement didactic learning and hands-on animal procedures when feasible.[23] Given the low incidence of EGC in the West, a modified stepwise approach is necessary. Both the European Society of Gastrointestinal Endoscopy and the American Society of Gastrointestinal Endoscopy core curricula recommend that ESD should be initially carried out in the rectum.[24,25] The authors have previously demonstrated that rectal ESD among Western centers is associated with an adequate safety profile and thereby a reasonable training approach, particularly given that recent studies have shown that experience in gastric ESD is not necessarily a prerequisite for colorectal ESD.[26,27] Yet, it should be emphasized that close supervision by an ESD expert is highly advisable, as untutored ESD training results in a steeper learning curve and higher risk for procedural adverse events.[28] Indirect assessment methods may potentially help circumvent the scarcity of available mentors. With technological innovations and increasing broadband availability, video-based live instruction could play an important role for the acquisition of ESD skills even with mentors in geographically distant locations.[22]

Technological innovation has and will continue to play a key role in the adoption of ESD as a mainstream procedure. Over recent years, the authors have seen an expanding array of different techniques and dedicated devices for ESD. The introduction of novel ESD knives with integrated submucosal injection capability and the development of new more durable injection solutions have resulted in lower procedural times.[29] Modifications to the conventional ESD technique, including submucosal tunneling ESD and the pocket-creation technique, have been shown to facilitate dissection by creating a stable working zone.[30] The need to maintain adequate visualization of the dissection plane during ESD has been recognized as an important rate-limiting step and one of the most difficult aspects of the procedure. Consequently, there have been several attempts to facilitate the procedure by using existing endoscopic tools and by developing traction devices and techniques to elevate the mucosal flap. External traction methods have included grasping forceps, using a second thin endoscope, double-channel endoscope, and peroral traction via a pulley system.[31–33] Internal traction techniques have included the clip-rubber band method, spring-action SO clip, the clip-in-line traction method, and the suture pulley technique.[34–37] Dedicated new retraction devices (ProdiGITraction Wire, Medtronic

Colorado) and endoluminal intervention platforms (DiLumen, Lumendi, Connecticut) have been specifically developed in the last few years with Western ESD in mind. More recently, a single-operator, through-the-scope retraction device with a 360° rotatable grasping forceps (TrackMotion, FujiFilm, Massachusetts) has been developed to facilitate real-time traction adjustment and triangulation during ESD. In all, these developments should help reduce the ESD learning curve and facilitate its implementation in Western routine practice.

In summary, the current evidence supports ESD as a mature endoscopic technique that can be safely and effectively performed at Western tertiary referral centers. Although technical demand and lack of proper reimbursement are current challenges to ESD in the West, the steady growth of available Western ESD mentors, suitable training pathways, and dedicated devices have significantly narrowed the gap of ESD practice between Asia and the West.

CLINICS CARE POINTS

- ESD is a mature technique commonly implemented in Asian countries for the resection of superficial neoplasia in the GI tract.
- Current evidence suggests that ESD can be safely and effectively performed at Western specialized centers.
- The introduction of viable multifaceted training pathways and the increasing availability of mentors have helped disseminate ESD in the West.
- Technical demand and lack of proper reimbursement are current challenges to ESD in the West.

DISCLOSURE

The authors have nothing to disclose.

REFERENCES

1. Yang D, Othman M, Draganov PV. Endoscopic mucosal resection vs endoscopic submucosal dissection for Barrett's esophagus and colorectal neoplasia. Clin Gastroenterol Hepatol 2019;17:1019–28.
2. McCarty TR, Bazarbashi AN, Hathorn KE, et al. Endoscopic submucosal dissection (ESD) versus transanal endoscopic microsurgery (TEM) for treatment of rectal tumors: a comparative systematic review and meta-analysis. Surg Endosc 2020;34:1688–95.
3. Nam MJ, Sohn DK, Hong CW, et al. Cost comparison between endoscopic submucosal dissection and transanal endoscopic microsurgery for the treatment of rectal tumors. Ann Surg Treat Res 2015;89:202–7.
4. Kotzev AI, Yang D, Draganov PV. How to master endoscopic submucosal dissection in the USA. Dig Endosc 2019;31:94–100.
5. Tsuji Y, Fujishiro M, Kodashima S, et al. Desirable training of endoscopic submucosal dissection: further spread worldwide. Ann Transl Med 2014;2:27–32.
6. Oda I, Odagaki T, Suzuki H, et al. Learning curve for endoscopic submucosal dissection of early gastric cancer based on trainee experience. Dig Endosc 2012;(Suppl 1):129–32.

7. Pasricha PJ, Hawari R, Ahmed I, et al. Submucosal endoscopic esophageal myotomy: a novel experimental approach for the treatment of achalasia. Endoscopy 2007;39:761–4.

8. Inoue H, Minami H, Kobayashi Y, et al. Peroral endoscopic myotomy (POEM) for esophageal achalasia. Endoscopy 2010;42:265–71.

9. Akintoye E, Kumar N, Olaitan I, et al. Peroral endoscopic myotomy: a meta-analysis. Endoscopy 2016;48:1059–68.

10. Yang D, Panna D, Zhang Q, et al. Evaluation of anesthesia management, feasibility, and efficacy of peroral endoscopic myotomy (POEM) for achalasia performed in the endoscopy unit. Endows Int Open 2015;3:E289–95.

11. Von Rental D, Inoue H, Minami H, et al. Peroral endoscopic myotomy for the treatment of achalasia: a prospective single center study. Am J Gastroenterol 2012; 107:411–7.

12. Stavropoulos SN, Model RJ, Friedel D, et al. The international per oral endoscopic myotomy survey (IPOEMS): a snapshot of the global POEM experience. Surg Endows 2013;27:3322–38.

13. Karallas P, Kazak D, Richter JE. Clinical practice update: the use of per-oral endoscopic myotomy in achalasia: expert review and best practice advice from the AGA institute. Gastroenterology 2017;153:1205–11.

14. Stavropoulos SN, Desilts DJ, Scott DJ, et al. Per-oral endoscopic myotomy white paper summary. Gastrointest Endosc 2014;80:1–15.

15. Inoue H, Shiwaku H, Iwakiri K, et al. Clinical practice guidelines for peroral endoscopic myotomy. Dig Endosc 2018;30:563–79.

16. Peery AF, Cools KS, Strassle PD, et al. Increasing rates of surgery for patients with nonmalignant colorectal polyps in the United States. Gastroenterology 2018;154:1352–60.

17. Moon N, Aryan M, Khan W, et al. Effect of referral pattern and histopathology grade on surgery for nonmalignant colorectal polyps. Gastrointest Endosc 2020;92:702–11.

18. Schlachterman A, Yang D, Goddard A, et al. Perspectives on endoscopic submucosal dissection training in the United States: Endoscopic submucosal dissection Endoscopic submucosal dissection survey analysis. Endosc Int Open 2018;6: E399–409.

19. Fuccio L, Hassan C, Ponchon T, et al. Clinical outcomes after endoscopic submucosal dissection for colorectal neoplasia: a systematic review and meta-analysis. Gastrointest Endosc 2017;86(1):74–86.

20. Draganov PV, Aihara H, Karasik MS, et al. Endoscopic submucosal dissection in North America: a large prospective multicenter study. Gastroenterology 2021; 160:2317–27.

21. Fleischmann C, Probst A, Ebigbo A, et al. Endoscopic submucosal dissection in Europe: results of 1000 neoplastic lesions from the German endoscopic submucosal dissection Registry. Gastroenterology 2021;161:1168–78.

22. Yang D, Wagh MS, Draganov PV. The status of training in new technologies in advanced endoscopy: from defining competence to credentialing and privileging. Gastrointest Endosc 2020;92:1016–25.

23. Khan R, Plahouras J, Johnston BC, et al. Virtual reality simulation training for health professions trainees in gastrointestinal endoscopy. Cochrane Database Syst Rev 2018;8:CD008237.

24. Pimentel-Nunes P, Pioche M, Albeniz E, et al. Curriculum for endoscopic submucosal dissection training in Europe: European Society of Gastrointestinal Endoscopy (ESGE) Position Statement. Endoscopy 2019;51:980–92.

25. Aihara H, Dacha S, Anand GS, et al. Core curriculum for endoscopic submucosal dissection (ESD). Gastrointest Endosc 2021;93:1215–21.
26. Yang D, Aihara H, Perbtani YB, et al. Safety and efficacy of endoscopic submucosal dissection for rectal neoplasia: a multicenter North American experience. Endosc Int Open 2019;7:E1714–22.
27. Probst A, Pommer B, Golger D, et al. Endoscopic submucosal dissection in gastric neoplasia – experience from a European center. Endoscopy 2010;42:1037–44.
28. Zhang X, Ly EK, Nithyanand S, et al. Learning curve for endoscopic submucosal dissection with untutored, prevalence-based approach in the United States. Clin Gastroenterol Hepatol 2020;18:580–8.
29. Zhou PH, Schumacher B, Yao LQ, et al. Conventional vs waterjet-assisted endoscopic submucosal dissection in early gastric cancer: a randomized controlled trial. Endoscopy 2014;46:836–43.
30. Keihanian T, Othman O. Colorectal endoscopic submucosal dissection: an update on best practice. Clin Exp Gastroenterol 2021;14:317–30.
31. Imaeda H, Hosoe N, Ida Y, et al. Novel technique of endoscopic submucosal dissection by using external forceps for early rectal cancer (with videos). Gastrointest Endosc 2012;75:1253–7.
32. Neuhaus H, Costamagna G, Deviere J, et al. ARCADE Group: endoscopic submucosal dissection (ESD) of early neoplastic gastric lesions using a new double-channel endoscope (the "R-scope"). Endoscopy 2006;38:1016–23.
33. Li CH, Chen PJ, Chu HC, et al. Endoscopic submucosal dissection with the pulley method for early-stage gastric cancer (with video). Gastrointest Endosc 2011;73:163–7.
34. Chen PJ, Chu HC, Chang WK, et al. Endoscopic submucosal dissection with internal traction for early gastric cancer (with video). Gastrointest Endosc 2008;67:128–32.
35. Parra-Blanco A, Nicolas D, Arnau MR, et al. Gastric endoscopic submucosal dissection assisted by a new traction method: the clip-band technique. A feasibility study in a porcine model (with video). Gastrointest Endosc 2011;74:1137–41.
36. Ritsuno H, Sakamoto N, Osada T, et al. Prospective clinical trial of traction device-assisted endoscopic submucosal dissection of large superficial colorectal tumors using the S-O clip. Surg Endosc 2014;28:3143–9.
37. Ge PS, Thompson CC, Jirapinyo P, et al. Suture pulley countertraction method reduces procedure time and technical demand of endoscopic submucosal dissection among novice endoscopists learning endoscopic submucosal dissection: a prospective randomized ex vivo study. Gastrointest Endosc 2019;89:117–84.

Building the Toolbox of Devices to Optimize a Practice in Submucosal Endoscopy

Rahil H. Shah, MD[a], Sunil Amin, MD[b],*

KEYWORDS

- Endoscopic submucosal dissection tools • Electrosurgical knives • Injection agents
- Traction devices • Electrosurgical knife accessories

KEY POINTS

- Endoscopic submucosal dissection (ESD) is a technically complicated procedure, and there are many tools developed to assist the endoscopist including: electrosurgical knives, caps, injecting agents, and traction devices.
- There are many types of electrosurgical knives (ie, needle type, insulated tip type, scissor type, and others) which may serve a single purpose or can be multifunctional to assist throughout the whole procedure.
- Injection agents are used to lift the layers and assist with visualization and safer dissection. They vary in availability, cost, and formulation and can range from normal saline to proprietary blends. The endoscopist should consider the level of submucosal lift, duration of lift, and potential to cause changes to histology.
- Traction devices are used to provide tension and stability to the endoscopist. They come in two broad categories of internal and external traction devices. The endoscopist should consider the direction of tension, cost, location in gastrointestinal (GI) tract, and spatial constraints when deciding which traction device to use.
- Closure devices, such as through the scope clips, over the scope clips, and suturing systems are important tools to have available for management of perforations and muscle injury. These will be discussed in another chapter in this collection.

 A video of double-clip traction method used during rectal ESD accompanies this article at http://www.giendo.theclinics.com.

[a] Department of Medicine, University of Miami/Jackson Memorial Hospital, 1611 Northwest 12th Avenue, C-600D, Miami, FL 33136, USA; [b] Division of Digestive Health and Liver Diseases, Department of Medicine, University of Miami, Miller School of Medicine at the University of Miami, 1120 Northwest 14th Street, Clinical Research Building, Suite 11145 (D-49), Miami, FL 33136, USA
* Corresponding author.
E-mail address: sunil.amin@med.miami.edu

Gastrointest Endoscopy Clin N Am 33 (2023) 15–28
https://doi.org/10.1016/j.giec.2022.09.001
1052-5157/23/© 2022 Elsevier Inc. All rights reserved.

giendo.theclinics.com

INTRODUCTION

Endoscopic submucosal dissection (ESD) is a complex procedure to remove early nonmetastatic lesions with precision and in a minimally invasive manner. ESD has many indications, but ideally it is used in situations where a neoplasm is confined to the mucosa without involvement of the submucosa or muscularis propria layer.[1] The advantage of ESD is that specimens can be presented *en-bloc* allowing for better margin analysis and integrity of architecture. ESD is more time-consuming and technically challenging than endoscopic mucosal resections.[1]

Technique

In general, ESD is composed of the following steps:

1. Marking: The perimeter of the lesion is marked by cautery using an electrosurgical knife.
2. Injection: A lifting agent is injected into to submucosa around the perimeter of the lesion.
3. Incision: The mucosa is incised and then cut circumferentially using an electrosurgical knife.
4. Dissection: The submucosa beneath the lesion is injected and dissected using an electrosurgical knife with the assistance of a cap and in some cases a traction device for visualization.
5. Hemostasis: Coagulating any potential bleeding vessels throughout and at the end of the procedure.

Each step of the process has a variety of tools available to the endoscopist. Owing to the complex nature of the procedure, there are many technical considerations the endoscopist must consider in their approach before starting an ESD. The authors discuss the tools of the trade and their respective pros and cons.

Electrosurgical Knife

The selection of which electrosurgical knife to use is a principal decision in ESD as it is the driving force behind the procedure. The choice of electrosurgical knife is vital as it may play a role in as few as one step to as many as all five steps in the procedure. There are a wide variety of electrosurgical knives on the market with unique characteristics differentiating one from another. When considering which electrosurgical knives to use, the endoscopist should consider location, size, position, and characteristics of the lesion to use the best electrosurgical knife for the job. **Table 1** lists all the knives, by manufacturer, with their corresponding intraprocedural functions[2] (**Fig. 1**).

Needle Tip and Hybrid/Water Jet

The needle tip knife is a multipurpose knife which can be used for marking, incision, and dissection. Many of the needle tip knives have a central lumen which allows for injection and irrigation. The needle tip electrosurgical knives include Olympus Dual Knife and Dual Knife J, Fujifilm Flush Knife NS and Flush Knife BT, PENTAX Splash-M knife, ERBE Hybrid Knife, Boston Scientific ProKnife, and Creo Medical's Speedboat.

The Olympus Dual Knife is manufactured in 1.5-mm length tips for thinner lumen organs (eg, esophageal and colon) and 2.0-mm length tips for thicker lumen organs (eg, stomach).[3] The Dual Knife J also comes in 1.5 and 2.0-mm length but has the added advantage of submucosal injection (with saline) within the same tool. It also has a knob shaped tip to prevent slipping and a dome cover to allow for smoother and safer

Table 1
Endoscopic submucosal dissection knives, with their corresponding functions, organized by manufacturer

Manufacturer	Brand Name	Marking	Injection	Mucosal Incision	Submucosal Dissection	Hemostasis
Boston Scientific	ProKnife	x	x	x	x	
Creo Medical	Speedboat	X	x	x	x	x
ERBE	HybridKnife (I-type, T-type, and O-type)	X	x	x	x	x
Fujifilm	Flush Knife NS (needle)	X	x	x	x	x
	Flush Knife BT (ball-tip)	X	x	x	x	x
	Clutch Cutter				x	x
Kachu	Fork Knife	x	x	x	x	x
Olympus	DualKnife	x		x	x	x
	DualKnife J	x	x	x	x	x
	IT knife, IT2, IT nano			x	x	x
	3-in-1 SB Knife			x	x	x
	HookKnife	x		x	x	x
	HookKnife J	x	x	x	x	x
	Triangle Tip	x		x	x	x
	Triangle Tip J	x	x	x	x	x
	FlexKnife	x		x	x	x
PENTAX	Splash-M knife	x	x	x	x	x
	Swanblade				x	
	Mucosectom				x	
Sumitomo Bakelite	SB Knife, SB Knife Short, SB Knife Jr	x			x	x

Adapted from Harlow C, Sivananthan A, Ayaru L, Patel K, Darzi A, Patel N. Endoscopic submucosal dissection: an update on tools and accessories. Therapeutic Advances in Gastrointestinal Endoscopy. January 2020.

manipulation. The Fujifilm Flushtip needle shaped (NS) and ball tip shaped (BTS) both offer functionalities for all portions of the ESD process from marking, lifting, injecting, dissecting, and coagulation. The Flushtip NS is needle-shaped with lengths of 1.5 and 2.0 mm, whereas the Flushtip BTS offers a ball tip shape.[4] The PENTAX Splash-M knife is similar to the Flushtip with the main difference being that the Splash-M Knife offers a metal plate on the distal sheath to achieve better hemostasis.[5] The ERBE HybridKnife also allows for irrigation and injection with a single knife.[6] The HybridKnife requires a jet lavage system (ERBEJET 2 System), which is powerful enough to penetrate the mucosa without a needle for lifting. It comes in three configurations. The I-type is straight without an added tip, the T-type has a non-insulated 1.6-mm diameter disk-shaped electrode at the tip, and the O-Type has a circular insulated tip. The Boston Scientific ProKnife comes in 1.5-, 2.0-and 3.0-mm length knives and has a channel in the center of its tip which allows for injection of their ORISE gel which is

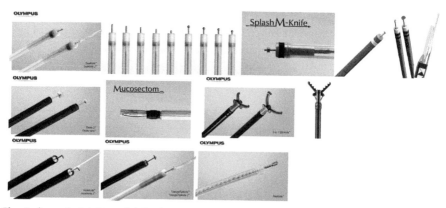

Fig. 1. (rows 1–4, left to right): Electrosurgical Knives Row 1: Olympus Dual Knife and Dual Knife J, Fujifilm Flush Knife NS (five needle tip sizes), Fujifilm Flush Knife BT (four needle tip sizes), PENTAX Splash-M Knife, Boston Scientific ProKnife, ERBE Hybrid Knife, Creo Medical Speedboat; Row 2: Olympus IT Knife 2, PENTAX Swanblade, PENTAX Mucosectom, Sumitomo Bakelite's SB Knife, Olympus 3-in-1 SB Knife, Olympus 3-in-1 SB Knife short, Fujifilm's Clutch Cutter; Row 3: Olympus HookKnife, Olympus Triangle TipKnife, Olympus FlexKnife. (*Courtesy of* Olympus, Fujifilm, PENTAX, Boston Scientific, © Erbe Elektromedizin GmbH, SB-Kawasumi Laboratories, Inc.)

a viscous lifting agent designed to provide long-lasting mucosal elevation.[7] The Creo Medical Speedboat offers a needle tool which allows for injection in addition to a bipolar radiofrequency and microwave energy to dissect, resect, and coagulate.[8]

Insulated Tip

The insulated tip knife was first introduced in the late 1990s[9] and has been widely used in ESD. They are defined by a ceramic (in most cases) insulator at the tip which helps reduce the risk of puncturing tissue and of perforations. One advantage of IT knives is the ability to perform safer resections of subepithelial tumors or lesions with fibrosis.[10] There is often poor visualization of the distal end of the knife in these situations; therefore, having a ceramic tip which will not cut or coagulate any tissue it is in contact with helps prevent blind cutting. Disadvantages of the insulated tip electrosurgical knives are related to maneuverability. Positioning is more difficult than with other knives and requires proper angulation of the knife to contact tissue, as the endoscopist depends on the shaft of the knife (rather than the tip) to drive the cutting process. This may potentially lead to the decreased current density and precision of cutting. The insulted tip electrosurgical knives cannot be used to make the initial incision, which requires using an additional electrosurgical knife for the initial steps. Examples of insulated tip electrosurgical knives include the Olympus IT knife 2 and IT knife nano, and the PENTAX Swanblade and Mucosectom.

The Olympus IT knife 2 has a 2.2-mm ceramic tip and a 4-mm knife length. It has an electrode on its proximal side of the tip to improve cutting in vertical and horizontal directions.[11] The IT knife nano has a 1.7-mm ceramic tip with a 3.5-mm knife length allowing easier maneuverability during ESD.[11] The nano is considered safer for esophageal and colorectal lesions with their thinner mucosa. The PENTAX Swanblade knife measures at 2.1 mm and has a sloped distal end to block the muscular layer. It also has a rotatable tip with optical marker for precise dissection.[12] The PENTAX Mucosectom's main differentiating feature is the addition of a longer knife measuring 2.5 and 5 mm which is designed to increase the speed of dissection.[13] The Swanblade and

Mucosectom are monofunctional and only allow for submucosal dissection (The PEN-TAX line of ESD knives is not available commercially in the United States).

Scissor/Grasping Type

The scissor knifes have the unique ability to grab tissue with their scissor shape and use monopolar high-frequency current to cut tissue. The blade is insulated, and the electrodes line the internal portion of the blade allowing for safer dissection. They allow the endoscopist to pull the tissue away from the plane and separate before cutting, which reduces the risk of perforations. In addition, these do not have injection functionality. Scissor type knives include Sumitomo Bakelite's (SB) Knife, SB Knife short, and SB Knife Jr 2, Olympus's 3-in-1 SB Knife, and Fujifilm's Clutch Cutter.

The SB Knife, SB Knife short, and SB Knife Jr 2 are indicated for stomach, esophagus, and colon, respectively. The SB Knife Jr 2 was released in 2011 with a slimmer structure allowing for less interference with the hood and working channel.[14] The Olympus 3-in-1 SB Knife comes in four configurations with varying forceps lengths (3.5, 6, and 7 mm), opening widths (4.5, 6, and 8 mm), and working lengths (1.95, 2.3, and 1.8 mm) suited for various techniques and locations.[15] The Olympus knife allows for mucosal incision, differentiating it from the other scissor knives. The Clutch Cutter comes in jaw lengths of 3.5 and 5.0 mm and its main advantage is a slightly thicker design which allows for improved hemostatic efficacy.[16]

Other Shaped Knives

Last, there are knives that do not neatly fit into these other categories and may be characterized by the shape of their knives. These include Olympus HookKnife, Hook-Knife J, Triangle TipKnife, Triangle TipKnife J and FlexKnife, and Kachu's Fork Knife.

The Olympus Hookknife has a tip which is bent at a right angle making an L shape.[17] This is useful for longitudinal and lateral dissection and allows for retraction of tissue as well. It has rotation movement as well (when not maximally extended). The Olympus Triangle Tip Knife has a non-insulated electrode at the tip extending 0.7 mm from the center in a triangular shape measuring 1.6 mm on each side. Dissection may be performed in all directions without the need for rotation.[18] The Olympus HookKnife J and Olympus Triangle Tip J both have saline injection capabilities. The Olympus FlexKnife has an adjustable braided loop design which can be adjusted to different lengths and allowing for dissection in all directions and suitable in all portions of the digestive tract.[19] The Kachu Fork Knife has two interchangeable knives, a fixed flexible snare and a forked knife, which has an inlet for injection and irrigation. The two knives can be changed by a switch on the main body. The flexible snare can be used for marking and making incisions, whereas the forked knife is more effective for dissection and coagulation.[20] (The Fork Knife is not available commercially in the United States.)

Electrosurgical Knife Accessories

Caps

Caps are transparent distal attachments that serve multiple purposes. They primarily serve to improve visualization during endoscopy.[21] During dissection, they work to keep the mucosa and resected tissue away from the camera lens. This also serves to improve dissection by increasing the distance between the submucosa and muscularis layers. The caps help provide a fixed distance from the mucosa and lumen, thereby increasing the safety of the procedure. They allow for stabilization of the operative field during external movements secondary to peristalsis, heartbeats, and respirations.[10] Many of these caps feature a side draining hole to prevent accumulation of fluids, blood in the cap. The hood can be emptied using the side draining port by lightly pressing against tissue which will drain the fluid out of the cap.

Caps come in various shapes which can assist the procedure in different ways (**Fig. 2A–C**). Olympus offers 10 different caps sizes (see **Fig. 2A**). They are all straight cylinders without narrowing, which improves visibility. PENTAX offers straight caps as well as caps with slits and holes for drainage (see **Fig. 2B**). Steris similarly offers the Reveal distal attachment caps that are straight caps with a single side hole for drainage ranging from 11.35 to 15.7 mm in diameter. Fujifilm on the other hand offers caps that taper distally (see **Fig. 2C**). The caps measure a diameter of 11.8 to 14.8 mm at the tip that attaches on the endoscope and then narrows distally to 8.0 mm.[22] Although this limits the field of view compared with the Olympus cap, it helps to wedge the layers and assists with dissection. The tapered cap also allows easier access to the submucosal space when a tunnel or pocket approach is chosen.

Injecting agents

ESD requires the injection of a fluid agent underneath the mucosa into the submucosal layer. This helps to increase safety by preventing perforations and thermal injury to the GI wall.[23] There are many different fluids which have been used in ESD as lifting agents including normal saline, hypertonic saline, hyaluronic acid (HA), glycerol, dextrose water, hydroxypropyl methylcellulose, fibrinogen mixture, hydroxyethyl starch, and proprietary blends such as ORISE and Eleview. The ideal injecting agent should provide a long-lasting cushion, be easy to inject, safe, inexpensive, readily available, and it should not cause any damage to the tissue or histopathological samples.

Injecting agents are required to have biologically inert dyes such as diluted indigo carmine or methylene blue, which assists in visualization during the procedure. Dyes can distinguish between muscle layer and submucosal layer. One very important function of dyes is to help the endoscopist identify muscularis propria injury, a potential harbinger of intraprocedural perforation.[24]

Normal saline is one of the most commonly used solutions as it is inexpensive, readily available, and safe. However, normal saline has one significant disadvantage in that there is relatively short tissue retention of the fluid relative to the more viscous solutions. The saline dissipates rapidly into the surround tissue, requiring continual readministration for suitable lift. Studies showed that normal saline cushions began to dissipate after 3 minutes, whereas other solutions (ie, HA) lasted 7 minutes without change.[25] Hypertonic saline has also been used due to the advantages that saline affords in addition to providing higher mucosal elevation than normal saline. However, one major disadvantage of hypertonic saline is that it causes local inflammatory reaction and tissue damage at the injection site.[24]

HA (in 0.1% and 0.4% formulations) has been shown to have greater mucosal elevation than normal saline. There are disadvantages including the lack of availability, expense, and difficulty with delivery due to the high viscosity.

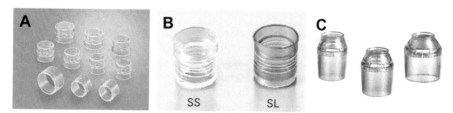

Fig. 2. Examples of various distal caps offered from (*A*) Olympus, (*B*) Fujifilm, (*C*) Pentax. (*Courtesy of* Olympus, Fujifilm, and Pentax.)

Glycerol is a hypertonic solution which allows for long-lasting elevation and is relatively inexpensive and readily available. As compared with dextrose, it does not cause histopathological damage. Dextrose solutions greater than 20% are not actually recommended due to this characteristic as well as impaired ulcer healing.[26]

Hydroxypropyl methylcellulose is a cellulose derivative with viscoelastic properties that can achieve long-lasting elevation with minimal tissue reaction.[27] Hydroxypropyl methylcellulose is cheaper than HA; however, it is a synthetic compound therefore, harbors a risk of antigen–antibody reactions.[28]

Hydroxyethyl starch is relatively safe, inexpensive, and readily available. Six percent hydroxyethyl starch has been used for submucosal lifting with longer retention than normal saline.[29] There are no significant disadvantages to its use.

Recently, preassembled solutions have entered the market, all of which have a blend of a proprietary solution with a dye component. Boston Scientific's ORISE gel was approved in 2018 by the food and drug administration (FDA) as a submucosal lifting agent. This agent is prepackaged in 10 cc syringes. Recently, the gel was associated with marked foreign body giant cell granulomatous reactions in the submucosa and muscularis propria.[30] In one study, 88% of resected samples using ORISE gel had deposition of an amorphous, pale, blue-gray fine granular material. Concern for misinterpretation during pathology assessment was raised if the pathologist was not aware of its use.[31] Moreover, ORISE gel mimics mucin on hematoxylin and eosin-stained histology which may lead to a misdiagnosis of mucinous adenocarcinoma unless proper stains are used (eg, Periodic acid–Schiff (PAS), and mucicarmine).[32] Eleview (Aries Pharmaceuticals Inc) is another proprietary blend designed to provide a duration of life up to 45 minutes. In contrast to ORISE gel, Eleview was not detectable on pathology.[33] Both are more expensive relative to the other solutions listed above.

Overall, there are many safe and effective options for injecting agents during submucosal dissection. Most endoscopists prefer a long-lasting viscous injectate over normal saline. The endoscopist should consider estimated time of procedure, costs, ease of access and potential harm to tissue, and the patient when choosing the ideal solution for ESD.

Traction devices

One important technique at the endoscopist's disposal when performing ESD is the use of traction to improve visualization and manipulation of tissue to improve safety and efficacy. An important consideration for the endoscopist when choosing a traction device is the direction of traction. Some traction devices are only able to provide traction in one direction, whereas others can be manipulated and provide traction in a range of directions, including proximally, distally, vertically, or diagonally. There are basic methods of obtaining traction such as gravity-assisted, pocket-creation method, buoyancy, and water pressure.[34] In addition to natural methods of obtaining traction, caps provide traction inherently once inserted underneath the mucosal layer. Of the cap options mentioned earlier, the tapered tip provides an advantage in wedging the layers compared with the straight cap. Often natural traction and cap traction are not enough and additional tools for traction are required.

Traction devices are broadly classified into external and internal traction devices. External traction devices include clip-in-line method, pulley method, sheath traction method, clip and snare method, Endo Trac, external forceps, double-scope method and magnetic anchor method. Internal traction devices include S-O clip method, ring thread, multiloop, traction wire, and double-clip and rubber band method. The authors discuss some of the most popular methods from those listed above.

External Traction Devices

External traction devices are those which the endoscopist manipulates the traction from outside the body. Broadly speaking, these are typically better served in esophageal, gastric, and rectal ESD, where there is more direct transmission of the endoscopist's movements.

To start, the original traction device first used in 2002 is the clip-with-line method (**Fig. 3**).[35] The endoscopist starts by making a circumferential incision. After removing the endoscope, they attach a line to a hemostatic clip which is already loaded in the accessory channel. Then, the endoscope is reinserted and the clip is deployed on the lesion allowing the endoscopist to pull on the line from outside of the body to provide varying levels of traction. This method is limited to unidirectional traction.

Many of the other external methods of traction delivery follow the general concept of the clip-in-line method with some modifications. A modification to the clip-and-line that allows movement in alternate directions is the pulley method. After placing the first clip on the lesion, a second clip is placed elsewhere in the lumen. This allows the endoscopist to create a pulley system allowing for traction in alternative directions. By using a more rigid sheath rather than a line the endoscopist may provide both pushing and pulling forces on the lesion. This is known as the sheath traction method. The external forceps method is another method for external traction. Instead of applying a clip to the lesion, forceps are driven in and placed on the lesion. This is accomplished by using a set of forceps in the accessory channel to drive a second set of forceps outside of the scope which attaches to the lesion. This allows for bidirectional traction and repositioning by releasing and regrasping the lesion.

Internal Traction Devices

Whereas external traction devices are depend on manipulation from outside of the patient's body, internal traction devices initiate and terminate inside the GI tract. Internal traction devices encompass a broad variety of technology from simple solutions using rubber bands to robotic-assisted traction delivery. Internal traction devices are preferred in colon and rectal ESD for their ability to provide local traction in narrower lumens. Examples of internal traction devices include Zeon Medical S-O Clip, multiloop suture, Medtronic ProdiGI traction wire (**Fig. 4A–C**), double clip and rubber band method (eg, Micro-Tech Endoscopy Elastic Traction Device) (see **Fig. 4A–C**), Lumendi DiLumen double-balloon system and EndoMaster endoluminal systems (see **Fig. 4A–C**).

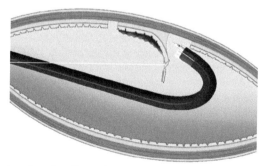

Fig. 3. A diagram showing the clip with line method where an endoclip is placed on the distal side of the lesion and traction is applied by pulling the line proximally. (Abe S, Wu SYS, Ego M, et al. Efficacy of Current Traction Techniques for Endoscopic Submucosal Dissection. Gut and Liver 2020;14:673-684.)

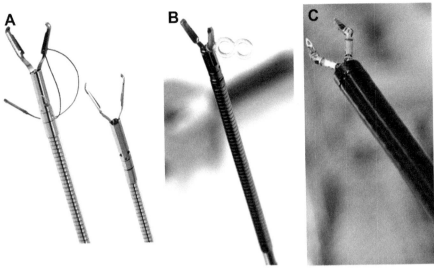

Fig. 4. (*A–C*) Examples of internal traction devices such as (*A*) Medtronic ProdiGI traction wire, (*B*) double-clip and rubber band method (eg, Micro-Tech Endoscopy Elastic Traction Device), (*C*) EndoMaster endoluminal systems. (Abe S, Wu SYS, Ego M, et al. Efficacy of Current Traction Techniques for Endoscopic Submucosal Dissection. Gut and Liver 2020;14:673-684.)

S-O Clip, Multiloop Suture, ProdiGi Traction Wire, and Double Clip and Rubber Band

The following methods all follow the same principle of creating traction by placing one hemostatic clip to the edge of the lesion and placing another hemostatic clip in another location within the GI lumen. These two clips are connected, which provides traction during ESD. The difference between each of these methods is what connects the two hemostatic clips. They can be connected by either a spring (S-O clip) (**Fig. 5**), thread (multiloop suture), wire (ProdiGi traction wire), or rubber bands (double clip and rubber band) (Video 1). The second clip can either be attached to the contralateral wall of the lumen or to the opposite side of the lesion.[36] Careful consideration for the site of attachment of the second clip should be given as the degree of traction provided will change as the dissection progresses and ultimately the clip will need to be removed. Adding additional clips or using removable devices may assist in changing the direction of traction at later stages of the procedure. If properly placed, it can provide sufficient traction throughout the whole procedure.

The Zeon Medical S-O clip developed in 2016 consists of a 5-mm spring attached to a hemoclip on one end with a 4-mm nylon loop on the other end.[37] The spring has higher elasticity than threads and rubber bands which can be easily adjusted for a large lumen to prevent lacerations of the mucosal flaps and slip-offs of breakage of the traction devices[34] (The Zeon Medical S-O clip is not available commercially in the United States). The ProdiGi traction wire offers wire lengths of 20 and 35 mm,[38] which would result in distances of 10 and 17.5 mm from clip to clip once secured. The Micro-Tech Elastic Traction Device consists of three interconnected elastic silicone bands (one 1.5 mm and two 3.3 mm bands).

The advantages of the methods listed above are that they do not require removal and reinsertion of the endoscope because the tools are designed to fit through the

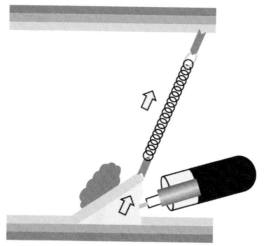

Fig. 5. A diagram showing the spring and loop method where an endoclip is placed on the distal side of the lesion and a second endoclip is anchored to the opposite side of the lumen, connected by a spring providing tension. (*From* Abe S, et al. Efficacy of Current Traction Techniques for Endoscopic Submucosal Dissection. *Gut Liver.* 2020;14(6):673-684.)

endoscope channel. In addition, they eliminate reliance on gravity to provide traction and are cost-effective.[39]

Double-Balloon System

The Lumendi double-balloon system (DiLumen) is composed of a polyurethane flexible over sheath with two independently inflatable balloons that slides over the endoscope.[40] The two balloons inflate proximal and distal to the lesion and are called the aft-balloon and fore-balloon, respectively. The sheath is 168 cm long and the balloons reach a diameter of 6 cm when maximally inflated.[40] The aft balloon provides endoscopic tip stability, whereas the fore balloon provides mucosal gripping, ability to flatten folds, straighten the lumen at the flexure, and tissue retraction.[40]

Endoluminal System

The EndoMaster endoluminal system is a novel robotic-assisted surgical system. These specialized endoscopes have two attachments at the distal end of their endoscopes which draw inspiration from laparoscopic and robotic surgeries. One attachment is a grasper with full range of motion and the other attachment is a probe for monopolar diathermy.[41] These are controlled by a user console like robotic surgery machines with two handles that control the two attachments. The system provides feedback to the endoscopist regarding pressure and tissue thickness.[42]

A recent systematic literature review on various types of traction devices concluded that multiple disparate endoscopic methods have the potential to improve tissue tension and facilitate visualization during ESD.[43] However, the study was not able to conclude that one traction method was superior and ultimately recommended a case-by-case selection based on lesion characteristics, endoscopic proficiency, and availability of resources.

Hemostasis Tools

Bleeding is a common and potentially serious complication of ESD. As shown in **Table 1**, nearly all knives have some capability for intraprocedural hemostasis. Typically, the hemostatic effect from knives is suitable for smaller oozing vessels but are not capable of managing larger vessel bleeds and require additional tools. The use of hemostatic clips is avoided when possible interprocedurally as they may lead to obstructed views and interfere with the procedure. Instead, hemostatic forceps (also known as coagulation graspers) are preferred. Examples include the Olympus Coagrasper and the PENTAX HemoStat-Y. These are shaped similarly to hot biopsy forceps with a wider surface area. The endoscopist uses the hemostatic forceps to grasp the bleeding site, tent the instrument away from the mucosa, then run a current for 1 to 2 seconds which leads to protein denaturation without burning tissue resulting in hemostasis. There will be a separate chapter in this series that will explain in greater detail the settings and mechanisms for these devices.

PuraStat is a synthetic hemostatic material. It has been shown to be effective in situations such as bleeding of small vessels, oozing from vascular anastomoses, and oozing from capillaries of the parenchyma and surround tissues of solid organs. It has also been shown to lead to a reduction of delayed bleeding following ESD in the colon.[44] It is prepared in a prefilled syringe and functions by self-assembling into a scaffold which mimics human extracellular matrix.[45] In addition, one advantage of PuraStat over other hydrogels is that it is broken down in approximately 30 days by enzymatic action which prevents swelling and compression of nearby structures. It has been shown to achieve hemostasis in less than 15 seconds.[44]

SUMMARY

As an endoscopic prepares for an ESD procedure, they should be aware of the various tools available at their disposal. With that knowledge at hand, they should approach each case as a unique entity that will be better suited with certain attributes. By focusing on location, characteristics, and anticipatory needs, the endoscopist may build the best toolbox for their case.

CLINICS CARE POINTS

- Trials comparing knives with injection capability to non-waterjet knives have shown that knives with injection capability reduce procedure time (43 vs 60.5 minutes) without significant differences in clinical outcomes or adverse events.[46]
- Trials comparing traction-assisted colorectal endoscopic submucosal dissection (ESD) to conventional ESD found that the use of traction results in shorter mean procedure time (51 vs 71 minutes), higher en bloc resection rate (99% vs 81%), and lower perforation rate (1.3% vs 4.3%).[47]
- There is a large learning curve for ESD which is improved using traction devices. Proficiency was achieved by trainees in 10 procedures with traction devices compared with 21 procedures in the control group.[48] Trainees in the traction device group have higher self-completion rates, dissection speeds, and en bloc resection rate.

DISCLOSURE

S. Amin is an advisor to Boston Scientific and Medtronic.

SUPPLEMENTARY DATA

Supplementary data related to this article can be found online at https://doi.org/10.1016/j.giec.2022.09.001.

REFERENCES

1. Rashid MU, Alomari M, Afraz S, et al. EMR and ESD: Indications, techniques and results. Surg Oncol 2022;101742. https://doi.org/10.1016/j.suronc.2022.101742, published online ahead of print, 2022 Mar 18.
2. Harlow C, Sivananthan A, Ayaru L, et al. Endoscopic submucosal dissection: an update on tools and accessories. Ther Adv Gastrointest Endosc 2020;13. 2631774520957220.
3. Corporation Olympus. ESD Devices | Endotherapy Devices in: Olympus Medical Singapore. 2022. Available at: https://olympusmedical.com.sg/products/all-products/endotherapy-devices/esd-and-emr/esd-devices/index.html. Accessed: April 19, 2022.
4. FujiFilm corporation. Treatment options for therapeutic endoscopy. 8. 2018. Available at: https://www.fujifilm-endoscopy.com/storage/app/media/products/files/ESD%20Brochure.pdf. Accessed: April 19, 2022.
5. Esaki M, Suzuki S, Hayashi Y, et al. Splash M-knife versus Flush Knife BT in the technical outcomes of endoscopic submucosal dissection for early gastric cancer: a propensity score matching analysis. BMC Gastroenterol 2018;18:35. https://doi.org/10.1186/s12876-018-0763-5.
6. Erbe USA. HybridKnife; 2017. Available at: https://us.erbe-med.com/fileadmin/user_upload/us-media/MKT505502_HybridKnife_OnePager_USA_0817.pdf. Accessed: April 19, 2022.
7. Boston Scientific Corporation. ORISE™ ProKnife Electrosurgical Knife. 2022. Available at: https://www.bostonscientific.com/en-US/products/endoluminal-surgery-devices/orise-proknife-electrosurgical-knife.html. Accessed: April 19, 2022.
8. CreoMedical. Speedboat inject in: CreoMedical. Available at: https://creomedical.com/speedboat-inject/. Accessed: April 19, 2022.
9. Mori G, Nonaka S, Oda I, et al. Novel strategy of endoscopic submucosal dissection using an insulation-tipped knife for early gastric cancer: near-side approach method. Endosc Int Open 2015;3(5):E425–31.
10. Choi HS, Chun HJ, Kim I. An unusual submucosal tumor of the stomach. Gastroenterology 2012;142(4):e11–2.
11. Corporation Olympus. IT Knife2 In: Knives ESD - Knives. 2022. Available at: https://medical.olympusamerica.com/products/knives/itknife2-kd-611l. Accessed: April 19, 2022.
12. PENTAX Medical. PENTAX Medical ESD Accessories. 2022. Available at: https://www.pentaxmedical.com/pentax/download/fstore/uploadFiles/Pdfs/Product%20Datasheets/EMEA_ACC_BR_Brochure_ESD_Accessories_02.2013.pdf. Accessed: April 19, 2022.
13. PENTAX Medical. ESD Accessories. 2022. Available at: https://www.pentaxmedical.com/pentax/en/95/36/ESD-Accessories. Accessed: April 19, 2022.
14. Shiratori Y, Ikeya T, Fukuda K. Introducing the newly developed SB Knife Jr 2: enhancing creative endoscopic submucosal dissection. Endoscopy 2021;53(9):E352–4.

15. Corporation Olympus. SB Knives in Products. 2022. Available at: https://medical.olympusamerica.com/products/sb-knives. Accessed: April 19, 2022.
16. Dohi O, Yoshida N, Terasaki K, et al. Efficacy of Clutch Cutter for Standardizing Endoscopic Submucosal Dissection for Early Gastric Cancer: A Propensity Score-Matched Analysis. Digestion 2019;100(3):201–9.
17. Corporation Olympus. HookKnife Electrosurgical Knife in Knives. 2022. available at: https://medical.olympusamerica.com/products/knives/hookknife-upper-length-kd-620lr. Accessed: April 19, 2022.
18. Corporation Olympus. Triangle Tip Electrosurigical Knife In: Knives. Available at: https://medical.olympusamerica.com/products/knives/triangle-tip-knife-kd-640l. Accessed: April 19, 2022.
19. Corporation Olympus. FlexKnife Electrosurgical Knife In: Knives. Available at: https://medical.olympusamerica.com/products/knives/flexknife-kd-630l.   Accessed: April 19, 2022.
20. Kim HG, Cho JY, Bok GH, et al. A novel device for endoscopic submucosal dissection, the Fork knife. World J Gastroenterol 2008;14(43):6726–32.
21. ASGE Technology Committee, Maple JT, Abu Dayyeh BK, et al. Endoscopic submucosal dissection. Gastrointest Endosc 2015;81(6):1311–25.
22. FujiFilm Group. ST Hoods In: ESD Devices. 2022. Available at: https://www.fujifilm.com/sg/en/healthcare/endoscopy/accessories/endoscopy-esd/st-hoodt. Accessed: April 19, 2022.
23. Uraoka T, Saito Y, Yamamoto K, et al. Submucosal injection solution for gastrointestinal tract endoscopic mucosal resection and endoscopic submucosal dissection. Drug Des Devel Ther 2009;2:131–8.
24. Castro R, Libânio D, Pita I, et al. Solutions for submucosal injection: What to choose and how to do it. World J Gastroenterol 2019;25(7):777–88.
25. Uraoka T, Fujii T, Saito Y, et al. Effectiveness of glycerol as a submucosal injection for EMR. Gastrointest Endosc 2005;61(6):736–40.
26. Fujishiro M, Yahagi N, Kashimura K, et al. Tissue damage of different submucosal injection solutions for EMR. Gastrointest Endosc 2005;62(6):933–42.
27. Feitoza AB, Gostout CJ, Burgart LJ, et al. Hydroxypropyl methylcellulose: A better submucosal fluid cushion for endoscopic mucosal resection. Gastrointest Endosc 2003;57(1):41–7.
28. Fujishiro M, Yahagi N, Kashimura K, et al. Comparison of various submucosal injection solutions for maintaining mucosal elevation during endoscopic mucosal resection. Endoscopy 2004;36(7):579–83.
29. Mehta N, Strong AT, Franco M, et al. Optimal injection solution for endoscopic submucosal dissection: A randomized controlled trial of Western solutions in a porcine model. Dig Endosc 2018;30(3):347–53.
30. Sun BL. Submucosal lifting agent ORISE gel causes extensive foreign body granuloma post endoscopic resection. Int J Colorectal Dis 2021;36(2):419–22.
31. Olivas AD, Setia N, Weber CR, et al. Histologic changes caused by injection of a novel submucosal lifting agent for endoscopic resection in GI lesions. Gastrointest Endosc 2021;93(2):470–6.
32. Yang D, Saulino D, Draganov PV. Histologic changes with a novel submucosal lifting gel for endoscopic resection: more than just a lift. Gastrointest Endosc 2022; 95(1):198.
33. Dong ZM, Fang J, Byrne KR, et al. Histologic mimics and diagnostic pitfalls of gastrointestinal endoscopic lifting media, ORISE™ gel and Eleview. Hum Pathol 2022;119:28–40.

34. Nagata M. Advances in traction methods for endoscopic submucosal dissection: What is the best traction method and traction direction? World J Gastroenterol 2022;28(1):1–22.

35. Oyama T, Kikuchi Y, Shimaya S, et al. Endoscopic mucosal resection using a hooking knife (hooking EMR) [in Japanese]. Stomach Intest 2002;37:1151–61.

36. Ge PS, Aihara H. A novel clip-band traction device to facilitate colorectal endoscopic submucosal dissection and defect closure. VideoGIE 2020;5(5):180–6. Published 2020 Mar 31.

37. Zeon Medical Inc. Countertraction CLIP. 2021. Available at: https://www. zeonmedical.co.jp/e/product_e/pdf/EX-010_Countertraction_CLIP_20211026. pdf. Accessed: April 19, 2022.

38. Medtronic. ProdiGI Traction Wire. 2021. Available at: https://www.medtronic.com/ content/dam/covidien/library/emea/en/product/Endoscopy%20Products/weu-prodigi-esd-traction-wire-sheet.pdf. Accessed: April 19, 2022.

39. Amin S, Sethi A. Embracing simplicity to improve outcomes in endoscopic submucosal dissection: Will it gain traction? Gastrointest Endosc 2021;94(2):344–6.

40. Sharma S, Momose K, Hara H, et al. Facilitating endoscopic submucosal dissection: double balloon endolumenal platform significantly improves dissection time compared with conventional technique (with video) [published correction appears in Surg Endosc. 2019 Jan 24. Surg Endosc 2019;33(1):315–21.

41. Tay G, Tan HK, Nguyen TK, et al. Use of the EndoMaster robot-assisted surgical system in transoral robotic surgery: A cadaveric study. Int J Med Robot 2018; 14(4):e1930.

42. Government of Singapore. EndoMaster In: National Research Foundation Prime Minister's Office Singapore. 2021. Available at: https://www.nrf.gov.sg/ innovation-enterprise/innovative-projects/health-and-biomedical-sciences/ endomaster. Accessed: April 19, 2022.

43. Tziatzios G, Ebigbo A, Gölder SK, et al. Methods that Assist Traction during Endoscopic Submucosal Dissection of Superficial Gastrointestinal Cancers: A Systematic Literature Review. Clin Endosc 2020;53(3):286–301.

44. 3-D Matrix Medical Technology. PuraStat In: 3-D Matric Medical Technology. 2022. Available at: https://3dmatrix.com/products/purastat/. Accessed: April 19, 2022.

45. Jhala D, Vasita R. A Review on Extracellular Matrix Mimicking Strategies for an Artificial Stem Cell Niche. Polym Rev 2015;55(4):561–95.

46. Huang R, Yan H, Ren G, et al. Comparison of O-Type HybridKnife to Conventional Knife in Endoscopic Submucosal Dissection for Gastric Mucosal Lesions. Medicine (Baltimore) 2016;95(13):e3148.

47. Fujinami H, Teramoto A, Takahashi S, et al. Effectiveness of S-O Clip-Assisted Colorectal Endoscopic Submucosal Dissection. J Clin Med 2021;11(1):141.

48. Mitsuyoshi Y, Ide D, Ohya TR, et al. Training program using a traction device improves trainees' learning curve of colorectal endoscopic submucosal dissection. Surg Endosc 2021. https://doi.org/10.1007/s00464-021-08799-y.

Understanding the Principles of Electrosurgery for Endoscopic Surgery and Third Space Endoscopy

Andrew A. Li, MD[a,b], Margaret J. Zhou, MD[a,b], Joo Ha Hwang, MD, PhD[a,b,*]

KEYWORDS

- Endoscopic surgery • Electrosurgery endoscopy • Submucosal endoscopy
- Electrosurgical generator units

KEY POINTS

- Understanding electrosurgical principles is important in endoscopic surgery to achieve the desired therapeutic effect, optimize patient outcomes, and prevent adverse events.
- Electrosurgical units (ESUs) provide settings with different properties that contribute to current density and tissue effect. Settings are adjusted based the desired tissue effect for different phases of a procedure.
- In addition to ESU settings, other factors, such as device properties, user technique, application time, and patient or tissue characteristics, also impact current density and tissue effect.
- Familiarity with concepts, such as current density, tissue effect, and the duty cycle and crest factor for each waveform, can help with understanding the various cutting and coagulation waveforms available on ESUs and selecting the appropriate setting for the desired therapeutic effect during endoscopic surgery.

INTRODUCTION
Overview of Electrosurgery and Physical Principles

Electrosurgery is the application of high-frequency electrical alternating current to biologic tissue to cut, coagulate, desiccate, and/or fulgurate. The technology of electrosurgery is widely used in many medical and surgical specialties, including gastrointestinal endoscopy. Within gastrointestinal endoscopy, there are a variety of applications including, biliary sphincterotomy, polypectomy, hemostasis, the ablation

[a] Division of Gastroenterology and Hepatology, Department of Medicine, Stanford University School of Medicine, Stanford, CA, USA; [b] 430 Broadway, Pavilion C-3rd Floor, GI Suite, Redwood City, CA 94063, USA
* Corresponding author. 300 Pasteur Drive, MC:5244, Palo Alto, CA 94305.
E-mail address: jooha@stanford.edu

Gastrointest Endoscopy Clin N Am 33 (2023) 29–40
https://doi.org/10.1016/j.giec.2022.07.001
1052-5157/23/© 2022 Elsevier Inc. All rights reserved.

of lesions, and endoscopic surgery. An understanding of the principles of electrosurgery is important to optimize patient outcomes for each of these applications and to prevent adverse events (eg, bleeding, perforation, or inadvertent damage to surrounding tissue). An understanding of several key concepts for electrosurgery is especially important in endoscopic surgery because of the extensive and dynamic use of electrosurgery to achieve the multiple desired tissue effects through different phases of each procedure (eg, marking, mucosal incision, submucosal dissection, hemostasis, and myotomy) while minimizing injury to nearby tissue.

DISCUSSION
Alternating Electrical Current and Tissue Effect

Applying electrical current to biologic tissue has several effects. With the application of direct current, there is an electrolytic effect where electrically charged molecules flow toward the opposite pole. With a rapid alternating current, such as that used in electrosurgical generator units (ESUs), the electrolytic effect is eliminated, and heat is produced through the intracellular oscillation of ionized molecules. This thermal effect is the basis of electrosurgery: high-frequency alternating current is used to directly generate heat within tissue, and the rapidity, amplitude, and depth of the heat generated determines the tissue effect.[1] By manipulating the properties of the rapidly alternating current and its application to the target tissue, different tissue effects are created. For example, with almost instantaneous heating to a high temperature (>100°C), water within cells quickly vaporizes and causes the cell membranes to burst, creating a cutting effect.[2] At lower temperatures (60°C), proteins are denatured, causing shrinking, drying, and devitalization of the tissue, which is used for coagulation or ablation of lesions. The relative balance of these two processes (cutting and coagulation) is referred to as the tissue effect.

A high frequency (>300 kHz) is used in ESUs to avoid neuromuscular effects that are seen at lower frequencies, such as shocking and electrocution. Because this frequency is in the AM radio range, this range of energy is also referred to as radiofrequency. Of note, electrosurgery is distinct from cautery, wherein electrical current is used to heat an element that is in turn used to cauterize tissue through heat conduction. This is different from electrosurgery in that heat rather than electrical current is passed to the tissue. Cautery is rarely used in gastrointestinal endoscopy, but examples include the heater probe.

Monopolar and Bipolar Devices

For circuits to conduct electricity, they must be closed. In electrosurgery, the patient is connected to a circuit containing the ESU through two electrodes, which is in turn grounded. These electrodes may take the form of monopolar devices paired with a return dispersive electrode, or bipolar devices that contain both electrodes (**Fig. 1**).

Most applications of electrosurgery in endoscopic procedures use monopolar devices, wherein one electrode is the device, such as a snare, endoscopic submucosal dissection knife, coagulation graspers, argon plasma probe, and so forth, and the other electrode is a return dispersive electrode. Colloquially, this is sometimes referred to as the "grounding pad," which is a misnomer, because the ESU is grounded, not the patient. Current flows from the ESU through the path of least resistance between the device and the dispersive electrode back to ESU to complete the electrical circuit. Because the surface area of the pad is orders of magnitude larger than the active device, the current density is extremely low at the pad site. Appropriate pad placement is critical to safely disperse the electrical energy and avoid an increase in skin

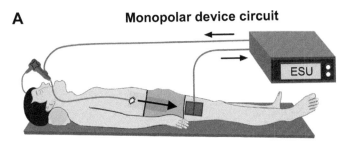

A   Monopolar device circuit

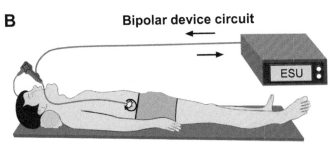

B   Bipolar device circuit

Fig. 1. Overview of electrosurgical generator units (ESU) and circuits. (*A*) Monopolar device circuits. In monopolar device circuits, current flows from the ESU to the device, which then flows through the target tissue and patient, and returns to the ESU through a return dispersive electrode. (*B*) Bipolar device circuits. In bipolar device circuits, there is no return dispersive electrode. Instead, current flows within the small area of tissue at the tip of the device, which contains active and return electrodes.

temperature under the pad (see discussion of safety). In contrast to monopolar devices, bipolar devices contain the active and return electrodes in the tip of the instrument. Electrical current flows within the small area of tissue without the need for a return dispersive electrode. An overview of the multiple different monopolar and bipolar devices used in endoscopic surgery is described elsewhere in this issue.

Current Density

The relative balance of cutting, devitalization, coagulation, and desiccation, or tissue effect, is determined by the magnitude of heat generated and the rapidity with which it is achieved. Although ESU manufacturers provide guidance and suggestive settings for common procedures, there are many factors beyond the generator that determine the tissue effect including device properties and operator technique.

The tissue effect is determined by ESU factors (eg, mode, waveform, and power settings), the device, user technique (eg, the surface area of the active electrode in contact with tissue, tension placed on tissue, velocity of the electrode), circuit impedance affected by patient and tissue characteristics (eg, water content, presence of coagulum, fibrosis, or fat content), and time of application. These many factors are summarized as affecting current density, or the intensity or concentration of current in an area of tissue; it is the key variable that determines the tissue effect. It is a measure of current concentration, defined as the current per unit area (**Fig. 2**).

Current density is important for achieving the desired tissue effect in the immediate vicinity of the active device, but also is important for safety considerations in terms of

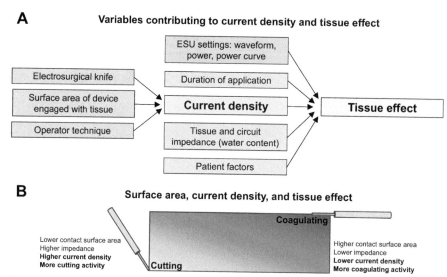

A   **Variables contributing to current density and tissue effect**

Fig. 2. Illustration of the factors that contribute to current density and tissue effect. (*A*) Current density is the principal factor in determining tissue effect. Many variables contribute to current density, including device selection, surface area of device used, technique, and electrosurgical generator unit settings. (*B*) Surface area, current density, and tissue effect. Illustrative example of how surface area affects current density, and thus tissue effect, even when the same device is used. If only the tip is in contact with tissue, there is higher current density and more of a cutting effect compared with if a broader area of the device is in contact with the target tissue resulting in lower current density and more of a coagulative effect.

minimizing thermal injury to nearby tissue. Mathematically, the temperature in tissue rises as a square of the current density, such that a current that almost instantaneously vaporizes water in a 1-mm^2 area, thereby cutting tissue, does not generate an appreciable effect on a 1-cm^2 area.[3]

Current density is affected by ESU settings (discussed later), but also the properties of the active device and user technique. For example, if a higher current density is desired to achieve more of a cutting effect rather than coagulation, options include changing the waveform to one with a higher duty cycle or lower crest factor (discussed in the next section) or using a smaller surface area to contact the tissue either through selection of a device with a thinner electrode or manipulating the device such that a smaller area is in contact with tissue (see **Fig. 2**B). This higher current density more rapidly heats the cells in contact with the active electrode to beyond 100°C, vaporizing the cells and cutting tissue with less heating of the immediately surrounding tissue leading to less coagulation effect. Conversely, if a lower current density is used, either through ESU settings, or a larger surface area of the active electrode contacting tissue (eg, with coagulation forceps), then tissue is heated slowly such that water is more gradually evaporated allowing for desiccation, coagulation, and fulguration of the tissue (see **Fig. 2**B). Moreover, beyond current density, user technique, such as tension on tissue, also alters the tissue effect.

Understanding Cut and Coagulation Settings

The rapidity and degree to which tissue is heated by electrical current determines the tissue effect, or the relative balance of cutting, coagulation, and desiccation of tissue.

Current density over time is the major factor in determining the tissue effect as discussed in the previous section.

The electrosurgical generator is an important aspect of the many factors that affect current density and tissue effect. Each ESU manufacturer has different settings, but the concepts that govern them are the same. Here, we provide a framework to better understand these different waveforms and settings, and their potential applications. There are sparse evidence-based data for the optimal waveform choice, so this is left to the physician's preference and experience based on the desired tissue effect.

Before discussing the continuum of cutting and coagulation currents, two key concepts for understanding the qualitative nature of waveforms warrant discussion. These are duty cycle and crest factor, which can provide a framework to understand several key properties of these waveforms (**Fig. 3**).

Duty cycle refers to the percentage of time that the energy is being actively delivered in each waveform. With a 100% duty cycle, the waveform is on for the full duration of time, whereas with a 6% duty cycle, the waveform is modulated such that energy is being delivered only 6% of the time and is off 94% of the time. These time intervals are modulated on the order of milliseconds. As discussed later, in general, higher percentage duty cycle waveforms produce more cutting and less coagulation tissue effect and lower percentage duty cycle waveforms produce more coagulation and less cutting for a given voltage. This is caused by the rapidity with which tissue is heated, wherein high duty cycle rapidly heats tissue compared with a low duty cycle waveform, wherein there is time between pulses of energy for heat to gradually rise and dissipate into nearby tissue, creating more gradual heating with a wider area of effect.

Crest factor is a term that refers to the peak voltage relative to the average voltage of a waveform (defined as peak voltage over the root-mean-squared average voltage). Higher voltage spikes can force current through desiccated tissue with high impedance adjacent to the active electrode, resulting in deeper tissue effect.

Fig. 4 lists cutting, coagulation, and blended currents for common waveforms with their associated duty cycle and crest factors.

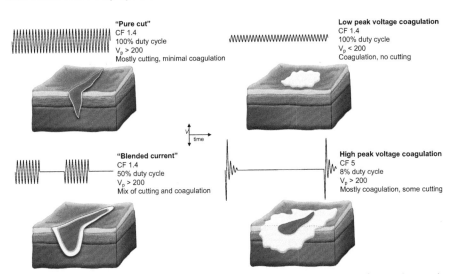

"Pure cut"
CF 1.4
100% duty cycle
$V_p > 200$
Mostly cutting, minimal coagulation

Low peak voltage coagulation
CF 1.4
100% duty cycle
$V_p < 200$
Coagulation, no cutting

"Blended current"
CF 1.4
50% duty cycle
$V_p > 200$
Mix of cutting and coagulation

High peak voltage coagulation
CF 5
8% duty cycle
$V_p > 200$
Mostly coagulation, some cutting

Fig. 3. Different waveforms produce different tissue effects based on crest factor, duty cycle, and voltage. CF, crest factor.

CUT	COAG		Crest Factor	Duty Cycle	Peak Volts
High Cut			1.4	100%	>200
Endo Cut			1.4	100% (cutting cycle)	>200
Dry Cut			2.7-3.8	30%	>200
	Swift Coag		5.4	8%	>>200
	PreciseSect		4.0 (dynamic)		>>200
	Forced Coag		6.0	8%	>>200
	Spray Coag		7.4	4%	>>>200
		Soft Coag	1.4	100%	<200

Fig. 4. Crest factor and duty cycle for common Erbe ESU waveforms.

Understanding cutting settings

A cutting current divides tissue by nearly instantaneously heating water within cells to greater than 100°C to create steam that bursts these cells' membranes. This is achieved by creating high current density along the leading edge of the electrode, typically though the use of a continuous (100% duty cycle, crest factor of ~1.4–1.6) high-frequency (>300 kHz) sine wave with a peak voltage greater than 200 Vp. This intensity of current is sufficient to create microelectric sparks between the active electrode and the target tissue that vaporizes cells and creates a microsteam layer, propagating the cutting effect.[4]

Although the term "pure cut" is sometimes used to refer to these waveforms, there is a layer of cells along the margin of the cut path that are heated less rapidly and not to the point of vaporization, but rather to the point of coagulation. The depth of this coagulated tissue is related to the peak voltage and surface area of the active electrode of the device. A higher peak voltage or a broader active electrode leads to a thicker margin of coagulation, whereas a lower peak voltage or thinner active electrode leads to a thinner margin of coagulation.

Most cutting waveforms are based on this 100% duty cycle setting. Some ESU manufacturers have created settings that introduce either pauses with no current (Olympus [Center Valley, PA], Genii [St. Paul, MN], and ConMed Pulse Cut [Utica, NY]) or alternating with a coagulating waveform (Erbe EndoCut I and Q [Marietta, GA]).

Blended cutting waveforms produce a tissue effect of cutting activity but with a greater depth of thermal injury and coagulation along the path of the electrode. This is achieved through modulation of the current with a lower duty cycle, typically ranging from 30% to 70%, and higher crest factor in the 1.8 to 3.8 range, as compared with a "pure" cutting current, which is 100% duty cycle and crest factor of about 1.4. The higher peak voltage (reflected by higher crest factor) and slower delivery of energy (reflected by lower duty cycle) allows current and heat generation to be delivered more deeply and slowly, respectively. Examples of this include Dry Cut (Erbe) or Blend Cut (Genii).

Understanding coagulation settings

Coagulation of tissue is achieved through the comparatively slow heating of tissue in close contact with the active electrode. Modern ESUs have various coagulation modes. With low duty cycle waveforms, the gradual heating of tissue is achieved by pulsing short bursts of energy with longer pauses between them. This results in the period delivery of current to create bubbling of cellular water content (wave on) and then steam release with cooling (wave off) repeated with each duty cycle, thereby desiccating and shrinking the cells, creating a coagulation effect.[5,6] However, these do have some electrosurgical cutting activity because of the voltage spikes, with peak voltages typically greater than 200 Vp, which are sufficient to create microsparks that cause cutting. Because of this, the conventional wisdom is that these waveforms are usually less suitable for precoagulation of large vessels, such as arteries, because they can be cut by the sparking before the vessel's edges are fully desiccated and coagulated. However, for small vessels and capillaries, it is often suitable because they are small enough in diameter to be sufficiently desiccated and coagulated before being cut by the sparking. Examples of these coagulation waveforms include Forced Coag, Spray Coag, and Swift Coag (Erbe Vio 3).

With low power (<200 Vp) pure sinusoidal waveforms (eg, Soft Coag, TouchSoft), a similar effect is achieved through the slower and gradual heating of the tissue. Although this is a 100% duty cycle waveform, the peak voltage is too low to generate the microsparks necessary for rapid vaporization and cutting tissue effect, in contrast to the low duty cycle high peak voltage waveforms described previously. The minimal cutting activity makes it a current more suitable for the coagulation of larger vessels, such as arteries. However, a limitation of this waveform is that because of the lower voltage, energy cannot be delivered as deeply when the tissue resistance is high after a coagulum has formed. Therefore, use of a device with a larger electrode surface area, such as hemostatic forceps (coagulation graspers), is needed to decrease current density and resistance to allow for sufficient coagulation, in addition to the coaptive properties of the forceps that decrease blood flow during coagulation reducing the heat sink effect of blood flow.

Most coagulation waveforms on modern ESU generators are variations of the low duty cycle, high peak voltage waveforms with high crest factors. Beyond the most common waveform with a 6% duty cycle (as in forced coagulation or pure coagulation), waveforms with a slightly higher duty cycle and lower crest factor offer more cutting activity and less thermal spread. Examples of these include Blend Coag or Swift Coag.[7,8]

Finally, a low duty cycle waveform with very high voltage waveform is used to induce arcing in a noncontact fashion. Very high voltages are required to ionize the mixed air between the electrode and tissue and therefore have high crest factors (>7–8) and may be named Spray Coagulation or fulgurate. Notably, this is a similar principle used in argon plasma coagulation (APC), but because of argon's more stable plasma, lower voltages can be used in APC as compared with mixed air. Although this setting has very high voltages, if the electrode is not in contact with the tissue, the current density at the level of the tissue is low as the current passes from the electrode, through air or CO_2 to a much larger surface area of target tissue; therefore, the current density is decreased and the current effectively coagulates vessels without deep penetration. However, if the electrode is in contact with the tissue, the very high voltage delivered directly to the tissue can result in very high current density resulting in deep penetration of current and resulting tissue effect. This setting should be used with caution. Also, this setting should be used with devices that are rated for high-voltage waveforms.

Practical Considerations

Cutting and coagulation waveforms exist on a continuum of the relative balance of cutting and coagulation activity, a large degree of which is captured with understanding the duty cycle and crest factor for each waveform.

In endoscopic surgery, considerations for which waveform to use depend on the desired tissue effect (eg, cutting, coagulation, or blend of both), tissue site and risk of thermal injury to adjacent tissue, the device used, user technique, and the many other factors that affect current density. Power settings are also affected by these considerations. In general, when the aim is to cut tissue, high current density is desired. If coagulation of vessels is the aim, a lower current density should be delivered to avoid prematurely cutting a vessel before it has been fully coagulated. For larger vessels, especially arteries, the use of coagulation graspers delivers lower current density (because of the large surface area of the electrode) and also coapts the vessel during the delivery of energy, decreasing blood flow and preventing a heat sink effect. Suggested settings for common applications in endoscopic surgery are listed in **Table 1**, but these must be individualized and potentially adjusted during the procedure to achieve the desired tissue effect and minimize risk of damaging nearby structures, bleeding, and perforation.

Safety

General safety features of electrosurgical generator units
ESU-related complications are rare; however, it is important to understand the potential risks. Historically, the most commonly reported patient injury with ESUs has been a skin injury at the site of the dispersive electrode, although to our knowledge this has not been reported with endoscopic procedures.[8,9] Other possible complications include burns from capacitive coupling (ie, a burn resulting from current transfer from the active electrode to a second conductive structure), interaction with implantable devices, or colonic gas explosion.[8-11]

Best practices when using ESUs include inspection of the ESU and power settings before activation, disconnecting the device from the active cord when not in use, placing the generator in "standby" mode if the procedure has not commenced, avoiding accidental activation of the electrode, handling tools by the plastic insulated areas, and never attempting to connect or disconnect accessories while current is flowing.[8,9,12] Most modern ESUs include a system that monitors contact quality between the patient and the dispersive pad when used with a split (ie, dual, or sensing) dispersive pad. This can trigger an alert if there is a change in contact (decreased surface contact, increased resistance to current) that could lead to heat dispersion on the patient's skin and a possible burn at the area of contact. This technology significantly reduces the risk of skin injury under the pad. It is thus highly recommended to use these safety features and a split pad.[9] In addition, it is important to always be aware of active electrodes to ensure the safety of patients and staff. A monopolar tool connected to a generator that is "on" is considered an active electrode and can potentially cause an electrosurgical injury if it is unintentionally activated.

Placement of dispersive electrodes
Dispersive electrode/pad placement is an important aspect of electrosurgery. When using a monopolar device, a dispersive electrode (grounding pad) is required to complete the electrical circuit. The current flows from the ESU to the treatment site via the device, through the patient's tissue to the dispersive electrode on the skin, and completes the circuit by flowing back to the generator.

It is crucial to train staff on best practices for the placement and management of dispersive pads. Proper pad placement includes placing pads as close as possible to the treatment site to allow for the shortest monopolar circuit, ensuring pad placement over areas with good blood supply, and avoiding placement over skin irregularities (scars, broken skin, excessive hair, or tattoos) or implants, because these can interfere with smooth current dispersion. Avoiding having vulnerable structures (eg, an implantable device) be placed between the active and dispersive electrode is also recommended. Ensuring the best possible contact between the skin and the entire dispersive pad is essential, and this is accomplished by using only fresh disposable pads with adherent gel, checking expiration dates of pads, and avoiding placing

Table 1
Suggested Erbe generator settings[a] for common applications in endoscopic surgery

Technique	Output Name	Power (W)	Cut Duration	Cut Interval	Effect	General Approach
Mucosal marking	Soft Coag	60–80			5	Coagulation setting.
	Forced Coag	10			1	Low power to avoid piercing through the muscularis mucosae.
	Spray Coag	10			1	Often performed with the knife tip retracted.
Mucosal incision	EndCut I	—	2–3	2–3	2–3	Cut setting.
	Dry Cut	60–80			2–5	Increase effect and/or cut interval if the tissue is more vascular.
Submucosal dissection	Forced Coag	30–50			2–3	Any cut or coagulation setting (other than Soft Coag) works for submucosal dissection.
	Precise Sect (Erbe VIO3)	40–60			—	Decreased surface area in contact with tissue increases current density and provides more dissection/cutting capability.
	Swift Coag	40–50			2–5	Coagulation of submucosal vessels requires lower current density to
	Spray Coag	40–50			1–2	coagulate the vessel while cutting through the vessel. If the vessel is large
	Dry Cut	30–40			3–5	or pulsating, use coagulation graspers to coagulate the vessel before
	EndoCut I	—	2–3	2–3	2–3	cutting across the vessel.
Myotomy	EndoCut I	—	2	2–3	2–3	EndoCut I with low effect or "tapping" of the pedal is effective for muscle with minimal vessels.
	Dry Cut	60–80			3–4	EndoCut I with higher effect (effect 3–4) or Dry Cut 80 W if the muscle is vascular.
Hemostasis	Soft Coag	60–80			5	Coagulation setting.
	Spray Coag	10			1	Low current density.
	Forced Coag	10			1	Coagrasper works best with Soft Coag resulting in low current density because of large surface area. Use for any arterial vessels. If using knife, increased surface area in contact with the vessel decreases current density and provides more coagulation capability.

[a] The Erbe VIO 300D and VIO3 have different power and effect settings. The suggestions are based on the power setting for the VIO3. The effect setting only applies to the VIO 300D.

pads over irregular skin surfaces.[9,12,13] These steps are important to allow for even dispersal of energy and to avoid a possible burn at the pad site. For endoscopic procedures, recommended areas for pad placement are on the flank or upper thigh, taking into consideration the aforementioned best practices for individual patients.[9]

Bowel preparation and explosion risk

There have been case reports of colonic gas explosion, characterized as rapid increase of temperature and pressure caused by sudden energy release leading to volume expansion of naturally occurring gases, such as hydrogen and methane that exist in the colon.[14] These cases have involved APC in the rectum or sigmoid, typically after enema preparation.[15] Prior studies have found that levels of hydrogen and methane may be lower after full bowel preparation for colonoscopy, such as with polyethylene glycol, compared with enema preparation for sigmoidoscopy.[16] Thus it has been posited that full bowel preparation may decrease the risk of colonic gas explosion. If electrosurgery must be performed on an unprepared colon, exchanging the colonic gas for carbon dioxide with repeated insufflation and suction may reduce the risk.

Electrosurgery with Implanted Devices

Implanted cardiac devices, including cardiac pacemakers and implantable cardioverter defibrillators, sense and react to electrical signals from the heart. Thus, they are subject also to sensing noncardiac electrical signals. Patients with these devices can undergo electrosurgery, but it is important to take adequate safety measures. The risk of device interference is variable depending on the type of interfering signal and the type and design of the device. Before the procedure, it is essential to obtain information about the device, indication for the device, the patient's underlying cardiac rhythm, and whether the patient is device dependent. All patients should undergo continuous cardiac rhythm monitoring throughout the procedure.[17,18]

Possible adverse effects of electrical interference from electrosurgery include inappropriate device programming because of signal misinterpretation by the device, inhibition of signal output, negative effects on battery life, or delivery of inappropriate shocks to the patient in the case of implantable cardioverter defibrillators.[18–20] Consultation with a cardiologist should be considered before a procedure in which electrosurgery is anticipated. Endoscopy units should have equipment for resuscitation, cardioversion, and defibrillation readily available, and all staff should be trained in protocols for managing patients with implantable devices. Consensus statements regarding management of patients with cardiac devices have been released by multiple societies including the American Society of Gastrointestinal Endoscopy and the Heart Rhythm Society/American Society of Anesthesiologists.[18,21]

Other implanted devices include implantable neurostimulators that deliver electrical stimulation to target nerve tissue for various conditions. These include gastric electrical stimulators for gastroparesis; deep brain stimulators for Parkinson disease; or other devices that can target areas including the spinal cord, cochlea, and bladder.[17] Most have an external control module that allows setting adjustment, including controlling the on/off status and electrical output.[22,23] Possible risks can include inhibition of neurostimulator device output or electrode heating. These risks may be able to be reduced by turning off the device before the procedure.

SUMMARY

An understanding of the basic principles of electrosurgery is important in endoscopic surgery to achieve the desired tissue effect through each portion of the procedure. Modern ESUs provide a variety of waveforms with different properties that contribute to current density over time and in turn, the tissue effect. Moreover, current density is also affected by factors beyond the ESU, including the device properties, user technique, and patient factors. A working knowledge of these principles is therefore essential in reducing risks and achieving the therapeutic effect.

CLINICS CARE POINTS

- Understanding electrosurgical principles used with electrosurgical units (ESUs) is important in endoscopic surgery to achieve the desired therapeutic effect, optimize procedural outcomes, and minimize adverse events.
- ESUs provide various settings with properties that contribute to current density and tissue effect. The tissue effect, or balance of cutting and coagulation, is determined by the magnitude and rapidity of heat generation by the electrical current.
- A working knowledge of concepts, such as current density and tissue effect, and knowledge of the duty cycle and crest factor for each waveform, can help with understanding the various cutting and coagulation settings available on ESUs.
- Current density is impacted by the duty cycle (percentage of time with active energy delivery), crest factor (measure of peak voltage), and surface area in contact with tissue. In general, cutting is best achieved with higher current density, whereas coagulation is best achieved with lower current density.
- In general, higher percentage duty cycle, lower crest factor, and decreased surface area contribute to a higher current density and greater cutting ability. However, these effects can vary depending on the clinical situation. ESU settings must be individualized and potentially adjusted to achieve the desired tissue effect at different phases in the procedure and minimize thermal injury to adjacent tissue.
- Although understanding properties of ESU settings is imperative, other factors, such as device properties, user technique, application time, and patient or tissue characteristics, are equally important in achieving the optimal therapeutic effect in endoscopic surgery.
- ESU-related complications are rare. However, it is important for the endoscopy team to understand best practices when using ESUs, such as optimal dispersive pad placement. When performing endoscopic surgery in patients with implanted devices, especially cardiac devices, it is essential to obtain information about the device and indication for the device.

DISCLOSURE

A. Li: No relevant disclosures. M.J. Zhou: No relevant disclosures. J.H. Hwang: Consultant for Olympus, Medtronic, Boston Scientific, Micro-Tech, and Lumendi.

REFERENCES

1. Tucker RD. Principles of electrosurgery. In: Sivak MV, editor. Gastroenterologic Endosc. 2000. p. 125–35.
2. Honig WM. The mechanism of cutting in electrosurgery. IEEE Trans Biomed Eng 1975;1:58–62.
3. Barlow DE. Endoscopic applications of electrosurgery: a review of basic principles. Gastrointest Endosc 1982;28(2):73–6.
4. Munro MG. Fundamentals of electrosurgery part I: principles of radiofrequency energy for surgery. In: Feldman L, Fuchshuber P, Jones DB, editors. The SAGES manual on the fundamental use of surgical energy (FUSE). New York: Springer; 2012. p. 15–59.

5. Morris ML. Electrosurgery in the gastroenterology suite: principles, practice, and safety. Gastroenterol Nurs 2006;29(2):126–32.

6. Morris ML, Hwang JH. Electrosurgery in therapeutic endoscopy. In: Chandrasekhara V, Elmunzer BJ, Khashab MA, et al, editors. Clinical gastrointestinal endoscopy. 3rd Edition. Philadelphia: Elsevier; 2019. p. 69–80.e62.

7. Singh N, Harrison M, Rex DK. A survey of colonoscopic polypectomy practices among clinical gastroenterologists. Gastrointest Endosc 2004;60(3):414–8.

8. Tokar JL, Barth BA, Banerjee S, et al. Electrosurgical generators. Gastrointest Endosc 2013;78(2):197–208.

9. Morris ML. Electrosurgery in the gastroenterology suite: principles, practice, and safety. Gastroenterol Nurs 2006;29(2):126–32, quiz 132-124.

10. Tucker R. Commentary on clinical applications of argon plasma coagulation in endoscopy. Gastroenterol Nurs 2007;30(2):129–30, author reply 130.

11. Spruce L, Braswell ML. Implementing AORN recommended practices for electrosurgery. AORN J 2012;95(3):373–84, quiz 385-377.

12. Rey JF, Beilenhoff U, Neumann CS, et al, (ESGE) ESoGE. European Society of Gastrointestinal Endoscopy (ESGE) guideline: the use of electrosurgical units. Endoscopy 2010;42(9):764–72.

13. Wright VC. Contemporary electrosurgery: physics for physicians. J Fam Pract 1994;39(2):119–22.

14. Ladas SD, Karamanolis G, Ben-Soussan E. Colonic gas explosion during therapeutic colonoscopy with electrocautery. World J Gastroenterol 2007;13(40): 5295–8.

15. Manner H, Plum N, Pech O, et al. Colon explosion during argon plasma coagulation. Gastrointest Endosc 2008;67(7):1123–7.

16. Monahan DW, Peluso FE, Goldner F. Combustible colonic gas levels during flexible sigmoidoscopy and colonoscopy. Gastrointest Endosc 1992;38(1):40–3.

17. Parekh PJ, Buerlein RC, Shams R, et al. An update on the management of implanted cardiac devices during electrosurgical procedures. Gastrointest Endosc 2013;78(6):836–41.

18. Dawes JC, Mahabir RC, Hillier K, et al. Electrosurgery in patients with pacemakers/implanted cardioverter defibrillators. Ann Plast Surg 2006;57(1):33–6.

19. Schulman PM, Treggiari MM, Yanez ND, et al. Electromagnetic interference with protocolized electrosurgery dispersive electrode positioning in patients with implantable cardioverter defibrillators. Anesthesiology 2019;130(4):530–40.

20. Fiek M, Dorwarth U, Durchlaub I, et al. Application of radiofrequency energy in surgical and interventional procedures: are there interactions with ICDs? Pacing Clin Electrophysiol 2004;27(3):293–8.

21. Crossley GH, Poole JE, Rozner MA, et al. The Heart Rhythm Society (HRS)/American Society of Anesthesiologists (ASA) Expert Consensus Statement on the perioperative management of patients with implantable defibrillators, pacemakers and arrhythmia monitors: facilities and patient management this document was developed as a joint project with the American Society of Anesthesiologists (ASA), and in collaboration with the American Heart Association (AHA), and the Society of Thoracic Surgeons (STS). Heart Rhythm 2011;8(7):1114–54.

22. Medtronic Inc. Digestive & Gastrointestinal Products: Information for Healthcare Professionals. Available at: www.medtronic.com/physician/gastroenterology. html. Accessed 31 March 2022.

23. Medtronic Inc. Neurological Products: Information for Healthcare Professionals. Available at: www.medtronic.com/physician/gastroenterology.html. Accessed 31 March 2022.

Training in Endoscopic Submucosal Dissection in the United States

The Current Paradigm

Cem Simsek, MD, Hiroyuki Aihara, MD, PhD*

KEYWORDS

- Endoscopic submucosal dissection • Training • Advanced endoscopy fellowship

KEY POINTS

- The traditional master-apprentice endoscopic submucosal dissection (ESD) training model in Japan is not practical in the United States; therefore, an alternative approach such as a prevalence-based model should be implemented.
- The ESD learning curve can be shortened with clinical observership, hands-on courses, simulation, and live animal model training.
- The trainees' competency in ESD should be assessed using clinical proficiency benchmarks such as en bloc resection rate, adverse event rate, and dissection speed.
- The new technologies and technical refinements might facilitate more widespread adoption of ESD in the United States.

INTRODUCTION

Endoscopic submucosal dissection (ESD) was developed in the late 1980s and is currently accepted in Japan as a gold-standard treatment of superficial gastrointestinal lesions.[1–4] ESD has several advantages over alternative treatments, such as higher en bloc resection rates allowing for accurate histopathologic evaluation and decreased local recurrence compared with endoscopic mucosal resection (EMR), reduced post-procedural morbidity and hospital stay compared with surgery.[5–8] However, in the United States, we are still seeing a delay in the adoption of ESD. One of the major obstacles causing this delay is the several issues associated with the ESD training. First, the number of gastric ESD cases suitable for the initial phase of the ESD training is limited in the United States because of the lower prevalence of gastric

Division of Gastroenterology, Hepatology and Endoscopy, Brigham and Women's Hospital, Harvard Medical School, Boston, MA, USA
* Corresponding author. Division of Gastroenterology, Hepatology and Endoscopy, Brigham and Women's Hospital, 75 Francis Street, Boston, MA 02115.
E-mail address: haihara@bwh.harvard.edu

Gastrointest Endoscopy Clin N Am 33 (2023) 41–53
https://doi.org/10.1016/j.giec.2022.07.003
1052-5157/23/© 2022 Elsevier Inc. All rights reserved.

cancer. Second, there is a scarcity of ESD experts to provide ESD training. Third, ESD is a complex and technically demanding procedure with a steep learning curve, preventing the training program from being incorporated into the 1-year advanced endoscopy fellowship.[1,9,10]

Despite the limitations listed above, it has become more evident that alternative training strategies can be sought based on the increasing number of evidence associated with ESD. Here in this review, we present a literature summary to provide an overview of the current paradigm of ESD training in the United States.

Currently Available Training Styles for Endoscopic Submucosal Dissection

In Japan, ESD training is conducted through a stepwise training program, the so-called master-apprenticeship model. In this model, first, the trainee starts learning the cognitive skills of ESD, such as pre-ESD endoscopic lesion evaluation, selection of ESD devices, electrocautery settings, and interpretation of pathology. Then, the trainee will undergo ex vivo ESD training under the supervision of ESD experts while assisting the experts in the clinical cases. It is followed by clinical hands-on training that typically begins with distal gastric lesions on the contra-gravity side of the stomach. Along with the improving proficiency, the trainee then progresses to the more technically challenging lesions in the proximal stomach and esophagus. Colorectal ESD is typically the final training step after achieving competency in gastric and esophageal ESD.[11]

This stepwise master-apprenticeship training pathway in Japan typically takes 3 to 4 years and cannot be directly applied to the United States due to the significant differences in the training system.[1,12–14] When developing the ESD training program in the United States, the initial phase should include ESD simulators, case observership, and ESD courses.[15]

Endoscopic submucosal dissection simulators and case observership

Several ESD simulators are currently available, including ex vivo animal tissue, live animal models, artificial simulators, and virtual reality simulators. The ex vivo animal models are the most preferred simulator for ESD training.

The ex vivo animal tissue provides essential components of ESD training, such as visual recognition of layers, the haptic feedback from the target tissue, and perforation management while allowing the trainee to use the same endoscopes and ESD devices as the clinical setting. The porcine stomach explant is the most widely used animal tissue based on the anatomical similarity to the human stomach (**Fig. 1A**). Kato and

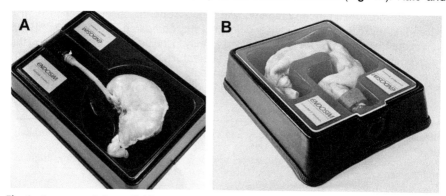

Fig. 1. A commercially available ex vivo tissue simulators used for ESD training. (*A*) Porcine stomach explant (EASIE-R3 Simulator) and (*B*) porcine colon explant (ColoEASIE-2 Simulator). (*Courtesy of* Endosim, LLC, Bolton, MA.)

colleagues[16] conducted a prospective ex vivo study analyzing the learning curves in ESD. This study included two trainee-level endoscopists without previous ESD experience and trained them using the ex vivo porcine stomach tissue. The lesions were simulated in six different areas, and each participant performed ex vivo ESD until the targeted resection outcomes were obtained. After a total of 30 ESD cases, 100% en bloc resection rates were obtained without perforation. Draganov and colleagues[17] compared the competency in ESD using the ex vivo animal tissue before and after a 5-week visit to high-volume ESD centers where the endoscopist observed 48 cases. After this observership, the procedure times were significantly reduced (32.7 $\pm$ 15.0 min vs 63.5 $\pm$ 9.8 min, $p < 0.001$).

Competency in gastric ESD is the benchmark before starting esophageal and colorectal ESD in Japan.[18–20] On the contrary, Iacopini and colleagues[21] evaluated the feasibility of ESD training starting with colorectal ESD without previous experience in clinical gastric ESD. In the study, first, the endoscopist did five unsupervised and one supervised ESD using the ex vivo porcine stomach. The endoscopist then visited a high-volume ESD center for 2 weeks for observership. Then, the endoscopist performed 30 rectal and 30 colon ESD cases over three years. The results showed that the en bloc resection rate increased to 80% after five cases, and the resection rate increased to 80% following 20 cases, along with the shorter procedure time. Gromski and colleagues[22] conducted a prospective study to determine the usefulness of ESD training using colorectal animal tissue explants (**Fig. 1B**). The study showed the composite score integrating procedure speed, en bloc resection rate, and perforation rate plateaued after nine training sessions. These data suggest that the colorectal ESD training could be safely conducted without prior experience in gastric ESD.

Despite the limited availability, live animal models are beneficial in ESD training as they include essential aspects of the ESD procedure, such as active bleeding and constant movement of the target tissue due to peristalsis and pulsation.[23] As shown by Chapelle and colleagues,[24] live animal models can be used for the initial training and would be helpful even with a short training period. They evaluated the effect of a 3-day ESD training on 14 trainees using the live porcine models. This study showed a significant improvement in the dissection speed between the first and second ESD procedures. In another study by Kuttner-Magalhaes and colleagues.[25] On 17 endoscopists without previous ESD experience, 70 ESD procedures were performed with a median number of 4 per participant. This study showed significant improvements in participants' skills reflected by increased mean dissection speed and en bloc resection rates.

Artificial simulators are also becoming available for ESD training. One of those simulators uses two layers of fabric connected with hook-and-loop fasteners, mounted in a resinoid stomach model.[26] The simulator is used with an insulated tip knife to pull and detach the fasteners, simulating the knife maneuvers to apply traction force during the submucosal dissection. The model also simulates bleeding control with red threads between the two fabrics representing submucosal vessels. The other recently developed artificial tissue model conducts electricity allowing for submucosal injection and electrocautery (Sunarrow Limited, Tokyo, Japan, **Fig. 2**).[27] These artificial ESD simulators do not require animal endoscopes and can be used in the endoscopy suite. This is one of the most significant advantages of these artificial models.

Virtual reality simulation is commonly used in surgical and endoscopic training. However, developing an ESD simulator could be challenging because of the complexity of the procedural steps. Nevertheless, there are efforts to apply the technology to ESD training[28] Although they show great promise, the benefits of virtual simulators in ESD training have not been fully studied yet.

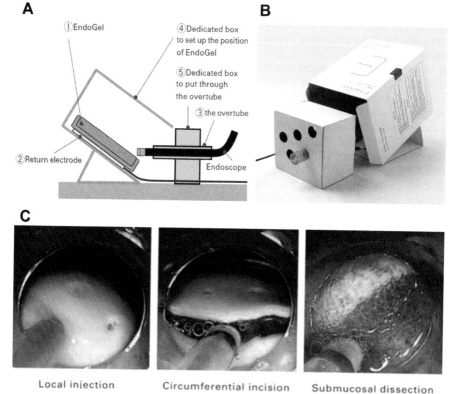

Fig. 2. An artificial ESD simulator made with nonbiological conductive material (EndoGel). (*A, B*) Setup of the ESD simulator with artificial tissue, return electrode, overtube, and two boxes. (*C*) Endoscopic images during the use of the simulator. Marking, injection, incision, and dissection can be performed. (*Courtesy of* Sunarrow, LTD, Tokyo, Japan.)

Endoscopic submucosal dissection courses

Hands-on training under the supervision of ESD experts is an essential component of the ESD training, providing a direct assessment, immediate feedback, and tailored hands-on instructions to the trainee. The ESD courses are often endorsed by societies or sponsored by industry and comprise one or more sessions of expert-tutored animal model training with varying participant-trainer ratios and depth of training. A recent study from the United States was conducted during two days of ESD course incorporating didactic lectures and hands-on sessions. Most of the participants had experience in EMR but limited exposure to ESD before the course. However, 44% of the participants reported performing clinical ESD cases following the course. Importantly, all these attending-level participants continued their training using ex vivo tissue and live animal models, additional ESD courses, and visiting high-volume centers. This study showed that a hands-on course in US settings is an essential step to engaging the trainees in ESD training.[24]

The limited number of ESD experts in the United States is one of the obstacles to ESD training. Utilizing the telemedicine approach in the early training phase might compensate for this limitation. A recent study evaluated remote proctorship at the beginning of the ESD training through reviewing and commenting on video recordings of ex vivo ESD procedures.[29] Two endoscopists completed 55 ESD procedures in an ex vivo animal model (endoscopist 1 performed 30 and endoscopist 2 performed 25); each procedure was recorded. The videos were sent to the expert endoscopist, who reviewed and gave written feedback. The expert also blindly scored the technical aspects of each procedure. After 23 and 25 cases, technical competency, defined as successful en bloc resection of three consecutive 3-cm lesions within 30 min, was reached. The study also reported that one of the endoscopists' initial eight clinical gastric and colonic ESD cases resulted in a 100% en bloc resection rate with no adverse events.[30]

Development of endoscopic submucosal dissection fellowship
ESD training in Japan typically starts at the end of the gastroenterology fellowship. The training continues for an additional three to four years while the trainees are junior faculty. On the contrary, the 1-year curriculum for the advanced endoscopy fellowship in the United States typically does not include dedicated ESD training.[13,31]

Ge and colleagues[32] implemented a 1-year ESD fellowship as a part of the advanced endoscopy fellowship. The trainee participated in 72 consecutive ESD cases with increasing exposure to ESD, observing/assisting 19 cases, partially performing 18 cases, and mainly performing 26 cases. At the end of the training period, the trainee achieved 84.7, 81.2, and 76.8% rates for en bloc, complete, and curative resections, although the vast majority of ESD cases were colorectal (57/72, 79.2%) and the majority of lesions (76.4%) were associated with mild (F1) or severe fibrosis (F2). A recent follow-up study reported the outcomes of the same trainee's 193 independent ESD cases performed over three years after the ESD fellowship. They reported higher en bloc, complete, and curative resection rates of 90.2%, 85.3%, and 77.5%. A resection speed of 9.0 cm²/h, used as a benchmark of procedural proficiency, was achieved after 62 cases.[33] Notably, this training model is different from the master-apprenticeship model, the organ-based stepwise training style. In this prevalence-based training model, the trainee was exposed to every ESD case starting from the early periods, and the degree of their involvement to assist, partially perform, or mainly perform was decided at the mentor's discretion (**Fig. 3**). ESD training can be implemented into the current structured training program in the United States, provided that an ESD expert and enough case volume are available.

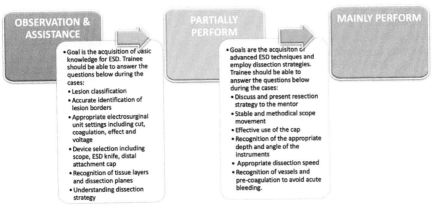

Fig. 3. Scheme showing the prevalence-based training model. (*Modified from* Ge, P.S., C.C. Thompson, and H. Aihara, *Development and clinical outcomes of an endoscopic submucosal dissection fellowship program: early united states experience. Surgical Endoscopy, 2019.* 34(2): p. 829-838.)

Competency Assessment in Endoscopic Submucosal Dissection

The trainees' competency needs to be assessed continuously during the training program. The ESD experts need to be familiar with the proficiency benchmarks to evaluate the trainees' skill levels as well as to set the next target of training steps. Moreover, this competency assessment can also be used to monitor the quality of ESD training, especially in the United States, where significant heterogeneity in ESD training still exists. There are several proposed benchmarks to evaluate the competency in ESD, such as en bloc resection rate over 90%, adverse event rate below 5%, curative resection rate over 80%, and dissection speed greater than 9 cm^2/hour.[34,35] These benchmarks are essential in allowing the trainees to be involved in more challenging cases.[36]

In terms of the number of cases to achieve competency in ESD, Oda and colleagues[37] evaluated the learning curves of 13 trainees over ten years in gastric ESD. They found that 30 and 40 cases are required to achieve proficiency for distal and proximal gastric ESD. Another study by Tsou and colleagues[38] evaluating the learning curve for esophageal ESD found that 30 cases are needed to achieve proficiency in esophageal ESD. The learning curves of endoscopists can vary depending on baseline endoscopic skills, previous training experience, and degree of supervision.[39] Therefore, the learning curve data from Japan may not be directly applicable to the United States. The study by Zhang and colleagues[15] analyzed the learning curve of a single US endoscopist over an eight-year of independent practice. The endoscopist, who had ten years of experience in interventional endoscopy, performed 540 ESD procedures during the study period without the supervision of ESD experts. The procedures were divided into 50 case blocks to analyze the number of cases required to achieve proficiency benchmarks. The study revealed en bloc resection rate plateaued at over 90% after 250 cases, and the R0 resection rate reached 95% at 400 cases. The learning curve thresholds in this study were significantly higher than the previously reported numbers from Japan. Potential reasons for this discrepancy are the absence of proctorship, prevalence-based practice with a higher frequency of right colonic lesions, and previously manipulated lesions. Another study from Europe evaluated the learning curve of a single endoscopist in colorectal ESD. The endoscopist had previous experience in 25 upper ESD and participated in a 3-week training at a high-volume ESD center. Over three years, the endoscopist performed 228 colorectal ESD, and the period was divided into six periods, each consisting of 38 cases. After completing 76 procedures, the en bloc resection rate was increased from 54.4% to 86.0%, and it was accompanied by a significant increase in the mean procedure speed of ≥9 cm^2/h.[40]

Another approach to evaluate the competency in ESD is to use the part-task endoscopy simulator. Thompson Endoscopic Skill Test (TEST) is an artificial simulator developed based on kinematic motion analysis to test and improve fundamental endoscopic skills. TEST includes five modules addressing different scope maneuvers: wheel control, retroflection, snare polypectomy, loop reduction, and torque. Each part-task is scored based on the time for completing the assigned task.[41,42] The scores in the TEST were proven to correlate with the skill levels in various endoscopic procedures validated by extensive assessment. The study by Tamai and colleagues[43] enrolled 23 endoscopists with different levels of procedural expertise. TEST scores were shown to be significantly correlated with the number of gastric ESDs performed ($r = 0.924$, $p < 0.01$), dissection speed ($r = -0.9$, $p < 0.01$), and self-completion rate (0.857, $p < 0.005$). This is a critical study that outlines the procedure numbers alone may not be enough to assess the proficiency in ESD, considering the individual differences in learning curves.

How Can We Improve the Learning Curve in Endoscopic Submucosal Dissection

ESD has constantly been evolving with the development of new techniques, devices, and tools for the past decade. Reducing the technical difficulty of ESD using these assistive techniques might be an alternative pathway to facilitate its adoption. These include pocket creation, submucosal tunneling, underwater ESD, hybrid ESD, and traction methods, which all have the potential to improve the learning curve.

In the pocket creation method, a small mucosal incision is first performed, followed by an expansion of the dissection plane underneath the lesion and then completion of the bilateral mucosal incision and submucosal dissection. This technique facilitates ESD by preventing the leakage of an injection solution, maintaining visualization of the muscle layer, and preserving traction inside the pocket.[44] Since its first description, the pocket creation method has been widely studied in various settings. In colorectal lesions, a recent meta-analysis including five studies with 1481 colorectal lesions showed that it achieved higher R0 and en bloc resection rates (odds ratio [OR]: 3.4, confidence interval [CI]: 1.3–8.9 and OR: 9.9, CI:2.7–36.2), and lower adverse events rates (OR: −0.6, CI: 0.3–1.0) as well as faster dissection (mean difference 11.5 min, CI: 3.1–19.9) compared with conventional ESD.[45] Another study, including 45 non-ampullary duodenal lesions, showed that the pocket creation method yielded higher R0 and en bloc resection rates, higher dissection speed, and lower perforation rate when compared with conventional ESD.[46]

Submucosal tunneling ESD is another modification of the standard technique. In this technique, anal and oral mucosal incisions are made and followed by submucosal dissection in a tunneling fashion underneath the lesion, and ESD is completed by bilateral mucosal incision and submucosal dissection.[47] Similar to the pocket-creation method, this technique stabilizes the endoscope within the tunnel, preserves the injection fluid, and maintains visualization of the submucosal layer.[48–50] Recent meta-analysis including 1161 esophageal lesions showed higher en bloc resection rates (OR:3.09, CI:1.54–3.96), and shorter procedure time (standard deviation [SD]: 0.49, CI: 0.16–0.83) compared with conventional technique.[51]

Underwater ESD is another modification of the standard ESD technique where CO_2 in the lumen is replaced by saline for better visualization based on the buoyancy effect and protection of the proper muscle layer against thermal damage. Underwater ESD can be combined with other techniques, although the current literature is limited.[52–56]

Hybrid ESD, defined as the combined endoscopic partial submucosal dissection and snare-assisted resection, is another strategy that could overcome the difficulties in the early learning curve. A meta-analysis comparing hybrid ESD with conventional technique showed shorter procedure times (mean difference: 18.45 min, CI: 6.21–30.70) and fewer adverse events (OR: 1.56, CI: 1.01–2.41) with no difference in recurrence or need for surgery; however, en bloc resection rates were lower with hybrid ESD (OR: 0.31, CI: 0.17–0.57).[57]

Traction methods mimic the "second hand" in surgery to apply countertraction to improve the visibility of the dissection plane and efficacy of tissue dissection. So far, various traction techniques have been developed, including clip-line, clip-band, clip-snare, spring-clip, suture-pulley, magnetic anchor, endoscope guided, two-point fixed, and external device-assisted strategies.[58–65] Traction methods improve the efficiency of ESD for both expert endoscopists and the trainees. This was well demonstrated by Mitsoyushi and colleagues[66] in a recent study evaluating the performance of trainees who were trained for colorectal ESD with or without using the traction technique. The study found that training with a clip-line traction technique contributed to the improvement of procedural success, increasing the self-completion rates (73.8% vs 58.8%), en bloc resection (100% vs 90%), and R0-resection (96% vs 83%) rates as well as the dissection speed (19.5 mm^2/min vs 15.9 mm^2/min). The learning curve for colorectal ESD has also improved with traction (10 vs 21 cases). Another traction technique, the "suture-pulley" method, was shown to shorten the procedure times and decrease the physical and mental efforts of an ESD expert.[67] A prospective study including 13 endoscopists with no ESD experience[68] showed that this technique significantly shortens the submucosal dissection time (8.4 ± 2.9 vs 47.2 ± 16.3 min) and reduces the mental and physical workloads in ESD. A recent meta-analysis compared traction-assisted ESD to conventional ESD on 2582 upper and lower lesions. The pooled estimates showed higher R0 resection rates (RD: 0.04, CI: 0.01–0.06), shorter procedure times (weighted mean difference = 20.35 min, CI: 13–27), and lower perforation rates (RD:0.03, CI:0.01–0.04).[69]

Robotic technology has long been an essential component of the surgical practice, but its utilization in endoluminal surgery has remained limited. Robotic surgery can overcome several issues in ESD, such as a single-channel endoscope limiting the number of device usage to one at a time, with limited degrees of freedom. As such, several bimanual robotic systems have been developed. One example is a robotic endoscopic system that incorporates a flexible robotically controlled endoscope and two working channels that can deploy mechanically controlled articulating instruments to the surgical site. In a randomized pilot study, de-Moura and colleagues[70] compared this robotic-assisted ESD with conventional ESD by including five endoscopists with no experience in conventional and robotic ESD. Robotic ESD decreased the total procedure (34.1 vs 88.6 min, p = 0.001) and submucosal dissection times (27.8 vs 79.4 min, p = 0.002). The perforation rate was significantly higher in the conventional ESD group. The endoscopists' efforts, evaluated by NASA Task Load Index, were also significantly lower in robotic ESD.

These robotic systems can potentially decrease the technical demand for ESD by enabling traction/countertraction and triangulation during the procedure. The robotic technology might bring a new paradigm with an improved procedural efficiency; however, the robotic system requires bimanual control, which interventional endoscopists are typically not familiar with. It would require a separate training program, and the significantly increased cost and resource utilization might also be obstacles to its adoption.

SUMMARY

The traditional ESD training system in Japan is highly proven to train expert-level endoscopists; however, applying this model to the US training program is not practical. The presented data support the alternative multifactorial pathways providing feasible and effective ways to pursue ESD training. The prevalence-based, multifactorial training program incorporating the current assistive techniques and technologies with increased involvement in the procedure depending on the trainees' competency levels is essential to successfully spreading and adopting ESD practice in the United States.

CLINICS CARE POINTS

- When developing a training program for ESD, consider incorporating the current assistive techniques and technologies to safely and effectively conduct the ESD training.

POTENTIAL CONFLICTS OF INTEREST

C. Simsek has no conflicts to disclose. H. Aihara is a consultant for Olympus America, Boston Scientific, and Fujifilm Medical Systems.

REFERENCES

1. Draganov PV, Wang AY, Othman MO, et al. aga institute clinical practice update: endoscopic submucosal dissection in the united states. Clin Gastroenterol Hepatol 2019;17(1):16–25.e1.
2. Friedland S. Endoscopic resection of duodenal adenomas: endoscopic mucosal resection or endoscopic submucosal dissection? Endoscopy 2015;47(02): 99–100.
3. Kunovský L. Endoscopic management of ampullary tumors: European Society of Gastrointestinal Endoscopy (ESGE) Guideline and Endoscopic management of superficial nonampullary duodenal tumors: European Society of Gastrointestinal Endoscopy (ESGE) Guideline. Gastroenterologie a Hepatologie 2021;75(4): 328–30.
4. Ono H, Yao K, Fujishiro M, et al. Guidelines for endoscopic submucosal dissection and endoscopic mucosal resection for early gastric cancer (second edition). Dig Endosc 2020;33(1):4–20.
5. McCarty TR, Bazarbashi AN, Hathorn KE, et al. Endoscopic submucosal dissection (ESD) versus transanal endoscopic microsurgery (TEM) for treatment of rectal tumors: a comparative systematic review and meta-analysis. Surg Endosc 2019;34(4):1688–95.
6. Nam MJ, Sohn DK, Hong CW, et al. Cost comparison between endoscopic submucosal dissection and transanal endoscopic microsurgery for the treatment of rectal tumors. Ann Surg Treat Res 2015;89(4):202–7.
7. Liu Q, Ding L, Qiu X, et al. Updated evaluation of endoscopic submucosal dissection versus surgery for early gastric cancer: a systematic review and meta-analysis. Int J Surg 2020;73:28–41.
8. Gotoda T, Kondo H, Ono H, et al. A new endoscopic mucosal resection procedure using an insulation-tipped electrosurgical knife for rectal flat lesions: report of two cases. Gastrointest Endosc 1999;50(4):560–3.
9. Barakat M, Ramai D, Cheung D, et al. Management of early gastric cancer meeting criteria for endoscopic resection: US population-based study. Endosc Int Open 2021;9(7):E989–93.
10. Peery AF, Cools KS, Strassle PD, et al. Increasing rates of surgery for patients with nonmalignant colorectal polyps in the united states. Gastroenterology 2018;154(5):1352–60.e3.
11. Gotoda T, Draganov PV. ESD training in the East. In: Fukami N, editor. Endoscopic submucosal dissection. Switzerland: Springer; 2015. p. 229–35.
12. Draganov PV, Coman RM, Gotoda T. Training for complex endoscopic procedures: how to incorporate endoscopic submucosal dissection skills in the West? Expert Rev Gastroenterol Hepatol 2014;8(2):119–21.
13. Aihara H, Dacha S, Anand GS, et al. Core curriculum for endoscopic submucosal dissection (ESD). Gastrointest Endosc 2021;93(6):1215–21.
14. Pimentel-Nunes P, Pioche M, Albéniz E, et al. Curriculum for endoscopic submucosal dissection training in Europe: european Society of Gastrointestinal Endoscopy (ESGE) Position Statement. Endoscopy 2019;51(10):980–92.

15. Zhang X, Ly EK, Nithyanand S, et al. Learning curve for endoscopic submucosal dissection with an untutored, prevalence-based approach in the united states. Clin Gastroenterol Hepatol 2020;18(3):580–588 e1.

16. Kato M, Gromski M, Jung Y, et al. The learning curve for endoscopic submucosal dissection in an established experimental setting. Surg Endosc 2012;27(1):154–61.

17. Draganov PV, Chang M, Coman RM, et al. Role of observation of live cases done by Japanese experts in the acquisition of ESD skills by a western endoscopist. World J Gastroenterol 2014;20(16):4675–80.

18. Ohata K, Nonaka K, Misumi Y, et al. Usefulness of training using animal models for colorectal endoscopic submucosal dissection: is experience performing gastric ESD really needed? Endosc Int Open 2016;4(3):E333–9.

19. Shiga H, Kuroha M, Endo K, et al. Colorectal endoscopic submucosal dissection (ESD) performed by experienced endoscopists with limited experience in gastric ESD. Int J Colorectal Dis 2015;30(12):1645–52.

20. Shiga H, Ohba R, Matsuhashi T, et al. Feasibility of colorectal endoscopic submucosal dissection (ESD) carried out by endoscopists with no or little experience in gastric ESD. Dig Endosc 2017;29(Suppl 2):58–65.

21. Iacopini F, Bella A, Costamagna G, et al. Stepwise training in rectal and colonic endoscopic submucosal dissection with differentiated learning curves. Gastrointest Endosc 2012;76(6):1188–96.

22. Gromski MA, Cohen J, Saito K, et al. Learning colorectal endoscopic submucosal dissection: a prospective learning curve study using a novel ex vivo simulator. Surg Endosc 2017;31(10):4231–7.

23. Küttner-Magalhães R, Dinis-Ribeiro M, Bruno MJ, et al. Training in endoscopic mucosal resection and endoscopic submucosal dissection: Face, content and expert validity of the live porcine model. United Eur Gastroenterol J 2018;6(4):547–57.

24. Chapelle N, Musquer N, Métivier-Cesbron E, et al. Efficacy of a three-day training course in endoscopic submucosal dissection using a live porcine model: a prospective evaluation. United Eur Gastroenterol J 2018;6(9):1410–6.

25. Küttner-Magalhães R, Dinis-Ribeiro M, Bruno MJ, et al. a steep early learning curve for endoscopic submucosal dissection in the live porcine model. Dig Dis 2021. https://doi.org/10.1159/000521429.

26. Chen M-J, Wang H-Y, Chang C-W, et al. A novel artificial tissue simulator for endoscopic submucosal resection training–a pilot study. BMC Gastroenterol 2016;16(1):1–8.

27. Sato H, Mizuno K-I, Sato Y, et al. Development and use of a non-biomaterial model for hands-on training of endoscopic procedures. Ann Translational Med 2017;5(8):182.

28. Cetinsaya B, Gromski MA, Lee S, et al. A task and performance analysis of endoscopic submucosal dissection (ESD) surgery. Surg Endosc 2019;33(2):592–606.

29. Bhatt A, Abe S, Kumaravel A, et al. Video-based supervision for training of endoscopic submucosal dissection. Endoscopy 2016;48(08):711–6.

30. Galvao Neto M, Jerez J, Brunaldi VO, et al. Learning process effectiveness during the COVID-19 pandemic: teleproctoring advanced endoscopic skills by training endoscopists in endoscopic sleeve gastroplasty procedure. Obes Surg 2021;31(12):5486–93.

31. American Society of Gastrointestinal Endoscopy International Pairing Program. 2022. Available at: https://www.asge.org/home/education/advanced-education-

training/international-programs/international-pairing-program. Accessed May 18, 2022.

32. Ge PS, Thompson CC, Aihara H. Development and clinical outcomes of an endoscopic submucosal dissection fellowship program: early united states experience. Surg Endosc 2019;34(2):829–38.

33. Ge PS, Raju GS, Chang GJ, et al. A tutored prevalence-based approach to endoscopic submucosal dissection training: mid-term results following completion of a us-based fellowship training program. Gastrointest Endosc, 2022;95:AB51.

34. Hotta K, Oyama T, Akamatsu T, et al. a comparison of outcomes of endoscopic submucosal dissection (ESD) for early gastric neoplasms between high-volume and low-volume centers: multi-center retrospective questionnaire study conducted by the nagano ESD study group. Intern Med 2010;49(4):253–9.

35. Oyama T, Yahagi N, Ponchon T, et al. How to establish endoscopic submucosal dissection in Western countries. World J Gastroenterol 2015;21(40):11209–20.

36. Pimentel-Nunes P, Dinis-Ribeiro M, Ponchon T, et al. Endoscopic submucosal dissection: European Society of Gastrointestinal Endoscopy (ESGE) Guideline. Endoscopy 2015;47(09):829–54.

37. Oda I, Odagaki T, Suzuki H, et al. Learning curve for endoscopic submucosal dissection of early gastric cancer based on trainee experience. Dig Endosc 2012;24:129–32.

38. Tsou Y-K, Chuang W-Y, Liu C-Y, et al. Learning curve for endoscopic submucosal dissection of esophageal neoplasms. Dis Esophagus 2016;29(6):544–50.

39. Yamamoto S, Uedo N, Ishihara R, et al. Endoscopic submucosal dissection for early gastric cancer performed by supervised residents: assessment of feasibility and learning curve. Endoscopy 2009;41(11):923–8.

40. Spychalski M, Skulimowski A, Dziki A, et al. Colorectal endoscopic submucosal dissection (ESD) in the West – when can satisfactory results be obtained? A single-operator learning curve analysis. Scand J Gastroenterol 2017;52(12):1442–52.

41. Jirapinyo P, Kumar N, Thompson CC. Validation of an endoscopic part-task training box as a skill assessment tool. Gastrointest Endosc 2015;81(4):967–73.

42. Thompson CC, Jirapinyo P, Kumar N, et al. Development and initial validation of an endoscopic part-task training box. Endoscopy 2014;46(09):735–44.

43. Tamai N, Aihara H, Kato M, et al. Competency assessment for gastric endoscopic submucosal dissection using an endoscopic part-task training box. Surg Endosc 2018;33(8):2548–52.

44. Hayashi Y, Sunada K, Takahashi H, et al. Pocket-creation method of endoscopic submucosal dissection to achieve en bloc resection of giant colorectal subpedunculated neoplastic lesions. Endoscopy 2014;46(Suppl 1 UCTN):E421–2.

45. Pei Q, Qiao H, Zhang M, et al. Pocket-creation method versus conventional method of endoscopic submucosal dissection for superficial colorectal neoplasms: a meta-analysis. Gastrointest Endosc 2021;93(5):1038–46.e4.

46. Miura Y, Shinozaki S, Hayashi Y, et al. Duodenal endoscopic submucosal dissection is feasible using the pocket-creation method. Endoscopy 2017;49(01):8–14.

47. Inoue H, Ikeda H, Hosoya T, et al. Submucosal endoscopic tumor resection for subepithelial tumors in the esophagus and cardia. Endoscopy 2012;44(3):225–30.

48. Lv X-H, Wang C-H, Xie Y. Efficacy and safety of submucosal tunneling endoscopic resection for upper gastrointestinal submucosal tumors: a systematic review and meta-analysis. Surg Endosc 2017;31(1):49–63.

49. Cao B, Lu J, Tan Y, et al. Efficacy and safety of submucosal tunneling endoscopic resection for gastric submucosal tumors: a systematic review and meta-analysis. Rev Esp Enferm Dig 2021;113(1):52–9.

50. Deprez PH, Moons LM, O'Toole D, et al. Endoscopic management of subepithelial lesions including neuroendocrine neoplasms: European Society of Gastrointestinal Endoscopy (ESGE) Guideline. Endoscopy 2022;54:412–29.

51. Zhang T, Zhang H, Zhong F, et al. Efficacy of endoscopic submucosal tunnel dissection versus endoscopic submucosal dissection for superficial esophageal neoplastic lesions: a systematic review and meta-analysis. Surg Endosc 2021; 35(1):52–62.

52. Despott EJ, Hirayama Y, Lazaridis N, et al. Saline immersion therapeutic endoscopy facilitated pocket-creation method for endoscopic submucosal dissection (with video). Gastrointest Endosc 2019;89(3):652–3.

53. Harada H, Murakami D, Suehiro S, et al. Water-pocket endoscopic submucosal dissection for superficial gastric neoplasms (with video). Gastrointest Endosc 2018;88(2):253–60.

54. Nagata M. Underwater endoscopic submucosal dissection in saline solution using a bent-type knife for duodenal tumor. VideoGIE 2018;3(12):375–7.

55. Rodríguez Sánchez J, úbeda Muñoz M, de la Santa Belda E, et al. Underwater hybrid endoscopic submucosal dissection in a rectal polyp: a case report of a new application of "underwater endoscopy". Revista Española de Enfermedades Digestivas 2017;110. https://doi.org/10.17235/reed.2017.5181/2017.

56. Yoshii S, Hayashi Y, Tsujii Y, et al. Underwater endoscopic submucosal dissection: a novel resection strategy for early gastric cancer located on the greater curvature of the gastric body. Ann Gastroenterol 2017;30(3):364.

57. Okamoto K, Muguruma N, Kagemoto K, et al. Efficacy of hybrid endoscopic submucosal dissection (ESD) as a rescue treatment in difficult colorectal ESD cases. Dig Endosc 2017;29:45–52.

58. Gotoda T, Oda I, Tamakawa K, et al. Prospective clinical trial of magnetic-anchor–guided endoscopic submucosal dissection for large early gastric cancer (with videos). Gastrointest Endosc 2009;69(1):10–5.

59. Hashimoto R, Hirasawa D, Iwaki T, et al. Usefulness of the S–O clip for gastric endoscopic submucosal dissection (with video). Surg Endosc 2017;32(2): 908–14.

60. Imaeda H, Hosoe N, Ida Y, et al. Novel technique of endoscopic submucosal dissection using an external grasping forceps for superficial gastric neoplasia. Dig Endosc 2009;21(2):122–7.

61. Yamada S, Doyama H, Ota R, et al. Impact of the clip and snare method using the prelooping technique for colorectal endoscopic submucosal dissection. Endoscopy 2015;48(03):281–5.

62. Yamasaki Y, Takeuchi Y, Uedo N, et al. Efficacy of traction-assisted colorectal endoscopic submucosal dissection using a clip-and-thread technique: A prospective randomized study. Dig Endosc 2018;30(4):467–76.

63. Yonezawa J, Kaise M, Sumiyama K, et al. A novel double-channel therapeutic endoscope ("R-scope") facilitates endoscopic submucosal dissection of superficial gastric neoplasms. Endoscopy 2006;38(10):1011–5.

64. Mortagy M, Mehta N, Parsi MA, et al. Magnetic anchor guidance for endoscopic submucosal dissection and other endoscopic procedures. World J Gastroenterol 2017;23(16):2883–90.

65. Aihara H, Ryou M, Kumar N, et al. A novel magnetic countertraction device for endoscopic submucosal dissection significantly reduces procedure time and minimizes technical difficulty. Endoscopy 2014;46(05):422–5.

66. Mitsuyoshi Y, Ide D, Ohya TR, et al. Training program using a traction device improves trainees' learning curve of colorectal endoscopic submucosal dissection. Surg Endosc 2021. https://doi.org/10.1007/s00464-021-08799-y.

67. Aihara H, Kumar N, Ryou M, et al. Facilitating endoscopic submucosal dissection: the suture-pulley method significantly improves procedure time and minimizes technical difficulty compared with conventional technique: an ex vivo study (with video). Gastrointest Endosc 2014;80(3):495–502.

68. Ge PS, Thompson CC, Jirapinyo P, et al. Suture pulley countertraction method reduces procedure time and technical demand of endoscopic submucosal dissection among novice endoscopists learning endoscopic submucosal dissection: a prospective randomized ex vivo study. Gastrointest Endosc 2019;89(1):177–84.

69. Lopimpisuth C, Simons M, Akshintala VS, et al. Traction-assisted endoscopic submucosal dissection reduces procedure time and risk of serious adverse events: a systematic review and meta-analysis. Surg Endosc 2022;36:1775–88.

70. de Moura DTH, Aihara DH, Jirapinyo P, et al. Robot-assisted endoscopic submucosal dissection versus conventional ESD for colorectal lesions: outcomes of a randomized pilot study in endoscopists without prior ESD experience (with video). Gastrointest Endosc 2019;90(2):290–8.

Endoscopic Submucosal Dissection in the Esophagus

Indications, Techniques, and Outcomes

Norio Fukami, MD, AGAF, FACG, MASGE, FJGES

KEYWORDS

- Esophageal squamous cell carcinoma • Barrett's-related neoplasm
- Early esophageal adenocarcinoma • Endoscopic resection
- Endoscopic submucosal dissection • Endoscopic mucosal resection

KEY POINTS

- Knowledge and experience with endoscopic evaluation of lesions with chromoendoscopy or advanced imaging modality are paramount in choosing treatment modality for the best outcomes.
- Primary endoscopic resection with curative intent is beneficial for superficial squamous neoplasm without suggestive changes for deep submucosal invasion, and it does not affect survival outcomes.
- Visible Barrett's dysplasia requires endoscopic resection. Endoscopic submucosal dissection (ESD) offers potential benefit over endoscopic mucosal resection (EMR) for larger lesions, multifocal high grade dysplasia (HGD) or cancer, or with significant nodularity.
- Postresection specimen processing is one of the most important steps of ESD.
- Stricture prevention should be considered after large circumferential resection and limited modalities are available to reduce the risk for significant stenosis.

INTRODUCTION

Early detection of neoplastic change in the esophagus is paramount in preventing esophageal cancer-related mortality. Once early cancer is detected, endoscopic resection (ER) offers detailed pathologic diagnosis and minimally invasive treatment to eradicate neoplastic change with lower morbidity compared with surgical therapy. Endoscopic submucosal dissection (ESD) is a new technique to remove mucosal lesions with a dedicated knife (or knives) by free-hand technique, which has become popular worldwide in the past decade. It offers the unique ability to control size, shape, and depth of ER removal in one piece (*en bloc*). With refinement of ESD techniques

Mayo Clinic College of Medicine and Science, Mayo Clinic Arizona, 13400 E Shea Boulevard, Scottsdale, AZ 85259, USA
E-mail address: Fukami.norio@mayo.edu

Gastrointest Endoscopy Clin N Am 33 (2023) 55–66
https://doi.org/10.1016/j.giec.2022.09.003
1052-5157/23/© 2022 Elsevier Inc. All rights reserved.

Abbreviations	
ER	Endoscopic resection
EMR	Endoscopic Mucosal Resection
ESD	Endoscopic Submucosal Dissection
AC	Adenocarcinoma
SCC	Squamous cell carcinoma
HGD	High Grade Dysplasia
MM	Muscularis Mucosae
SM	Submucosa
LVI	Lymphovascular invasion
LNM	Lymph Node Metastasis
GEJ	Gastroesophageal Junction
APC	Argon Plasma Coagulator
EUS	Endoscopic Ultrasound

and reported excellent outcomes, wider application of ESD is now accepted in treating early neoplastic lesions in the esophagus. In this article, indications, techniques, and outcomes of esophageal ESD will be discussed.

INDICATIONS

The dominant histologic type of esophageal cancer shifted from squamous cell carcinoma (SCC) to adenocarcinoma (AC) in the United States. AC is predominantly found in Caucasians, whereas SCC is the dominant type in Blacks and Asians.[1] AC is commonly associated with a presence of Barrett's esophagus and eradication therapy for dysplastic Barrett's esophagus has reduced the incidence of esophageal AC.[2,3] For eradication therapy, nodular lesions or visible lesions in the Barrett's esophagus is recommended to be removed endoscopically by ER. Squamous cell cancer metastasizes to lymph nodes even in the early luminal invasive stage (invasion to muscularis mucosae [MM]; m3 stage), and removal of earlier disease (m1–m2; high-grade dysplasia or invasive only to lamina propria) by ER is considered to be curative if margins are negative.[4–6]

Endoscopic mucosal resection aided by band or cap are useful techniques to perform ER, however, it is limited by the precision on the area and the size of resection. Margin-negative resection is often possible for lesions less than 1 cm (10 MM) but becomes less successful if lesions are larger.[7] For SCC, 15 MM cutoff has been suggested at expert centers with excellent technique.[8] ESD offers the ability to resect a wider area even in the setting of irregular shape. It also offers better pathologic evaluation that translates to better stratification of the patient for further treatment and surveillance.

SQUAMOUS CELL CARCINOMA

There is no effective screening program in the United States, and the finding of squamous dysplasia is mostly an incidental finding during upper endoscopy. An increase in vascular pattern, which is reflective of abnormal intrapapillary capillary loops, would be detected on white light endoscopy. Detailed inspection is important because features of large granularity, nodule, depression, or ulceration indicate MM–SM invasion or deeper pathologic condition.[9,10] Advanced imaging and virtual chromoendoscopy to enhance the vascular pattern are increasingly used to demarcate the lesion and are helpful to determine the T stage.[11,12] Lugol chromoendoscopy is of a great help to delineate the margins of the lesion vividly; however, the major role is now being replaced by digital chromoendoscopy.[11,13,14]

ER is effective for flat lesions with smaller sizes. Both band-EMR and cap-EMR are effective. Cap-EMR using oblique caps (hard and soft) increases the size of the resection but the use of cap-EMR requires submucosal (SM) lifting and training on the proper technique to reduce the risk for perforation. Ensuring the negative margin reduces the need for close endoscopic follow-up. ESD is beneficial and suitable for larger lesions or nodular lesions that are not well captured by EMR offering higher likelihood to obtain negative margins.[6–8,15]

Curative resection is defined by negative resection margins with minimum risk for lymphatic or vascular spread. Those lesions include squamous low-grade and high-grade dysplasia and early cancers that only invades to lamina propria (m1–m2) without lymphovascular invasion (LVI). Once SCC invades MM, it has similar metastatic risk as one with shallow SM invasion (m3–SM1). SM invasion is considered shallow (SM1) if the invasion depth is less than 200 μm.[16] Due to the endoscopic and endosonographic limitation to separate m1–m2 from m3–SM1, ER is a beneficial tool to provide a precise pathologic stage that may offer curative resection.[4–6] Any nodularity within squamous cell dysplasia is suggestive of m3 disease or deeper and the indication for ER should be carefully sought.

ADENOCARCINOMA

Dysplastic change within Barrett's esophagus is an indicator of a risk for a presence or a development of AC. Nodular or visible dysplasia should be removed by ER to obtain a pathologic diagnosis recommended by multiple societies.[2,3,17] EMR is effective for smaller lesions as described in squamous cell neoplasia, and ESD has gained popularity and is accepted to be more effective than ER if lesions are more complex (larger, nodular, and multifocal).[6,15,17]

Intramucosal AC has very low risk for lymph node metastasis (LNM) and ER is considered curative if there is no poorly differentiated component and without LVI. There are lymphatic channels within the lamina propria and there is duplication of the MM at distal esophagus, which makes the pathologic diagnosis challenging. Invasion into the connective tissue between MM layers are considered to be the same as MM invasion,[18] and it is important to recognize the presence of duplication because we have seen incorrect pathologic staging of T2 when the second layer of MM had invasion on the slide.

SM invasion is considered shallow (SM1) if the invasion depth is less than 500 μm. Shallow invasion (SM1) with no risky features such as poor differentiation, single-cell invasion, or LVI is considered as a low-risk lesion for LNM and careful surveillance can be an option rather than to offer esophagectomy with lymph node dissection.[19]

In summary, m1–m2 squamous cell dysplasia/carcinoma and m1–SM1 HGD/AC with no risky features are considered as a good indication for ER and often curative if margin-negative resection is achieved. An m3–SM1 SCC is considered as relative indication because its LNM risk increases. However, upfront ER with subsequent therapy per pathologic findings was shown to have similar outcomes as upfront surgery for SCC without signs of deep invasion (SM2-3 or T2)[20] and therefore, ER can be considered as a first-line therapy for lesions amenable for complete ER. If ER is applied as cancer resection, margin-negative resection is important to offer adequate local therapy and cure. Thus, pretreatment (resection) assessment and determination of method of ER is paramount. ESD offers precise margin determination and more effective negative margin resection for lesions more than 1 cm and should be considered as preferred method for all complex lesions.[6,15,17]

OTHER LESIONS (GRANULAR CELL TUMOR, LEIOMYOMA ARISING FROM MM, AND OTHERS)

ESD is reported to be useful in removing some subepithelial tumors. If the tumor is separated from muscularis propria (MP) layer by SM tissue, ESD is possible. ESD offers similar benefit of offering en bloc and R0 resection of tumors. Endoscopic ultrasound (EUS) is beneficial in identifying the clear SM layer that separates tumor from the MP layer before proceeding with ESD.

ANATOMY

The esophagus is a tubular organ that is easily approachable with an upper endoscope. SM dissection can be rather effortless because it is aided by the natural angle of approach that is nearly parallel to the esophageal wall. Two unique features are to be clearly understood. The esophageal muscle layer is thin, as in the colonic wall, and it lacks serosa, which is usually a protective layer for perforation or leak.

If the gastric cardia is included in the treatment area, approaching the cardia is always easier in retroflexion rather than a straight view approach. The cardia harbors penetrating vessels supplied from the left gastric artery and additional care is needed not to prematurely cut this vessel without adequate coagulation to avoid significant bleeding.

PREOPERATIVE/PREPROCEDURE PLANNING

Regular preprocedural preparation for EGD is sufficient. Water irrigation with the endoscope is ideal for an efficient ESD procedure and a use of an appropriate attachment cap is required. If the lesion involves gastroesophageal junction (GEJ) or cardia, the approach to the distal part of lesion may require a retroflexed view and selecting an endoscope with full retroflexion capability should be selected. It is important to consider patients with squamous neoplasms and ones with Barrett's-related neoplasms separately, as the latter often have thick mucosa and SM fibrosis. Preplanning on ESD methods (eg, conventional or tunneling) and a preparation of tools for traction are advisable (eg, string or snare and clips).

PREPARATION AND PATIENT POSITIONING

For esophageal ESD, general endotracheal anesthesia is ideal to prevent aspiration, to control respiratory rate and volume, and to control heart rate. Patient may be in the left lateral decubitus position similar to a diagnostic procedure or in the supine position. Routine use of a warm blanket and a sequential compression device for a possibly long ESD procedure is recommended by this author.

PROCEDURAL APPROACH

ESD in the esophagus deserves special attention. Esophagus is a tubular organ, and SM dissection is rather straightforward. However, the esophagus lacks a serosal layer outside that usually prevents leaks and also facilitates closure when perforation occurs. Therefore, deep SM dissection should be avoided unless clinically necessary due to fibrosis or suspected cancer invasion into SM layer. Moreover, GEJ is often included in the resection area, which demands different approaches and techniques.

ESD methods include (1) a traditional method where a circumferential mucosal incision is performed and SM dissection is completed afterward and (2) a tunneling method where the distal and proximal mucosal incision are made and dissected down to SM layer, and then the SM dissection is completed from the proximal to distal end creating a tunnel.[21] Lateral mucosal incisions and subsequent SM dissection are performed. The tunneling method does not necessarily require traction method because traction is maintained by the residual tissue at the lateral sides of the lesion while the endoscope with cap is pushed forward. Traction method is very useful for the traditional method to facilitate SM dissection reducing adverse events. Simple clip and line technique or clips with snare technique would create traction to expose the SM layer facilitating dissection.[22]

Due to the proximity to greater vessels, heart, and diaphragm, extraesophageal movement can be complicating factors and those are best managed by anesthesia care with endotracheal intubation.

Tools:
a. Attachment cap or hood: Straight or cone/tapered shaped. Straight cap usually suffices.
b. Endoscope: One with water jet function is ideal.
c. Knife and scissors: Tip-knife with/without water jet capability, insulated-tip knife, and/or scissors-type device.
d. Injection fluid: Long-lasting fluid with dye (normal saline is not recommended for initial injection. However, saline solution is often used for additional injections via the knife during SM dissection).
e. Traction method: Clip and string or clip with snare.

Step 1: Mark 5 MM outside the lesion with the tip of a knife. Some use argon plasma coagulator (APC) probe; however, this adds additional cost.

Step 2: Determine the technique to be used: Conventional versus tunneling method.

Step 3: Mucosal incision at distal margin.

a. ESD within the esophagus
Incision at distal margin is done in a straight view position.
Injection of the fluid is to be done distal to the markings, and then mucosal incision is performed at or slightly proximal to the peak of the injected mound. It is important to incise down into the middle of SM layer but not down to expose the MP. The depth ensures recognition of the end point during SM dissection.
b. ESD for a lesion that includes the GEJ or the cardia
An incision in the cardia is best performed in a retroflexed position. A gradual incision from mucosal to SM is performed here because there is an abundant vascular network in SM layer at cardia. Coagulation of bleeding points or vessels needs to be done frequently to avoid ongoing blood loss and contamination of the dissection field with blood. Insulated tip knife works well in the cardia in retroflexion because the MP layer approaches more perpendicular to the knife when SM dissection progresses toward the Z line. An IT 2 knife needs to be used with caution so as not to make it parallel to the MP layer in order to avoid thermal damage or incision into the MP with the triangle electrode that is attached to the insulated tip.

Step 4: Mucosal incision at proximal margin.
Injection of the fluid is performed 5 MM *proximal* to the markings, and same process described in Step 3 (a) is repeated. The incision starts at the top or proximal to the peak of the injection mound.

Step 5: SM dissection and lateral mucosal incision.

a. Conventional method

Lateral mucosal incision is performed after additional fluid injection at the incision line outside the line created by marking. The dependent side (to gravity) should be incised first. With using a tip-knife, a proximal to distal direction is safer because the knife moves toward the lumen away from MP. With an insulated-tip knife, a distal to proximal movement works best. The full lateral mucosal incision beyond the MM should be completed to free up the lesion on both sides.

SM dissection begins at the proximal incision gradually moving distally. Once an adequate mucosal flap is created, a traction method may be used. The proximal edge is captured with a clip attached to the string or snare to provide traction. Two or more clips are recommended to secure the attachment to the snare.[23] Completion of SM dissection to free up the lesion is done by conducting SM dissection with either a tip-knife, insulated-tip knife, or scissor-type knives.

b. Tunneling method

SM dissection is performed from the proximal end to distal end until a tunnel is created. The width of dissection should be adequate to allow scope tip maneuvers but it is best to avoid expanding the tunnel width to the full width of the lesion.

Once a tunnel is created, the lateral mucosal incisions are done as in Step 5 (a). Then, the remaining SM layer at the sides are dissected from inside toward outside widening the tunnel or taking off the SM layer alternating one side to other side starting at proximal end moving distally. With an insulated-tip knife, SM dissection may be performed from the distal end moving proximally or follow the process described above.

c. Coagulation of vessels

Preemptive coagulation of vessels should be done whenever possible. Coagulation forceps with low voltage coagulation (SoftCoag) can be used to seal the vessel before dissection, or the knife can be used with low-energy coagulation mode (forced coagulation effect 1, 10 W, or very low wattage spray coagulation). Isolation of vessels by dissecting surrounding SM fibers (trimming) is an effective way to enhance the sealing effect of the vessels.

Step 6: Preemptive coagulation on vessels after resection.

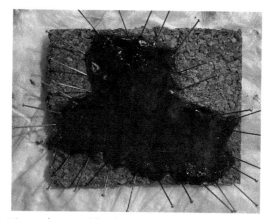

Fig. 1. C1M5 Barrett's esophagus with adenocarcinoma (IIa + IIc lesion) immediately after resection. Tissue was placed cut surface down and pinned on the cork board. Use of short thin clothing pin is recommended. Tissue should be stretched to the original shape while placing the pin.

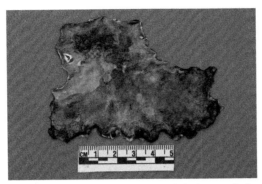

Fig. 2. After formalin fixation. Photo documented before coloring the margin and sectioning for future reference.

Exposed vessels at the resection bed should be coagulated by coagulation forceps to reduce post ESD bleeding. Thermal damage must be reduced by pulling the grasped tissue off the MP when applying coagulation energy. Air bubbles signify adequate temperature increase and signals the end of treatment.

Step 7: Preparation of tissue specimen.

Resected tissue is best retrieved with a net to prevent damage to the tissue. The lesion should be pinned on the cork around the resection edge for a proper orientation of the section and a precise evaluation of the margins and the depth of invasion (**Figs. 1** and **2**). Discussion with a pathologist and pathology technician in the processing room is extremely helpful to set up proper processing of ESD specimens.

RECOVERY AND REHABILITATION

Post ESD care consists of dietary modification, observation status (outpatient vs admission), and the use of antibiotics. Diet will be restricted to clear liquids or nil per os (NPO) depending on the risk for bleeding and perforation. We often allow patients to have clear liquids on the day of the procedure to continue for 1 or 2 days depending on the size and location of the resection. Risk of bleeding is highest within 48 hours, and if there no bleeding during that time, the diet can be safely advanced. High doses of proton pump inhibitors should be prescribed for the initial 6 to 8 weeks to reduce chemical irritation and can be reduced to once daily afterward for patients with Barrett's-related neoplasm. Administration of antibiotics is not routine and is only advisable with evidence of intraprocedural MP injury or perforation. This author has been managing patients undergoing ESD as same day surgery patients unless patients have severe medical conditions (ie, cardiopulmonary, severe renal disease, or on anticoagulation or antithrombotic agent, which requires to be resumed soonest after ESD). Outpatient management is combined with a follow-up phone call on the next day to monitor patient's status.

OUTCOMES

The goals of the ER for esophageal lesions are to obtain tissue diagnosis and pathologic T stage, thus predicting the risk for recurrence and/or metastatic disease, and also to provide cure from the disease. Adverse events should be considered for any invasive treatments to weigh benefits against risks compared with other therapeutic modalities such as esophagectomy.

Successful technical outcomes of ER are defined by a resection of the lesion in one piece (*en bloc* resection) and ER of lesion with negative lateral and deep margins (R0 resection). Moreover, successful clinical outcomes are defined by the risk of local recurrence, and risk of metastatic recurrence (curative resection), and rates and degree of the adverse events.

a. Tissue resection and cancer risk assessment

Precise pre-ER staging of the tumor is often difficult and the separation of the T1a from T1b is challenging given the thinness of each layer in the esophagus. EUS allows more reliable separation of the T stage than computed tomographic scan, and EUS is recommended if there is no evidence of metastatic disease but separating T1a from T1b can be suboptimal.[24-28] Therefore, ER is a more definitive tool to provide pathologic T stage for early-stage cancer when endoscopic examination does not suggest deeper invasion. EUS confirmation may be beneficial to exclude tumor invasive to the MP or deeper (T2 or deeper). ER should be done not only to obtain pathologic diagnosis in this case but to aim for curative resection because the first resection is the best chance to obtain clear margins without prohibitive scarring.

Successful resections were achieved in most cases at the completion of ESD. Meta-analysis of published data on Barrett's ESD described ESD rates as follows: en bloc resection rate 96%, R0 resection 74.5%, and curative resection 64.9%.[29] Other systematic review and meta-analysis comparing EMR and ESD for esophageal cancer including both SCC and AC, from both East and West showed significantly high en bloc, R0, and curative resection rate for ESD with OR of 36.32, 4.77, and 9.74, respectively.[7] In this study, there was no difference was seen in outcomes between EMR and ESD for lesions less than 10 MM size.

Curative resection is defined by en bloc, margin-negative (R0) resection with very low risk for nodal and metastatic recurrence (ie, mucosal cancer or shallow SM invasion with no poor differentiation and no LVIs – see *indication section*). The risks for nodal and metastases differs between SCC and AC. SCC is known to spread to lymph nodes in the early tumor stage. Epithelial and cancer invasion into lamina propria (m1 and m2) are acceptable as low-risk invasion depth. Invasion to muscularis mucosae (MM) and shallow SM invasion up to 200 μm (m3 and SM1) are considered to have higher LNM up to 16% to 26.1%,[12,16,30] and thus, it is considered as a relative indication for ER because there would be higher risk for recurrence but ER may be of benefit if patients are at high risk for undergoing other therapy such as surgery or chemoradiation therapy.

There was a concern about ER being used as a therapeutic modality for SCC that may be invasive to MM or superficial SM because when pathologic evaluation later proved it to be noncurative, ER may adversely affect efficacy of subsequent treatment outcomes. Several studies tried to answer this question. In retrospective studies and a separate meta-analysis, survival outcomes did not differ between the patients who underwent primary ER compared with patients who underwent esophagectomy for T1b SCC.[20,31,32] In a propensity score–matched cohort study by Min and colleagues, the authors demonstrated that primary ER for T1 lesions with/without subsequent adjuvant surgery or chemoradiation achieved similar survival outcomes as primary surgery.[20] This study reinforced the appropriateness of ER as the primary therapeutic attempt providing pathologic diagnosis to stratify patients for further treatments.

Multiple societies recommend ER for any visible dysplastic nodule within Barrett's esophagus.[2,3,33] ER with pathologic evaluation offers definitive pathologic diagnosis and the risk stratification. Further eradication of remaining Barrett's epithelium is universally recommended to reduce metachronous HGD or cancer within the residual Barrett's. The risk of metastatic spread of shallow SM invasion without high-risk signs was reported to be similar to T1a cancer[19] but the criteria is not accepted universally as curative resection criteria in the West, and further clarification on the risk of the patient group is needed. Multidisciplinary discussion is recommended to create the local institutional clinical pathway. A patient-centered approach that involves the patient for decision-making is ideal.

b. Adverse events

Most significant adverse events are bleeding, perforation, and resultant esophageal stricture. AE rates were reported as 1.8% for bleeding and 1.5% for perforation in meta-analysis[29] and compared with those for EMR, the bleeding rate was similar but perforation risk was higher (OR 2.47), especially for SCC.[7] Intraprocedural bleeding is almost always controllable during the procedure. Delayed bleeding can occur manifesting as fainting, hematemesis, and melena. Most commonly, patients develops nausea with subsequent hematemesis. Urgent endoscopy is necessary to achieve hemostasis and interventional radiology intervention is rarely required. Delayed perforation may require surgical intervention; however, a temporary fully covered esophageal stent can be placed to attempt to seal the leak. Endoscopic suture application may be of help if the perforation site is near or below GEJ. Exposed MP layer in the tubular esophagus would not hold clips or suture because the esophagus lacks serosa and attempts to apply such devices into the exposed MP layer should be avoided. Preemptive fully covered esophageal stent placement may be considered to reduce post ESD bleeding and leak.

Steroid injection or oral high-dose steroid administration were reported to reduce the risk of stenosis.[34–38] Steroid injection is effective in preventing stricture after ESD for squamous-related neoplasms but does not seem so effective after ESD for Barrett's related neoplasms likely due to coexisting acid and nonacid reflux. Strictures start to manifest around 3 weeks after ESD, and preemptive dilations are effective to maintain the esophageal diameter and to prevent dysphagia.[39]

SUMMARY

Esophageal ESD is highly effective in the removal of large areas in one piece (en bloc), offering the benefit of complete removal of neoplasms with negative margin. ESD steps are relatively established and standardized. Proper procedural planning and effective use of tools are paramount to achieve high clinical success and to reduce complications.

CLINICS CARE POINTS

- General endotracheal anesthesia is ideal for esophageal endoscopic submucosal dissection (ESD) for the best control of airway, respiratory effort, and cardiac movement to facilitate the procedure.
- Detailed inspection on the target lesion with the use of advanced imaging is the most critical first procedural step to plan and aim for successful resection with the proper techniques.
- The tubular esophagus lacks a protective serosal layer and submucosal dissection should be performed well above muscularis propriae to prevent muscle exposure or injury.
- Submucosal tissue is a protective layer to prevent leaks and to receive steroid injection for the prevention of stenosis. This author recommends dissection at SM2 layer (middle layer of submucosal [SM] layer) unless SM invasion of cancer is suspected.
- Pathologic evaluation is the key factor for the clinical success of ESD. Proper processing of the tissue needs to be established in the gastrointestinal (GI) laboratory and in the pathology

laboratory before the start of ESD practice.

DISCLOSURE

Author has relationship as consultant to the companies below: Creo Medical, Boston Scientific.

REFERENCES

1. Corona E, Yang L, Esrailian E, et al. Trends in Esophageal Cancer Mortality and Stage at Diagnosis by Race and Ethnicity in the United States. Cancer Causes Control 2021;32(8):883–94.
2. Sharma P, Shaheen NJ, Katzka D, et al. AGA Clinical Practice Update on Endoscopic Treatment of Barrett's Esophagus With Dysplasia and/or Early Cancer: Expert Review. Gastroenterology 2020;158(3):760–9.
3. Shaheen NJ, Falk GW, Iyer PG, et al. Diagnosis and Management of Barrett's Esophagus: An Updated ACG Guideline. Am J Gastroenterol 2022;117(4): 559–87.
4. Kitagawa Y, Uno T, Oyama T, et al. Esophageal cancer practice guidelines 2017 edited by the Japan Esophageal Society: part 1. Esophagus 2019;16(1):1–24.
5. Kitagawa Y, Uno T, Oyama T, et al. Esophageal cancer practice guidelines 2017 edited by the Japan esophageal society: part 2. Esophagus 2019;16(1):25–43.
6. Pimentel-Nunes P, Libanio D, Bastiaansen BAJ, et al. Endoscopic submucosal dissection for superficial gastrointestinal lesions: European Society of Gastrointestinal Endoscopy (ESGE) Guideline - Update 2022. Endoscopy 2022;54(6): 591–622.
7. Han C, Sun Y. Efficacy and safety of endoscopic submucosal dissection versus endoscopic mucosal resection for superficial esophageal carcinoma: a systematic review and meta-analysis. Dis Esophagus 2021;34(4).
8. Kawashima K, Abe S, Koga M, et al. Optimal selection of endoscopic resection in patients with esophageal squamous cell carcinoma: endoscopic mucosal resection versus endoscopic submucosal dissection according to lesion size. Dis Esophagus 2021;34(5).
9. Ebi M, Shimura T, Yamada T, et al. Multicenter, prospective trial of white-light imaging alone versus white-light imaging followed by magnifying endoscopy with narrow-band imaging for the real-time imaging and diagnosis of invasion depth in superficial esophageal squamous cell carcinoma. Gastrointest Endosc 2015; 81(6):1355–61.e2.
10. Shimamura Y, Ikeya T, Marcon N, et al. Endoscopic diagnosis and treatment of early esophageal squamous neoplasia. World J Gastrointest Endosc 2017;9(9): 438–47.
11. Inoue H, Kaga M, Ikeda H, et al. Magnification endoscopy in esophageal squamous cell carcinoma: a review of the intrapapillary capillary loop classification. Ann Gastroenterol 2015;28(1):41–8.
12. Oyama T, Inoue H, Arima M, et al. Prediction of the invasion depth of superficial squamous cell carcinoma based on microvessel morphology: magnifying endoscopic classification of the Japan Esophageal Society. Esophagus 2017;14(2): 105–12.

13. Costa-Santos MP, Ferreira AO, Mouradides C, et al. Is Lugol necessary for endoscopic resection of esophageal squamous cell neoplasia? Endosc Int Open 2020;8(10):E1471–7.
14. Yip HC, Chiu PW. Endoscopic diagnosis and management of early squamous cell carcinoma of esophagus. J Thorac Dis 2017;9(Suppl 8):S689–96.
15. Draganov PV, Wang AY, Othman MO, et al. AGA Institute Clinical Practice Update: Endoscopic Submucosal Dissection in the United States. Clin Gastroenterol Hepatol 2019;17(1):16–25 e11.
16. Japan Esophageal S. Japanese Classification of Esophageal Cancer, 11th Edition: part I. Esophagus 2017;14(1):1–36.
17. Ishihara R, Arima M, Iizuka T, et al. Endoscopic submucosal dissection/endoscopic mucosal resection guidelines for esophageal cancer. Dig Endosc 2020; 32(4):452–93.
18. Estrella JS, Hofstetter WL, Correa AM, et al. Duplicated muscularis mucosae invasion has similar risk of lymph node metastasis and recurrence-free survival as intramucosal esophageal adenocarcinoma. Am J Surg Pathol 2011;35(7): 1045–53.
19. Manner H, Pech O, Heldmann Y, et al. The frequency of lymph node metastasis in early-stage adenocarcinoma of the esophagus with incipient submucosal invasion (pT1b sm1) depending on histological risk patterns. Surg Endosc 2015; 29(7):1888–96.
20. Min YW, Lee H, Song BG, et al. Comparison of endoscopic submucosal dissection and surgery for superficial esophageal squamous cell carcinoma: a propensity score-matched analysis. Gastrointest Endosc 2018;88(4):624–33.
21. Linghu E, Feng X, Wang X, et al. Endoscopic submucosal tunnel dissection for large esophageal neoplastic lesions. Endoscopy 2013;45(1):60–2.
22. Oyama T. Counter traction makes endoscopic submucosal dissection easier. Clin Endosc 2012;45(4):375–8.
23. Shimamura Y, Inoue H, Ikeda H, et al. Multipoint traction technique in endoscopic submucosal dissection. VideoGIE 2018;3(7):207–8.
24. Krill T, Baliss M, Roark R, et al. Accuracy of endoscopic ultrasound in esophageal cancer staging. J Thorac Dis 2019;11(Suppl 12):S1602–9.
25. Ajani JA, D'Amico TA, Bentrem DJ, et al. Esophageal and Esophagogastric Junction Cancers, Version 2.2019, NCCN Clinical Practice Guidelines in Oncology. J Natl Compr Canc Netw 2019;17(7):855–83.
26. Thosani N, Singh H, Kapadia A, et al. Diagnostic accuracy of EUS in differentiating mucosal versus submucosal invasion of superficial esophageal cancers: a systematic review and meta-analysis. Gastrointest Endosc 2012;75(2):242–53.
27. Yoshinaga S, Oda I, Nonaka S, et al. Endoscopic ultrasound using ultrasound probes for the diagnosis of early esophageal and gastric cancers. World J Gastrointest Endosc 2012;4(6):218–26.
28. Qumseya BJ, Bartel MJ, Gendy S, et al. High rate of over-staging of Barrett's neoplasia with endoscopic ultrasound: Systemic review and meta-analysis. Dig Liver Dis 2018;50(5):438–45.
29. Yang D, Zou F, Xiong S, et al. Endoscopic submucosal dissection for early Barrett's neoplasia: a meta-analysis. Gastrointest Endosc 2018;87(6):1383–93.
30. Akutsu Y, Uesato M, Shuto K, et al. The overall prevalence of metastasis in T1 esophageal squamous cell carcinoma: a retrospective analysis of 295 patients. Ann Surg 2013;257(6):1032–8.

31. Lee HD, Chung H, Kwak Y, et al. Endoscopic Submucosal Dissection Versus Surgery for Superficial Esophageal Squamous Cell Carcinoma: A Propensity Score-Matched Survival Analysis. Clin Transl Gastroenterol 2020;11(7):e00193.
32. Liu Z, Zhao R. Endoscopic Submucosal Dissection vs. Surgery for Superficial Esophageal Squamous Cancer: A Systematic Review and Meta-Analysis. Front Oncol 2022;12:816832.
33. Standards of Practice C, Wani S, Qumseya B, et al. Endoscopic eradication therapy for patients with Barrett's esophagus-associated dysplasia and intramucosal cancer. Gastrointest Endosc 2018;87(4):907–31.e9.
34. Hashimoto S, Kobayashi M, Takeuchi M, et al. The efficacy of endoscopic triamcinolone injection for the prevention of esophageal stricture after endoscopic submucosal dissection. Gastrointest Endosc 2011;74(6):1389–93.
35. Hanaoka N, Ishihara R, Takeuchi Y, et al. Intralesional steroid injection to prevent stricture after endoscopic submucosal dissection for esophageal cancer: a controlled prospective study. Endoscopy 2012;44(11):1007–11.
36. Takahashi H, Arimura Y, Okahara S, et al. A randomized controlled trial of endoscopic steroid injection for prophylaxis of esophageal stenoses after extensive endoscopic submucosal dissection. BMC Gastroenterol 2015;15:1.
37. Yamaguchi N, Isomoto H, Nakayama T, et al. Usefulness of oral prednisolone in the treatment of esophageal stricture after endoscopic submucosal dissection for superficial esophageal squamous cell carcinoma. Gastrointest Endosc 2011;73(6):1115–21.
38. Probst A, Ebigbo A, Markl B, et al. Stricture Prevention after Extensive Endoscopic Submucosal Dissection of Neoplastic Barrett's Esophagus: Individualized Oral Steroid Prophylaxis. Gastroenterol Res Pract 2019;2019:2075256.
39. Ezoe Y, Muto M, Horimatsu T, et al. Efficacy of preventive endoscopic balloon dilation for esophageal stricture after endoscopic resection. J Clin Gastroenterol 2011;45(3):222–7.

Endoscopic Submucosal Dissection in the Stomach and Duodenum

Techniques, Indications, and Outcomes

Sarah S. Al Ghamdi, MBBS, FRCPC[a],
Saowanee Ngamruengphong, MD[b],*

KEYWORDS

- Endoscopic submucosal dissection • Endoscopic resection • Stomach • Duodenum
- Early gastric cancer • Dysplasia

KEY POINTS

- Gastric endoscopic submucosal dissection (ESD) is well established for management of early gastric cancer (EGC).
- Diagnosis of EGC relies on adequate endoscopic assessment involving lesion size, histopathology, presence of ulceration, and depth of invasion.
- Absolute indications for endoscopic resection of EGC are if patients are presumed to have a less than 1% risk of lymph node metastasis, and long-term outcomes are similar to those with surgical gastrectomy.
- Several novel traction devices and strategies have been developed to facilitate ESD, including elastic band-assisted traction, double scope method, and multiloop traction.
- Duodenal ESD is more technically difficult and requires ESD expertise in other locations.

INTRODUCTION

Endoscopic resection (ER) techniques of gastric and duodenal neoplasms include endoscopic mucosal resection (EMR) and endoscopic submucosal dissection (ESD). These techniques have become first-line options for management of noninvasive lesions.[1] ESD allows for en bloc resection irrespective of lesion size and for those with high risk features of submucosal invasion (SMI) to allow for accurate

a Division of Gastroenterology and Hepatology, Department of Medicine, King Abdulaziz University, Jeddah, PO Box 80215, Saudi Arabia; b Division of Gastroenterology and Hepatology, Department of Medicine, King Abdulaziz University, Building 10, 2nd Floor, PO Box 80215, Jeddah 21589, Saudi Arabia
* Corresponding author.
E-mail address: sngamru1@jhmi.edu

Gastrointest Endoscopy Clin N Am 33 (2023) 67–81
https://doi.org/10.1016/j.giec.2022.07.005
1052-5157/23/© 2022 Elsevier Inc. All rights reserved.

histopathological assessment. This article discusses the indications, techniques, and outcomes of gastric and duodenal ESD.

GASTRIC ENDOSCOPIC SUBMUCOSAL DISSECTION
Background

Gastric cancer ranks the sixth most common malignant tumor and the fourth leading cause of cancer-related mortality worldwide.[18] Because of the frequently late disease diagnosis, 5-year survival of gastric cancer is about 32%.[19] Several histologic classifications for phenotypes of gastric carcinogenesis exist, such as the revised Vienna classification[20,21] and the World Health Organization classification. The most adhered to terminology comprises low-grade dysplasia (LGD), high-grade dysplasia (HGD), noninvasive carcinoma (carcinoma in situ), and intramucosal carcinoma (invasion into lamina propria or muscularis mucosa). The histologic entity of early gastric cancer (EGC) was based on the observation that gastric cancer of this type had a favorable prognosis, with a 5-year survival greater than 90%.[22] EGC is defined as invasive gastric adenocarcinoma confined to the mucosa or submucosa, irrespective of lymph node metastasis (LNM) (T1, any N as per American Joint Commission on Cancer classification[23]). Prognosis largely depends on the presence of LNM, which occurs in 2% to 5% of EGCs that are confined to the mucosa and increases to 10% to 25% when submucosal invasion is present.[24,25]

Treatment of EGC previously centered around surgical resection (gastrectomy and lymphadenectomy) to ensure complete resection. Currently, ER is standard of care for the treatment of EGC with negligible risk for LNM given their lesion size and are amenable to resection en bloc, owing to similar oncological outcomes. En bloc resection is crucial, as precise histopathological diagnosis is essential for risk assessment of LNM and to prevent the potential risk of local recurrence after piecemeal resection.[26] In well selected cases, endoscopic management has significant advantages over surgery, as it is less morbid and organ preserving. To ensure good outcomes of ER, knowledge regarding diagnosis and indications and long-term surveillance are critical. ER techniques include EMR and ESD. EMR was first reported in 1984 and has been widely accepted as an effective treatment for EGC. However, en bloc resection by EMR is limited in larger-sized lesions (>2 cm). ESD was pioneered for EGC in 1999 by Gotoda and colleagues.[27] ESD enables higher en bloc resection with lower local recurrence rates compared with EMR.[28,29]

DIAGNOSTIC STRATEGIES OF SUPERFICIAL GASTRIC NEOPLASIA

Appropriate lesion selection requires endoscopic diagnosis and assessment of high-risk features for SMI and is critical to help determine the best resection strategy. This includes assessment of lesion morphology, surface architecture, and vessel patterns that require endoscopic expertise and advanced technology. Most modern endoscopes contain optical diagnostic techniques using blue-light imaging (BLI) such as narrow-band imaging (NBI) or image-enhanced endoscopy (i-SCAN), combined with high-definition white-light imaging (HD-WLE). Dye-based chromoendoscopy (CE) using contrast dyes such as methylene blue (MB) or indigo carmine also plays a role in visual analysis. Dye and blue light imaging are complementary techniques as they provide subtly different information on surface integrity.

The Japanese Society of Gastroenterology (JGES) and Japanese Gastric Cancer Association (JGCA) jointly advocate the magnifying endoscopy simple diagnostic algorithm for gastric cancer (MESDA-G).[2] This algorithm involves determining whether a demarcation line (DL) is present between the mucosal lesion and the background

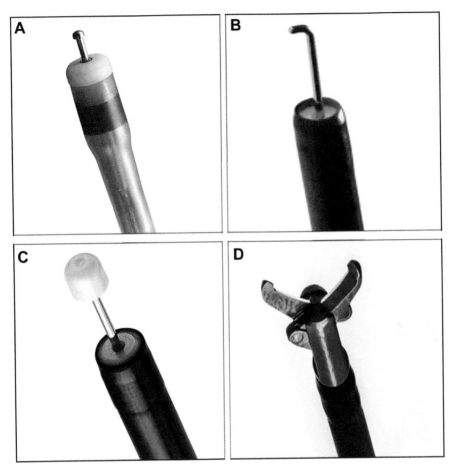

Fig. 1. Examples of ESD knives. (*A, B*) Needle-type knives. (*C*) Insulated-tip type knife. (*D*) Scissor-type knife. (*Courtesy of* Olympus, Center Valley, Pennsylvania.)

mucosa. If a DL is absent, the lesion is diagnosed as noncancerous. If a DL is present, an irregular microvascular (MV) pattern and/or an irregular microsurface (MS) pattern should be evaluated. If both an irregular MV pattern and an irregular MS pattern are absent, the lesion is diagnosed as noncancerous; if either pattern is present, the lesion is diagnosed as cancerous. The vessels plus surface (VS) classification is also used for the analysis of magnifying endoscopic findings.[3] The characteristic findings of high-grade dysplasia or early gastric cancer (EGC) are the presence of a clear DL between noncancerous and cancerous mucosa, and the presence of an irregular MV pattern and/or irregular MS pattern within the DL. Depth of tumor invasion is usually determined by lesion characteristics on conventional endoscopy. When depth of tumor invasion as measured using conventional endoscopy is uncertain, endoscopic ultrasound (EUS) occasionally has a role in adjunct to this method.

Techniques of gastric endoscopic submucosal dissection

ESD techniques have greatly evolved since their introduction in the early 2000s. Proper planning and careful lesion assessment are imperative to choose the most appropriate technique and to ensure adequate resection margins.[4] A standard high-

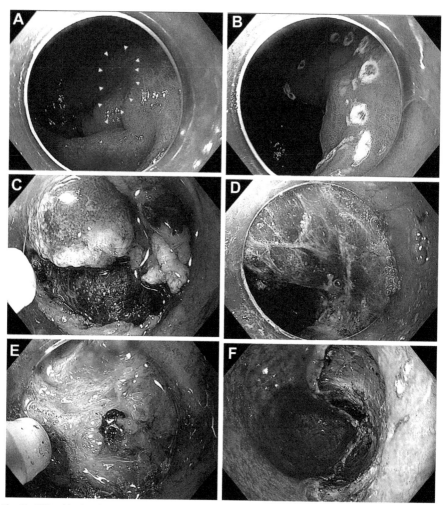

Fig. 2. ESD of lesion in gastric antrum. (*A*) Endoscopic assessment of 30 mm depressed lesion with no obvious ulceration. (*B*) Circumferential marking of lesion. (*C*) Circumferential incision. (*D*) Submucosal dissection. (*E*) Submucosal fibrosis during submucosal dissection. (*F*) Final ESD defect.

definition video gastroscope with magnification and image-enhanced technology is typically used. An auxiliary water jet channel is necessary to help enhance visualization. Normal saline is preferred over water to maintain effective electrosurgical dissection. The use of a transparent plastic distal attachment cap or hood aids in stabilization of scope position during submucosal dissection. A reliable electrosurgical unit is crucial, as ESD depends on safe and accurate electric current throughout the procedure. Carbon dioxide insufflation should be used for ESD procedures as it significantly reduces abdominal pain and analgesic usage compared with air insufflation.[5] Electrosurgical knives are used for mucosal incision and submucosal dissection. These are broadly categorized into needle type, insulated tip type, and scissor-type knives (**Fig. 1**), with some having an added water jet channel to minimize instrument exchanges during the procedure.

Generally, the steps of ESD include marking, submucosal injection, mucosal incision, submucosal dissection, and hemostasis[6] **(Fig. 2)**. The margins of gastric lesion become indistinct after submucosal injection, necessitating circumferential marking (see **Fig. 2A**). Preprocedural marking of gastric lesions is therefore essential to facilitate the mucosal incision and ensure adequate lateral resection margins. Marking should be performed about 5 mm outside the lesion, with small gaps between each mark (see **Fig. 2B**). Occasionally, margins of EGC are difficult to delineate on initial endoscopic evaluation.

Indigo carmine chromoendoscopy assists margin delineation before ESD. Magnifying endoscopy with narrow-band imaging can also be used and has been found to successfully delineate margins in over 70% of cases that initially show unclear margins.[7] Alternatively, biopsies of the surrounding normal-appearing mucosa can be taken to confirm horizontal margins. After marking the lesion, submucosal injection is performed using a viscous solution. Mucosal incision is then performed using a needle-type ESD device beginning at the near or far side, depending on type of knife and preferred ESD technique (see **Fig. 2C**). Mucosal incision can be completed by a needle-type or insulated-type knife. The incision should traverse the muscularis mucosa and reach the submucosa. The conventional ESD technique begins with completion of a circumferential incision, whereas the pocket creation method begins with a partial mucosal incision on the near/oral side of the lesion.[8] The partial incision is typically one-third to one-half of the lesion circumference and is followed by submucosal

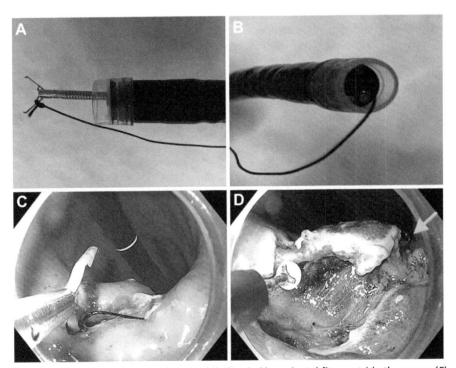

Fig. 3. Clip-with-line traction technique. (*A*) Clip tied by a dental floss outside the scope. (*B*) The clip is pulled back into the scope while the dental floss remains alongside the scope. (*C*) The clip is deployed on the edge of the lesion. (*D*) Improved visualization of the submucosal layer after pulling on the line from the oral side to place traction on the mucosal flap.

dissection underneath the lesion prior to completion of the mucosal incision. The pocket creation method has been found to facilitate ESD by helping to stabilize the scope position.[9] Submucosal dissection is then performed using either a needle-type or insulated-type knife (see **Fig. 2**D,E). The latter method is beneficial in gastric lesions owing to the thick nature of gastric submucosa. During submucosal dissection, the submucosal space is expanded using an injection solution. The optimal layer for dissection is the deep submucosa just above the muscularis propria. This provides a thicker specimen that may reduce the chance of vertical margin involvement, especially in EGC with submucosal invasion. During submucosal dissection, large penetrating submucosal vessels should be prophylactically coagulated using the dissection knife or coagulation forceps.

Several novel traction devices and strategies have been developed to facilitate ESD and have been found to result in shorter procedure time, improved R0 resection rates, and lower risk of perforation when compared with conventional ESD without traction.[10] Clip line traction is the most commonly used traction technique in gastric ESD.[11] A clip-with-line can be easily assembled by attaching a string (eg, dental floss or silk surgical suture) to a standard endoscopic clip (**Fig. 3**). An endoclip is inserted into the accessory channel of the endoscope, and a nylon string or dental floss is tied to 1 arm of the clip by a surgeon's knot (see **Fig. 3**A). Before intubation of the esophagus, the endoclip is withdrawn inside the channel to avoid trauma during insertion of the endoscope (see **Fig. 3**B). When the scope reaches the lesion, the clip is deployed to the oral edge of the lesion (see **Fig. 3**C), and the line is pulled gently in the oral direction by the endoscopist or an assistant for traction (see **Fig. 3**D). Other traction methods include elastic band-assisted traction, a double scope method, and a novel multiloop traction device.[12]

Closure of ESD defects can be technically difficult using standard endoscopic clips. Several endoscopic suturing techniques were devised and have been clinically applied to mucosal defects after gastric ESD. These include the Overstitch suturing system (Apollo Endosurgery, Incorporated, Austin, Texas),[13] the through-the-scope X-tack suturing system (Apollo Endosurgery, Incorporated),[14] both of which are available in the United States. Also available in Japan are the endoscopic ligation technique with O-ring closure[15] and the double-arm bar suturing system and endoscopic hand-suturing (EHS) using the through-the-scope type flexible needle holder (Olympus Company, Ltd., Tokyo)[16]. These were found to provide reliable closure and potentially decrease the risk of delayed postoperative bleeding.

Following en bloc resection, the specimen is retrieved and pinned onto a flat board. This is to ensure appropriated histopathologic evaluation to ensure adequate endoscopic resection. Important parameters that should be reported include lesion size, the presence of ulceration, histologic cellular type, differentiation, involvement of lateral and vertical margins, depth of invasion, and lymphovascular invasion. Standardized reporting is important to confirm curative resection.[17]

Preoperative Assessment

In order to determine whether ER (ESD or EMR) is indicated, it is necessary to determine histopathological type, lesion size, presence of ulceration, and depth of invasion. Histopathological type is determined through histopathological examination of a biopsy specimen obtained during endoscopy. Lesion size as assessed during endoscopic evaluation is frequently inaccurate, so final measurements are determined from the resected specimen. The presence of ulceration (either active ulceration or an ulcer scar) is also assessed at preoperative endoscopy. Active ulceration refers to open ulcers with adherent white exudates and is histopathologically deeper than the muscularis mucosa. Superficial erosions are not included, as these are histopathologically confined to the surface epithelium. A healing or scarred ulcer contains mucosal folds or rugae converging on 1 point and is also considered ulceration. Depth of invasion is generally assessed using conventional endoscopy with or without dye spraying. Characteristic features of SMI include irregular or nodular surface protrusion or depression, deep ulcer with marked marginal elevation, fusion of converging folds, and abrupt cutting or clubbing of converging folds. Several studies determined that the overall accuracy of conventional endoscopy in terms of distinguishing lesions with and without SMI was about 62% to 78%.[30,31]

EUS can also be used as an adjunct to aid in determining the depth of invasion. Various reports on the diagnostic ability of EUS to distinguish T stage have been published. EUS staging is typically performed using a radial or miniprobe. In 1 prospective study, the accuracy of miniprobe EUS was significantly higher than that of radial EUS (79.5% vs 59.6%, $P<.001$), but did not differ significantly from that of conventional endoscopy (79.0%). A meta-analysis that included 54 studies and 5601 patients with gastric cancer undergoing disease staging with EUS revealed that this was highly accurate in differentiating T1-2 from T3-4 gastric cancer.[32] Furthermore, EUS had a high sensitivity and low specificity for differentiating T1a and T1b gastric cancer.[33,34] In a meta-analysis of 20 studies (n = 3321) on accuracy of EUS in differentiating between T1a (mucosal) versus T1b (submucosal) gastric cancers, the summary sensitivity and specificity were 0.87 (95% confidence interval [CI] 0.81–0.92) and 0.75 (95% CI 0.62–0.84), respectively.[32]

In 2019, the American Gastroenterological Association (AGA) recommended that ESD should be considered as first-line therapy for visible, endoscopically resectable, superficial gastric neoplasia.[35] The European Society of Gastrointestinal Endoscopy (ESGE) recommends ER for the treatment of gastric superficial neoplastic lesions that possess a low risk of lymph node metastasis.[36] Moreover, JGES, in collaboration with JGCA guidelines, define absolute and expanded criteria for endoscopic resection of EGC.[1]

Indications of Gastric Endoscopic Submucosal Dissection

According to the 2021 JGES guidelines, lesions are considered absolute indications for endoscopic resection if they are presumed to have a less than 1% risk of LNM and long-term outcomes similar to those with surgical gastrectomy. Absolute indications for endoscopic resection include differentiated type adenocarcinomas without ulcerative findings (UL-), of which the depth of invasion is clinically diagnosed as intramucosal (cT1a), and cT1a undifferentiated type adenocarcinomas when the diameter is less than 2 cm (**Fig. 4**). For lesions with ulcerative findings (UL+), absolute indications include cT1a differentiated type and a diameter of 3 cm or less.[1] Of note, in the first version of these guidelines, lesions categorized as expanded indications according to tumor-related factors have been integrated into absolute indications in the 2021 guidelines.

Several factors are taken into consideration when determining the most appropriate resection strategy. These include patient comorbidities, likelihood of LNM, cost, local expertise, and expected disease-free survival. This decision requires a multidisciplinary approach involving gastroenterologists, surgeons, oncologists, pathologists, and radiologists. For EGC lesions that meet absolute criteria for endoscopic resection, current consensus is that ER should be the standard of care to avoid unnecessary surgical intervention. EMR and ESD are both reasonable options for lesions less than 1 cm in size, as long as en bloc resection can be achieved. For larger lesions, the indistinct lesion margins and relative thickness of the gastric mucosa make ESD superior to

Depth of invasion	Ulceration	Differentiated		Undifferentiated	
T1a (M)	UL (-)	≤2cm	>2cm	≤2cm	>2cm
		Absolute indication for EMR/ESD	Absolute indications for ESD	Relative indication	
	UL (+)	≤3cm	>3cm		
		Absolute indication for ESD	Relative indications		
T1b (SM)		Relative indications			

Fig. 4. Classification of indications for endoscopic resection of EGC according to tumor-related factors. UL (−) no ulceration, UL (+) ulceration present; M, intramucosal cancer; SM, submucosally invasive cancer. (*Adapted from* Ono H, Yao K, Fujishiro M, et al. Guidelines for endoscopic submucosal dissection and endoscopic mucosal resection for early gastric cancer (second edition). *Dig Endosc* 2021;33(1):4-20.)

EMR. Although there are no randomized controlled trials comparing therapeutic outcomes between gastric EMR and ESD, a meta-analysis found that better en bloc resection rates are achieved with ESD than with EMR.[29] It has also been reported that for lesions larger than 1 cm, en bloc resection rates are significantly lower for EMR than for ESD.[37,38]

There have been no randomized controlled trials comparing ESD and surgery for EGC to date. However, a systematic review and meta-analysis that included 18 retrospective studies found that ESD had several benefits over surgery, including shorter procedure time, shorter hospital stay, lower risk of procedure-related death, and lower risk of overall complications.[39] ESD was also found to be more cost effective and had better quality of life. However, ESD had a lower rate of en bloc resection, curative resection, and a higher rate of local recurrence. Another recent propensity score-matched study on 84 patients from a tertiary referral center compared short- and long-term outcomes between surgery and ESD.[40] The study showed comparable results in terms of overall and disease-free survival between both approaches during a 5-year follow up period. Regarding lesions within the expanded criteria (which have been integrated into absolute indications in the most recent 2021 JGES guidelines[1]), surgery has traditionally been the treatment of choice. A multicenter retrospective study from South Korea of patients treated with ESD or surgical resection within the expanded criteria over a 2-year period showed shorter procedure times and hospital stay in the ESD group.[41] However, the 5-year cancer recurrence rate was higher in the ESD group, and the 5-year disease-free survival rate was higher in the surgical group.

Undifferentiated histology has a higher rate of LNM compared witho differentiated histology, reaching up to 10.6% in SM1 lesions.[1] A multicenter retrospective study from 18 centers in Korea compared between ESD and surgery for curative resection of undifferentiated type EGC within expanded indications; ESD showed comparable overall and 5-year survival to surgery.[42] However, the recurrence rate was higher in the ESD group than the surgery group. Appropriate lesion selection is therefore critical for expanded criteria to establish noninferior outcomes.

Evaluation of Curability

Evaluation of endoscopic curability is based on local factors and risk factors for LNM. A risk-scoring system name the eCura system[43] was developed to help predict LNM using 5 factors including lymphatic invasion, tumor size greater than 3 cm, vertical margin involvement, venous invasion, and submucosal invasion greater than 500 mm. This model may help treatment decision in patients who do not meet curative criteria for ER of EGC, which is referred to as eCura C-2 in the latest guidelines. Based on these criteria, ER is considered curative when all of the following conditions are fulfilled: en bloc resection, predominantly differentiated type histology (or predominantly undifferentiated with long diameter measuring ≤2 cm) with no ulcerative findings, pT1a, negative horizontal and vertical margins, and absence of lymphovascular infiltration. In lesions with ulcerative findings, only predominantly differentiated type, pT1a lesions with a long diameter of no more than 3 cm are considered for endoscopic curability A or eCuraA.[1] Lesions that are resected en bloc, are no more than 3 cm in long diameter, predominantly of the differentiated type, and satisfy the following criteria: pT1b1(SM1) (within <500 μm from the muscularis mucosae), with negative margins and no lymphovascular invasion are considered endoscopic curability B (eCuraB). Curability can be expected in these lesions.

Noncurative resection (or endoscopic curability C, eCuraC) is subclassified into 'eCuraC-1 and 'eCuraC-2. When eCuraC lesions are differentiated-type lesions and fulfill other criteria to be classified into either eCuraA or eCuraB but are either not resected en bloc or have positive horizontal margins, they are considered eCuraC-1. All other eCuraC lesions are considered eCuraC-2 and require additional surgery with lymph node dissection following ER because of the risk of metastasis and recurrence. However, additional gastrectomy with lymphadenectomy in all these patients may be excessive, as LNM was seen in only 2.2% to 11%.[38,44–46] Less-invasive function-preserving surgery and further less invasive treatment such as ER with chemotherapy is therefore considered in patients who prefer to avoid additional gastrectomy. A systematic review and meta-analysis that included 24 studies comprising 3877 patients (311 of whom had LNM) aimed to identify the prevalence and risk factors of LNM in patients with noncurative resection after endoscopic resection for EGC.[47] The study found that the most notable pathologic factors associated with LNM in patients with noncurative resection were lymphatic invasion and lymphovascular invasion.

Post-treatment Follow-Up

Following curative gastric ESD, scheduled endoscopic surveillance is recommended. ESGE suggests an endoscopy after 3 to 6 months and then annually.[36] Following ESD of ulcerated, submucosal, or undifferentiated tumors, a staging abdominal CT should be considered. After piecemeal resection or presence of positive lateral margins not meeting criteria for surgery, an endoscopy with biopsies is recommended at 3 and 9 to 12 months and then annually.

Outcomes of Gastric Endoscopic Submucosal Dissection

Although most outcome data originate from the East, several studies support the feasibility and safety of ESD in the West as long as an adequate learning curve is accomplished.[48] Overall, long-term outcomes have been found to be comparable to Eastern data.[40,49] Local recurrence rates ranged from 0% to 1.8% for absolute indications, and 0.9% to 7% for expanded indications.[49] Metachronous gastric cancer occurred in 3% to 20.2% of lesions with absolute indications, and 1.9% to 25.4% of lesions with expanded indications for ER.

Metastatic recurrence occurred in 0.2% to 0.6% of lesions, all of which were within expanded indications. A systematic review and meta-analysis compared outcomes from 13 retrospective studies between absolute indication and expanded indication groups. The expanded indication group had lower rates of en bloc resection (93.6% vs 97.0%, P<.0001) and complete resection (87.8% vs 95.8%, P<.00001) than the absolute indication group.[50] Local recurrence rates were lower in the absolute indication group than in the expanded indication group (0.6% vs 1.5%, P=.03).

In a prospective multicenter cohort study from 12 centers in Korea,[51] authors found that 5-year disease-free survival was not significantly different between the curative and noncurative group, but 5-year overall survival was significantly higher in the curative group. Local recurrence and metachronous rates were not different between curative and noncurative groups, but the rate of distant metastasis was significantly higher in the noncurative resection group.

DUODENAL ENDOSCOPIC SUBMUCOSAL DISSECTION
Background

Duodenal polyps are identified in as many as 4.6% of upper endoscopies.[52] They are commonly defined on the basis of their location–either in the duodenal bulb, ampullary, or periampullary region or distal duodenum. Most duodenal polyps are non-neoplastic (eg, inflammatory or regenerative/hyperplastic) and occur in the duodenal bulb. Neoplastic lesions such as adenomas are more commonly found in the second portion of the duodenum and may involve the ampullary area. Approximately 60% of nonampullary adenomas are associated with familial adenomatous polyposis (FAP) or MUTYH-associated polyposis (MAP), while sporadic duodenal adenomas are found in only 0.3% to 0.5% of upper endoscopies. EMR is a safe and effective technique for most nonampullary duodenal adenomas.

Duodenal ESD is also technically difficult because of its unique anatomic features. The risks include intraprocedural complications, delayed bleeding, and perforation.[49] With the advances in devices and techniques, duodenal ESD has been more feasible and safer.

Indications and Outcomes

The 2019 AGA clinical practice update states that duodenal ESD should be limited to endoscopists with extensive experience in performing ESD in other locations.[35] To date, there are no randomized studies assessing duodenal ESD versus EMR outcomes. However, EMR has been reported to be an effective therapeutic option in sporadic nonampullary duodenal tumors.[53] En bloc resection is preferred, as piecemeal resection may lead to a non-negligible recurrence rate of 0% to 37%.[54] A systematic review and meta-analysis that included 14 studies and 794 patients assessed the characteristics and outcomes of ESD and EMR procedures for nonampullary superficial duodenal tumors.[55] The authors found that duodenal ESD for nonampullary lesions may achieve higher en bloc and R0 resection rates than EMR. ESD had a greater intraoperative and delayed perforation rate compared with EMR. The impact on local recurrence remains uncertain and requires further prospective studies.

The rate of intraoperative perforation in duodenal ESD was reported to be 6.0% to 31.6%, while the rate of delayed perforation was 1.5% to 4.8%, both significantly higher than with gastric ESD.[56] The largest study to date revealed that additional intervention is only required in 3.1% of cases with perforation, similar to the rate following perforation in gastric ESD.[57] Complete mucosal closure diminished the need for additional intervention. The rate of delayed bleeding was reported to be 0.0% to 18.4%. A meta-analysis revealed that complete closure of the mucosal defect following duodenal ESD significantly reduced delayed bleeding.[58]

Techniques of Duodenal Endoscopic Submucosal Dissection

Basic techniques of ESD in the duodenum are largely similar to ESD in other locations. Several other techniques have been described to facilitate ESD in the duodenum. The water pressure method is performed after filling the duodenal lumen with normal saline while the mucosal flap is opened to improve visualization of the submucosa by the water stream from the water jet function. A prospective study also found that the water pressure method and using an ESD knife with waterjet function significantly shortened procedure times for duodenal ESD.[59] The water pressure method also significantly reduced the intraprocedural perforation rate. ESD techniques are continuously evolving as uptake continues to expand worldwide.

The pocket-creation method (PCM) is an attractive alternative technique for duodenal ESD as it allows stability at the tip of the endoscope even in difficult locations such as at the duodenal angles. In a study that evaluated the safety and usefulness of PCM for duodenal ESD, PCM was associated with higher en bloc resection rate, faster dissection speed, and lower rates of perforation.[9]

The use of scissor-type knives in duodenal ESD has been reported to decrease intraoperative perforation. In a retrospective study by Dohi and colleagues,[60] the intraoperative perforation rate was significantly lower in the ESD group using the Clutch Cutter knife (Fujifilm Medical, Tokyo) than in the group using Flush knife (0% vs 13.5%, respectively, $P=.014$).

Complete closure of duodenal ESD defects was found to reduce delayed complications including bleeding and perforation. Techniques include closure with clips, clips with string or endoloop, over-the-scope clips, and shielding with a polyglycolic acid sheets and fibrin glue.[61] In the event of duodenal perforations, a study by Fukuhara and colleagues showed the utility of endoscopic retrograde cholangiopancreatography (ERCP) with placement of nasobiliary and nasopancreatic drains to protect the site from the damaging effect of bile and pancreatic juice. Placement of nasobiliary and nasopancreatic drains was especially important for lesions in the descending part of the duodenum near the papilla of Vater.[57]

SUMMARY

ESD is the only endoscopic treatment that can reliably achieve R0 resection of precancerous lesions and mucosal cancer of the entire gastrointestinal tract regardless of their size or shape. Gastric ESD is well established for management of EGC and has promising outcomes and a good safety profile. Further studies assessing long-term outcomes will allow for more thorough risk stratification of patients who would benefit from gastric ESD over surgery. Duodenal ESD remains a more challenging procedure with a higher risk profile, even in the most experienced hands. Future studies are needed to evaluate the most effective and feasible techniques to prevent adverse events. Prospective studies are still needed to determine if ESD can become integrated into the standard of care of duodenal lesions.

CLINICS CARE POINTS

- For ESD in the stomach and duodenum, appropriate lesion selection using endoscopic diagnosis and assessment of high-risk features for SMI is critical.
- Endoscopic resection using ESD is standard of care for the treatment of EGC with negligible risk for lymph node metastasis.
- ER is considered curative when all of the following conditions are fulfilled: en bloc resection, predominantly differentiated type histology (or predominantly undifferentiated with long diameter measuring ≤2 cm) with no ulcerative findings, pT1a, negative horizontal and vertical margins, and absence of lymphovascular infiltration.

- Due to its technical difficulty, duodenal ESD should be limited to endoscopists with extensive experience in performing ESD in other locations.

DISCLOSURES

S.S. Al Ghamdi: none to declare. Saowanee Ngamruengphong is a consultant for Boston Scientific.

REFERENCES

1. Ono H, Yao K, Fujishiro M, et al. Guidelines for endoscopic submucosal dissection and endoscopic mucosal resection for early gastric cancer (second edition). Dig Endosc 2021;33(1):4–20.
2. Muto M, Yao K, Kaise M, et al. Magnifying endoscopy simple diagnostic algorithm for early gastric cancer (MESDA-G). Dig Endosc 2016;28(4):379–93.
3. Yao K, Anagnostopoulos GK, Ragunath K. Magnifying endoscopy for diagnosing and delineating early gastric cancer. Endoscopy 2009;41(5):462–7.
4. Ahmed Y, Othman M. EMR/ESD: techniques, complications, and evidence. Curr Gastroenterol Rep 2020;22(8). https://doi.org/10.1007/S11894-020-00777-Z.
5. Kim SY, Chung JW, Park DK, et al. Efficacy of carbon dioxide insufflation during gastric endoscopic submucosal dissection: a randomized, double-blind, controlled, prospective study. Gastrointest Endosc 2015;82(6):1018–24.
6. Nishizawa T, Yahagi N. Endoscopic mucosal resection and endoscopic submucosal dissection: technique and new directions. Curr Opin Gastroenterol 2017; 33(5):315–9.
7. Nagahama T, Yao K, Maki S, et al. Usefulness of magnifying endoscopy with narrow-band imaging for determining the horizontal extent of early gastric cancer when there is an unclear margin by chromoendoscopy (with video). Gastrointest Endosc 2011;74(6):1259–67.
8. Mori G, Nonaka S, Oda I, et al. Novel strategy of endoscopic submucosal dissection using an insulation-tipped knife for early gastric cancer: near-side approach method. Endosc Int Open 2015;3(5):E425–31.
9. Miura Y, Shinozaki S, Hayashi Y, et al. Duodenal endoscopic submucosal dissection is feasible using the pocket-creation method. Endoscopy 2017;49(1):8–14.
10. Lopimpisuth C, Simons M, Akshintala VS, et al. Traction-assisted endoscopic submucosal dissection reduces procedure time and risk of serious adverse events: a systematic review and meta-analysis. Surg Endosc 2022;36(3): 1775–88.
11. Abe S, Wu SYS, Ego M, et al. Efficacy of current traction techniques for endoscopic submucosal dissection. Gut Liver 2020;14(6):673–84.
12. Matsui H, Tamai N, Futakuchi T, et al. Multi-loop traction device facilitates gastric endoscopic submucosal dissection: ex vivo pilot study and an inaugural clinical experience. BMC Gastroenterol 2022;22(1):1–8.
13. Kantsevoy SV, Bitner M, Mitrakov AA, et al. Endoscopic suturing closure of large mucosal defects after endoscopic submucosal dissection is technically feasible, fast, and eliminates the need for hospitalization (with videos). Gastrointest Endosc 2014;79(3):503–7.
14. Zhang LY, Bejjani M, Ghandour B, et al. Endoscopic through-the-scope suturing. VideoGIE 2022;7(1):46.

15. Nishiyama N, Kobara H, Kobayashi N, et al. Efficacy of endoscopic ligation with O-ring closure for preventing gastric post- ESD bleeding under antithrombotic therapy: A prospective observational study. Endoscopy 2022. https://doi.org/10.1055/A-1782-3448.

16. Goto O, Kaise M, Iwakiri K. What's new with endoscopic treatments for early gastric cancer in the "post-ESD era". Digestion 2022;103:92–8.

17. Ono H, Yao K, Fujishiro M, et al. Guidelines for endoscopic submucosal dissection and endoscopic mucosal resection for early gastric cancer. Dig Endosc 2016;28(1):3–15.

18. Sung H, Ferlay J, Siegel RL, et al. Global cancer statistics 2020: Globocan estimates of incidence and mortality worldwide for 36 cancers in 185 countries. CA Cancer J Clin 2021;71(3):209–49.

19. Cancer facts & figures 2021. American Cancer Society's (ACS), National Cancer Institute's Surveillance, Epidemiology, and End Results (SEER) program. 2021. Available at: https://www.cancer.org/content/dam/cancer-org/research/cancer-facts-and-statistics/annual-cancer-facts-and-figures/2021/cancer-facts-and-figures-2021.pdf. Accessed March 1, 2022.

20. Schlemper RJ, Riddell RH, Kato Y, et al. The Vienna classification of gastrointestinal epithelial neoplasia. Gut 2000;47(2):251–5.

21. Kushima R. The updated WHO classification of digestive system tumours—gastric adenocarcinoma and dysplasia. Der Pathol 2021;43(1):8–15.

22. Green PHR, O'Toole KM, Slonim D, et al. Increasing incidence and excellent survival of patients with early gastric cancer: experience in a United States medical center. Am J Med 1988;85(5):658–61.

23. Amin M, Edge S, Greene F, et al. AJCC cancer staging manual. In: American Joint Commission on Cancer. 8th edn. New York: Springer; 2017.

24. Kwee RM, Kwee TC. Predicting lymph node status in early gastric cancer. Gastric Cancer 2008;11(3):134–48.

25. Lee KS, Oh DK, Han MA, et al. Gastric cancer screening in Korea: report on the national cancer screening program in 2008. Cancer Res Treat 2011;43(2):83–8.

26. Gotoda T, Ono H. Stomach: endoscopic resection for early gastric cancer. Dig Endosc 2021. https://doi.org/10.1111/DEN.14167.

27. Gotoda T, Kondo H, Ono H, et al. A new endoscopic mucosal resection procedure using an insulation-tipped electrosurgical knife for rectal flat lesions: report of two cases. Gastrointest Endosc 1999;50(4):560–3.

28. Lian J, Chen S, Zhang Y, et al. A meta-analysis of endoscopic submucosal dissection and EMR for early gastric cancer. Gastrointest Endosc 2012;76(4):763–70.

29. Park YM, Cho E, Kang HY, et al. The effectiveness and safety of endoscopic submucosal dissection compared with endoscopic mucosal resection for early gastric cancer: a systematic review and meta-analysis. Surg Endosc 2011;25(8):2666–77.

30. ONO H. Endoscopic diagnosis of the depth of cancer invasion for gastric cancer. Stom Intest 2001;36:334–40.

31. Choi J, Kim SG, Im JP, et al. Endoscopic prediction of tumor invasion depth in early gastric cancer. Gastrointest Endosc 2011;73(5):917–27.

32. Mocellin S, Marchet A, Nitti D. EUS for the staging of gastric cancer: a meta-analysis. Gastrointest Endosc 2011;73(6):1122–34.

33. Tsujii Y, Kato M, Inoue T, et al. Integrated diagnostic strategy for the invasion depth of early gastric cancer by conventional endoscopy and EUS. Gastrointest Endosc 2015;82(3):452–9.

34. Park CH, Park JC, Chung H, et al. A specific role of endoscopic ultrasonography for therapeutic decision-making in patients with gastric cardia cancer. Surg Endosc 2016;30(10):4193–9.

35. Draganov PV, Wang AY, Othman MO, et al. AGA Institute clinical practice update: endoscopic submucosal dissection in the United States. Clin Gastroenterol Hepatol 2019;17(1):16–25.e1.

36. Pimentel-Nunes P, Dinis-Ribeiro M, Ponchon T, et al. Endoscopic submucosal dissection: European Society of Gastrointestinal Endoscopy (ESGE) guideline. Endoscopy 2015;47:829–54.

37. Suzuki H, Takizawa K, Hirasawa T, et al. Short-term outcomes of multicenter prospective cohort study of gastric endoscopic resection: "real-world evidence" in Japan. Dig Endosc 2019;31(1):30–9.

38. Kikuchi S, Kuroda S, Nishizaki M, et al. Management of early gastric cancer that meet the indication for radical lymph node dissection following endoscopic resection: a retrospective cohort analysis. BMC Surg 2017;17(1). https://doi.org/10.1186/S12893-017-0268-0.

39. Liu Q, Ding L, Qiu X, et al. Updated evaluation of endoscopic submucosal dissection versus surgery for early gastric cancer: a systematic review and meta-analysis. Int J Surg 2020;73:28–41.

40. Quero G, Fiorillo C, Longo F, et al. Propensity score-matched comparison of short- and long-term outcomes between surgery and endoscopic submucosal dissection (ESD) for intestinal type early gastric cancer (EGC) of the middle and lower third of the stomach: a European tertiary referral center experience. Surg Endosc 2021;35(6):2592–600.

41. Ryu SJ, Kim BW, Kim BG, et al. Endoscopic submucosal dissection versus surgical resection for early gastric cancer: a retrospective multicenter study on immediate and long-term outcome over 5 years. Surg Endosc 2016;30(12):5283–9.

42. Ahn JY, Kim YII, Shin WG, et al. Comparison between endoscopic submucosal resection and surgery for the curative resection of undifferentiated-type early gastric cancer within expanded indications: a nationwide multi-center study. Gastric Cancer 2021;24(3):731–43.

43. Hatta W, Gotoda T, Oyama T, et al. A scoring system to stratify curability after endoscopic submucosal dissection for early gastric cancer: "eCura system. Am J Gastroenterol 2017;112(6):874–81.

44. Son SY, Park JY, Ryu KW, et al. The risk factors for lymph node metastasis in early gastric cancer patients who underwent endoscopic resection: is the minimal lymph node dissection applicable? A retrospective study. Surg Endosc 2013; 27(9):3247–53.

45. Yamada S, Hatta W, Shimosegawa T, et al. Different risk factors between early and late cancer recurrences in patients without additional surgery after noncurative endoscopic submucosal dissection for early gastric cancer. Gastrointest Endosc 2019;89(5):950–60.

46. Kawata N, Kakushima N, Takizawa K, et al. Risk factors for lymph node metastasis and long-term outcomes of patients with early gastric cancer after noncurative endoscopic submucosal dissection. Surg Endosc 2017;31(4):1607–16.

47. Hatta W, Gotoda T, Kanno T, et al. Prevalence and risk factors for lymph node metastasis after noncurative endoscopic resection for early gastric cancer: a systematic review and meta-analysis. J Gastroenterol 2020;55(8):742–53.

48. Catalano F, Mengardo V, Trecca A, et al. The impact of experience on short- and long-term outcomes on gastric ESD: a Western series. Updates Surg 2019;71(2): 359–65.

49. Nishizawa T, Yahagi N. Long-term outcomes of using endoscopic submucosal dissection to treat early gastric cancer. Gut Liver 2018;12(2):119–24.
50. Peng LJ, Tian SN, Lu L, et al. Outcome of endoscopic submucosal dissection for early gastric cancer of conventional and expanded indications: systematic review and meta-analysis. J Dig Dis 2015;16(2):67–74.
51. Kim SG, Park CM, Lee NR, et al. Long-term clinical outcomes of endoscopic submucosal dissection in patients with early gastric cancer: a prospective multicenter cohort study. Gut Liver 2018;12(4):402.
52. Kővári B, Kim BH, Lauwers GY. The pathology of gastric and duodenal polyps: current concepts. Histopathology 2021;78(1):106–24.
53. Navaneethan U, Hasan MK, Lourdusamy V, et al. Efficacy and safety of endoscopic mucosal resection of non-ampullary duodenal polyps: a systematic review. Endosc Int Open 2016;4(6):E699.
54. Kakushima N, Tanaka M, Takizawa K, et al. Treatment for superficial non-ampullary duodenal epithelial tumors. World J Gastroenterol 2014;20(35):12501.
55. Pérez-Cuadrado-Robles E, Quénéhervé L, Margos W, et al. ESD versus EMR in non-ampullary superficial duodenal tumors: a systematic review and meta-analysis. Endosc Int Open 2018;6(8):E998.
56. Hatta W, Koike T, Abe H, et al. R E V I E W Recent approach for preventing complications in upper gastrointestinal endoscopic submucosal dissection. DEN open 2021;2(1):e60.
57. Fukuhara S, Kato M, Iwasaki E, et al. Management of perforation related to endoscopic submucosal dissection for superficial duodenal epithelial tumors. Gastrointest Endosc 2020;91(5):1129–37.
58. Kato M, Ochiai Y, Fukuhara S, et al. Clinical impact of closure of the mucosal defect after duodenal endoscopic submucosal dissection. Gastrointest Endosc 2019;89(1):87–93.
59. Kato M, Takatori Y, Sasaki M, et al. Water pressure method for duodenal endoscopic submucosal dissection (with video). Gastrointest Endosc 2021;93(4):942–9.
60. Dohi O, Yoshida N, Naito Y, et al. Efficacy and safety of endoscopic submucosal dissection using a scissors-type knife with prophylactic over-the-scope clip closure for superficial non-ampullary duodenal epithelial tumors. Dig Endosc 2020;32(6):904–13.
61. Takimoto K, Imai Y, Matsuyama K. Endoscopic tissue shielding method with polyglycolic acid sheets and fibrin glue to prevent delayed perforation after duodenal endoscopic submucosal dissection. Dig Endosc 2014;26:46–9.

Endoscopic Submucosal Dissection in the Colon and Rectum

Indications, Techniques, and Outcomes

Amyn Haji, MA, MBBChir, MSc, MD, FRCS

KEYWORDS

- Endoscopic submucosal dissection (ESD) • Colorectal polyps

KEY POINTS

- Accurate endoscopic diagnosis using magnification endoscopy is the key for decision-making on treatment of colorectal polyps.
- Endoscopic submucosal dissection (ESD) for colorectal lesions should be offered to polyps that have higher risk of submucosal invasion.
- Successful training in colorectal ESD requires knowledge of endoscopic diagnosis, colorectal endoscopic anatomy, strategy for resection, and awareness of management of complications.

INTRODUCTION

Endoscopic submucosal dissection (ESD) is a procedure, which is accepted worldwide for resection of colorectal lesions, and its presence is increasing in western practice. The complexity of the procedure requires a robust training program in order to minimize complications, notably perforation and bleeding. Recently, the position statement from the European Society of Gastrointestinal Endoscopy (ESGE)[1] addressed many of these training issues and produced guidelines to support the uptake of ESD in western practice. It is of paramount importance that accurate assessment of colorectal polyps is undertaken with careful endoscopic diagnosis in order to identify those lesions that are suitable for en bloc resection by ESD. This article addresses endoscopic diagnosis using advanced endoscopic imaging, indications, and decision-making for ESD, its technical aspects and surgical planning with appropriate strategy, and finally reviewing current outcomes in the literature.

Department of Colorectal Surgery, King's College Hospital, Denmark Hill, London SE5 9RS, United Kingdom
E-mail address: amynhaji@nhs.net

Gastrointest Endoscopy Clin N Am 33 (2023) 83–97
https://doi.org/10.1016/j.giec.2022.08.001
giendo.theclinics.com
1052-5157/23/Crown Copyright © 2022 Published by Elsevier Inc. All rights reserved.

ENDOSCOPIC DIAGNOSIS

It is imperative that an accurate endoscopic diagnosis is undertaken in order to identify lesions that are suitable for ESD. Guidelines have been introduced from both the Japanese Gastrointestinal Endoscopy Society (JGES)[2] and ESGE[3] indicating the importance of identifying high-risk lesions that would benefit from en bloc resection. An initial endoscopic examination with good technique is needed in order to detect lesions by using appropriate inflation and deflation during examination, changing the position of the patient and performing appropriate J maneuvers (retroflexion) in the right colon and in the rectum to identify subtle flat lesions and areas of faint redness that may indicate potential polyps with submucosal invasion.

Multimodal endoscopic examination has been shown to be superior for detection of high-grade dysplasia and early cancer than other cross-sectional imaging such as computerized tomography or MRI for rectal polyps.[4] Indeed, this is more useful than biopsy as the latter needs to be targeted accurately from the precise areas of suspected early invasive cancer in order to make an accurate judgment. In addition, this process creates submucosal fibrosis, which can make subsequent en bloc resection and submucosal dissection more challenging. In our institution, the following measures are undertaken for detailed assessment of colorectal polyps before decision-making regarding of whether techniques of endoscopic mucosal resection (EMR) or ESD or indeed full thickness resection and laparoscopic surgery are appropriate.

Steps for detailed endoscopic assessment.

1. Gentle irrigation of the surface of the lesion in order to wash all areas of fecal debris and mucous plugs. Ideally, an irrigation pump is used with reduced pressure so that there is limited surface trauma to the colorectal polyp in order to minimize bleeding.
2. Morphology of the polyp according to Paris classification[5] is carefully assessed and this is outlined in **Fig. 1**. Most lesions referred for ESD are lateral spreading tumors (LST) that can be subdivided into granular (G) or nongranular (NG). LST-G can be further subdivided into homogeneous (H) and multinodular (MN) types. In addition, LST-NG is also subdivided into a flat type (F) and a pseudo-depressed (PD) type. This morphologic classification is important because the risk of submucosal invasion increases as polyps progress from G to NG, and indeed, there are more occurrences of multifocal invasion and submucosal fibrosis with LST-NG. **Table 1** shows our institutional data regarding the risk of submucosal invasion for the different subtypes and this is compared with the Japanese literature.[6]
3. Magnification endoscopy ($\times$80–130 zoom) and super magnification with endocytoscopy (EC; $\times$500 zoom) have been used for careful assessment of pit pattern and vascular pattern in order to make an accurate endoscopic diagnosis without biopsy. In our practice, we would use magnification narrow band imaging (NBI) to assess the vascular pattern initially according to the Japanese NBI expert team classification (JNET[7]; **Fig. 2**). JNET type 2A has a regular vascular pattern suggestive of benign adenomas. JNET type 2B has an irregular vascular pattern, and this should be evaluated further with chromoendoscopy with either indigo carmine (0.4%) or crystal violet 0.05% to give an accurate Kudo pit pattern diagnosis.[8] **Fig. 3** shows the different pit patterns along with their predicted histologic diagnosis. Vi pit pattern indicates either of high-grade dysplasia (intramucosal cancer) or the presence of early submucosal invasion, whereas Vn pit identifies lesions that require surgical resection in most cases due to deep submucosal invasive cancer. Furthermore, Vi is subdivided into Vi low-grade with well-defined regular borders and Vi high grade with irregular margins (**Fig. 4**) corresponding to an endoscopic diagnosis of high-grade dysplasia and early submucosal invasion, respectively.

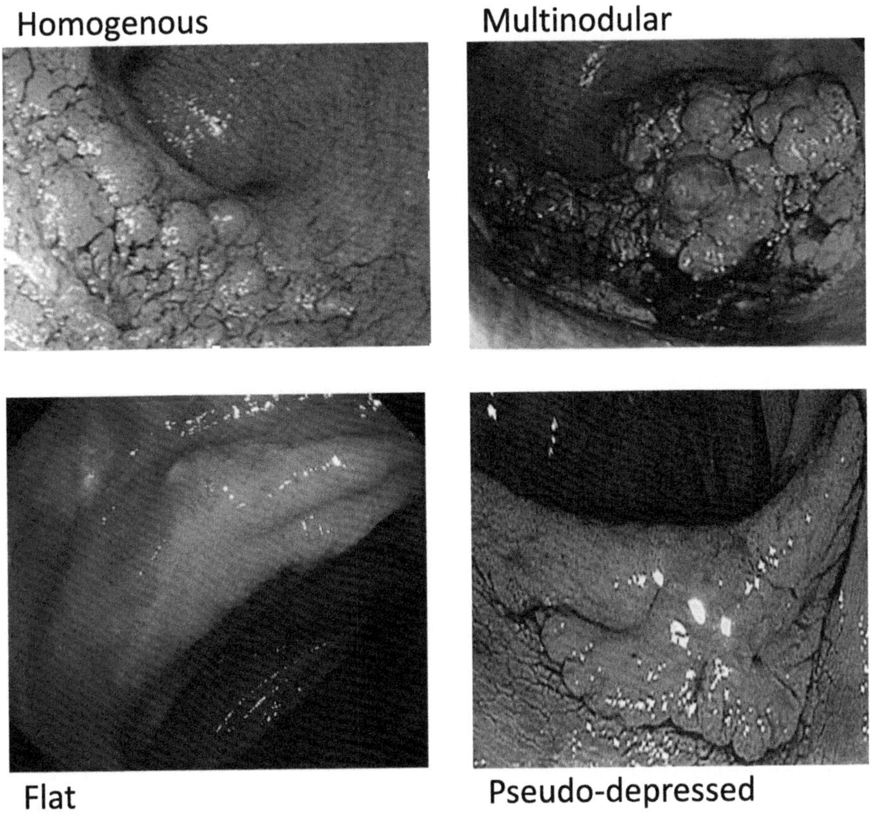

Homogenous

Multinodular

Flat

Pseudo-depressed

Fig. 1. LSTs.

This detailed examination of type V pit pattern is clearer with crystal violet rather than indigo carmine.

There are cases where the endoscopic diagnosis is difficult, and there is uncertainty regarding the histologic prediction. In such cases, super magnification with EC can be used. This requires staining with both 0.1% methylene blue and 0.05% crystal violet in order to stain both the nuclei and the cytoplasm. **Fig. 4** shows the EC classification

Table 1 Risk of submucosal invasive cancer within lateral spreading tumors		
LST	King's Data (%)	Kobayashi et al (%)[a]
G—Homogenous	0.8	3
G—MN	8	11
NG—Flat type	12	14
NG—PD type	18	36

[a] Predictors of invasive cancer of large laterally spreading colorectal tumors: A multicenter study in Japan. Open JGH 2020 (4): 83-89.

	Type 1	Type 2A	Type 2B	Type 3
Vessel pattern	Invisible	Regular calibre and distribution	Irregular calibre and distribution	Loose areas
Surface pattern	Similar to su... ...osa	Regular	Irregular	Amorphous areas
Predicted histology	Hy... ses...	Lo... ...sia	Hi... ...sia / e... ...al in...	De... ...ca...

Fig. 2. JNET classification.

developed by Professor Kudo at Showa University, Yokohama with the images being very similar to that seen on true histologic examination[9] (**Fig. 5**). Utilization of optical biopsy techniques are favored because this provides real-time endoscopic diagnosis without biopsy and subsequent fibrosis of the lesion. Further adjuncts to the endoscopic assessment include high-frequency mini probe ultrasound[10] introduced during the index colonoscopy through the working channel of the colonoscope in order to evaluate the depth of the colorectal polyps. The different layers of the colonic wall are imaged, and one can ensure that there is no deeper invasion into the muscularis propria before embarking on a trial ESD (**Fig. 6**). This can be particularly useful for colonic lesions in order to ensure that the lesion is favorable with no adverse features or deeper submucosal invasion thereby avoiding a long complex ESD procedure.

ASSESSMENT OF COLORECTAL ANATOMY

The strategy for endoscopic resection during ESD requires precise planning in order to maximize efficiency and minimize complications. During the initial assessment, it is important to view the polyp in all patient positions. This would mean that the patient needs to be turned from left lateral to supine to right lateral and indeed prone

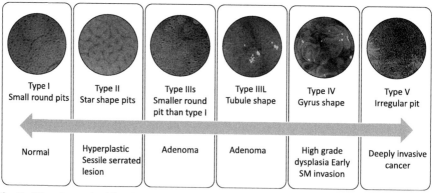

Type I Small round pits	Type II Star shape pits	Type IIIs Smaller round pit than type I	Type IIIL Tubule shape	Type IV Gyrus shape	Type V Irregular pit
Normal	Hyperplastic Sessile serrated lesion	Adenoma	Adenoma	High grade dysplasia Early SM invasion	Deeply invasive cancer

Fig. 3. Pit pattern classification.

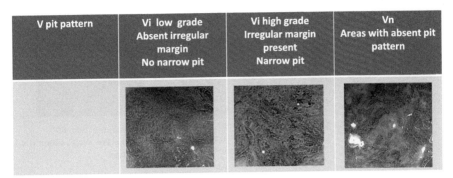

V pit pattern	Vi low grade Absent irregular margin No narrow pit	Vi high grade Irregular margin present Narrow pit	Vn Areas with absent pit pattern

Fig. 4. V pit pattern.

positioning in order to identify the most favorable approach. Fluid is irrigated during such assessment so that we can identify the areas of the colon and rectum that are retroperitoneal and those that are antimesenteric. For example, in evaluating rectal lesions, if patients are in the supine position and the lesion is in the pool of fluid, then we know this is a posterior lesion and, therefore, on the mesorectal side. However, if the lesion is on the opposite side to the pool of fluid (antigravity), then it is an anterior lesion. A perforation during such a procedure may be intraperitoneal particularly in women as the pouch of Douglas often descends lower anteriorly. This assessment using fluid to identify the gravity side of the lesion, and the antigravity part helps in the decision-making for the steps of the dissection. The antigravity section is often easier because the submucosal plane is more open when compared with the gravity side. Therefore, if the gravity position is not easily accessible by the scope when turning the patient, it is important to dissect this area first because this will get increasingly difficult with ongoing dissection of the easier antigravity side. In addition, because the length of the procedure increases, there is worsening colorectal spasm that often makes the oral side of the lesion more difficult to access. One should therefore contemplate making the oral incision earlier in these circumstances.

The assessment report should not only contain a detailed description of the polyp including morphology, JNET and pit pattern diagnosis but also the relevant colorectal anatomy and the strategy for endoscopic resection. In this manner, more appropriate scheduling of patience can occur with a limited number of unexpected events.

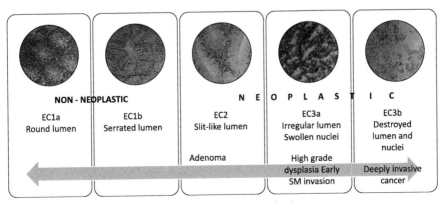

Fig. 5. EC classification. (*Courtesy* of Yuichi Mori, MD, PhD.)

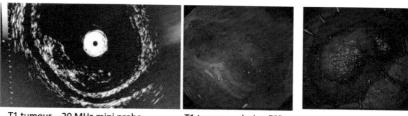

T1 tumour – 20 MHz mini probe

T1 tumour – during ESD
Submucosal invasion but
clear plane

En bloc resection, R0
1200 micrometres submucosal
Invasion

Fig. 6. Miniprobe ultrasound during colorectal ESD.

INDICATIONS FOR ENDOSCOPIC SUBMUCOSAL DISSECTION

The Kings' algorithm for decision-making and treatment of colorectal polyps is outlined in **Fig. 7**. Patients with polyps that have a Vi pit pattern or LST-NG are absolute indications for colorectal ESD. LST-G (MN) has a higher risk of submucosal invasion and should also be treated by en bloc resection. In addition, lesions that have significant fibrosis either due to previous manipulation by biopsy or attempted snare resection, lesions in patients with inflammatory bowel disease or previous radiotherapy, all

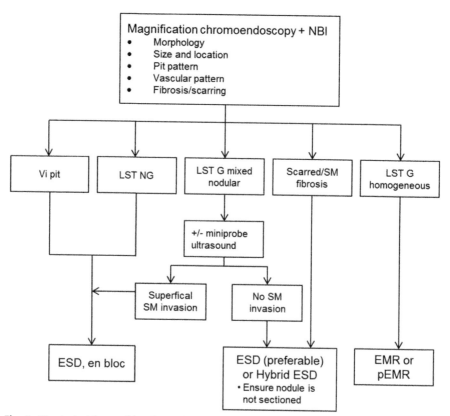

Fig. 7. King's decision-making for endoscopic resection.

require treatment with ESD if technically feasible. This is similar to the guidance produced by the JGES.[2]

There is some debate regarding patients that have LST-G (H) because the risk of submucosal invasion is less than 1%.[6] Therefore, in western practice, many of these patients are treated with piecemeal EMR techniques particularly if patients have existing comorbidities.

There are several considerations when adopting a piecemeal EMR. In Japanese practice, ESD is used to treat polyps that cannot be treated with en bloc EMR and these are often those with lesion size greater than 2 to 3 cm. There is some evidence that risk of submucosal invasion increases with size and recurrence after piecemeal EMR and has been shown to be between 10% and 30% in the literature.[11] The Australian data[12] suggests that the use of snare tip coagulation to treat the edges reduces recurrence significantly in good quality wide field EMR and should be adopted. We have also shown that there is 13% residual adenoma at the edges when sampled using the EndoRotor device (Interscope, Interscope, Inc, USA) after piecemeal EMR.[13] This provides some histologic evidence and a rationale for using ablative techniques on the margins of the EMR scar. The second consideration is in relation to surveillance after endoscopic resection. It should be noted that patients after piecemeal EMR potentially require more visits for follow-up colonoscopy due to the higher recurrence rate.[14] Therefore, the decision between EMR and ESD for patients with LST-G H type needs to be considered carefully in conjunction with the patient's comorbidities and the expertise of the endoscopist, and discussed with the patients so that they are suitably counseled before making a decision regarding the procedure.

ENDOSCOPIC SUBMUCOSAL DISSECTION TECHNIQUE

The usual practice in our institution is to initially perform a colonoscopy without a distal attachment before embarking on commencing the ESD procedure. This allows for appropriate irrigation and cleansing of the proximal colon as well as washing the lesion appropriately to minimize the fecal debris and mucus before the resection. Once this has been established, a distal attachment is placed (Fuji ST hood) on the end of the endoscope. The conical shape of the attachment allows for easier access to the submucosal space, whereas the straight type distal attachments allow for wider views (**Fig. 8**). The steps of the procedure, particularly for training, have been subdivided into appropriate subsections so that they allow for a standardized robust approach

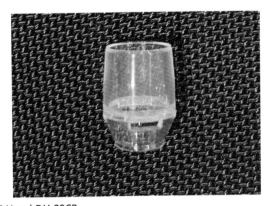

Fig. 8. Fujifilm ST Hood DH-29CR.

to the majority of cases and also allow for endoscopists at different stages of the training to perform different sections of the dissection. This process is outlined in **Fig. 9** and the steps are detailed below.

1. Injection using a 23-gauge needle using gelofuscine or volpex (colloid) mixed with indigocarmine solution to ensure that this is a light blue color that is not too dark so that a newspaper print can be read through the transparency. This shade of solution allows for easy visualization of the muscle layer and vessels in the submucosal layer, and the fluid is injected on the anal side of the lesion.
2. The rate of injection by the assistant needs to be slow initially until there is an increase in the submucosa and then can increase in speed ensuring that the assistant counts the number of millilitres introduced, and the rate of lifting of the submucosal space is at the same speed as the counting. This also avoids a submucosal hematoma forming with an initial forceful injection.
3. ESD knives are manufactured either as needle type or with a ball/wider tip and endoscopists often choose one that supports their technique. In our institution, we use a 1.5 to 2-mm knife that can be irrigated through (flush knife). The flushing solution is normal saline with indigocarmine at the same concentration as the injection solution.
4. Mucosal incision (Effect 2, cut interval 2, cut duration 2-ERBE Vio 300D [ERBE Vio 300D, ERBE Elektromedizin, Gemany]) and trimming is undertaken using the flush knife on the anal side of the lesion starting one cap distance away from the margin of the polyp. This is increased to 2 cap distances if there are areas of fibrosis in patients that have recurrent polyps or previous treatment. The submucosal space is entered and submucosal tunneling is undertaken through to the central part of the lesion until arriving at a distance beyond the oral edge of the lesion. If vessels are encountered during the dissection, they are treated with the following algorithm: (1) all arterial vessels are coagulated with a bipolar grasper before division with the knife and (2) venous structures are divided using the knife as follows. If the vein is larger than the diameter of the knife, then a low effect on low wattage (Effect

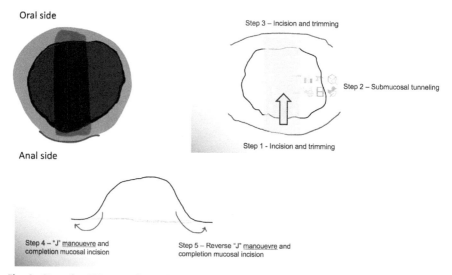

Fig. 9. Steps for ESD tunneling of colorectal lesion.

1, 10 W – ERBE Vio 300D) is applied, which allows for appropriate precoagulation as the blood-stained structure in which the color changes to white with a noticeable "boiling effect" of the current. The vein can then be divided with the knife. Smaller veins can be divided directly using forced coagulation (Effect 2, 40W – ERBE Vio 300D).

5. Incision and trimming on the oral side is now performed so that the submucosal central tunnel can meet from beneath the lesion to break through to the oral side. This creates a self-retracting polyp similar to a bridge over water.

6. The next stage is to dissect the 2 lateral margins. The mucosal incisions are initially created on the lateral edges of the polyp followed by dissection from the inside of the submucosal tunnel to the outside in order to dissect the 2 lateral pillars. This maneuver is termed the J maneuver on the left and the reverse J maneuver on the right.

7. Copious irrigation of the scar is undertaken with water to ensure that the base is clearly evaluated for visible vessels and muscular defects. In addition, this irrigation of the scar may help ensure that polyp seedlings are not present from the trauma of submucosal dissection.

8. Patients who are on antiplatelet or other anticoagulants usually have their mucosal defect closed either using clips or endoscopic suturing using the Apollo overstitch device (Apollo Overstitch device, Apollo Endosurgery Inc., USA). It is important to adhere to surgical principles and achieve a tension free repair and closure of the defect. On occasions, where this is not possible, a hemostatic agent can be applied to the base in order to reduce the risk of delayed bleeding (eg, Purastat, three-dimensional matrix). Nonetheless, it is important to identify the visible vessels on the scar and treat these prophylactically using the bipolar forceps (Haemostat, Pentax Medical [PENTAX Europe GmbH, Hamburg, Germany]).

9. Withdrawal of the specimen after procedure requires careful manipulation in order to minimize the risk of trauma or fragmentation during extraction. Smaller lesions can often be removed using an endoscopic net to capture the polyp and withdraw through the anal canal easily. Polyps larger than 5 cm often are removed using careful suction into the distal attachment and withdrawal into the low rectum followed by gentle assistance using a rectal digital examination alongside the scope in order to have some anal dilatation while carefully withdrawing the polyp alongside the inserted index finger. Alternatively, a proctoscope can be inserted into the anal canal and low rectum, which can provide assistance to evacuate the contents of the rectum and the dissected polyp.

"J" Maneuver and Traction

Access of the lesion during a J maneuver (retroflexed scope) should be assessed early on during the procedure. In many circumstances, particularly in the right colon, stability is improved in this position allowing access to the oral side, enabling earlier mucosal incision and trimming. If this position proves to provide good access, the submucosal dissection is continued until technically feasible.

In some scenarios, if access to the submucosal plane is challenging and the lesion continues to be on the gravity side due to the concavity of the colorectum and pooling of fluid, traction can be used to assist opening up the submucosal plane with better visualization. There are 2 techniques that we currently use in our institution. The first relates to a clip flap technique[15] (**Fig. 10**) where a clip is placed on the mucosal edge of the polyp on the anal side, and this allows the clip to be an extension of the polyp enabling the distal attachment to apply countertraction against the clip itself.

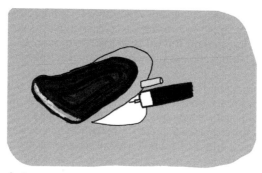

Fig. 10. Clip flap technique.

Furthermore, a clip and line technique[16](**Fig. 11**) can also be used in the distal colon, whereby countertraction is applied using either some dental floss or surgical suture. In the circumstances whereby the line is too long due to a proximal location of the lesion in the colon, one can use a loop on the clip, which is then used as a purchase for the second clip to apply countertraction to the opposing mucosal surface.

Dealing with Fibrosis

Prior biopsy, attempted endoscopic resection, or inflammatory conditions of the bowel can induce fibrosis in the submucosal layer. In addition, LST-NG lesions also naturally have fibrosis in the submucosal layer. Careful planning of the approach to the fibrosis is the key for successful resection of these lesions. Our practice is to start the mucosal incision 2 cap (distal attachment) distances away from the area of fibrosis and access the submucosal space in an area devoid of such fibrosis. This ensures that an adequate flap is created in normal tissue and allows easier traction with a sufficient tunnel in order to treat the fibrotic area. The technique of dissection is slightly different in that the tip of the knife is used for applying diathermy carefully so that vessels are not divided inadvertently with deeper penetration of the knife.

Regular injection using the flushing knife and appropriate traction is also used to tackle fibrosis. It may require multiple approaches in areas of relatively normal submucosa from all sides of the lesion before tackling a stubborn fibrotic region adherent to the muscular layer. In such circumstances, dealing with such an area at the end of the procedure is advantageous because this area offers a higher risk of perforation. If perforation were to occur then we know that the procedure is nearly complete and the perforation can be closed in a timely manner.

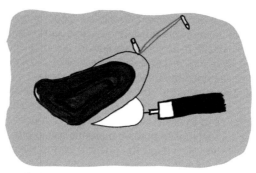

Fig. 11. Clip and line technique.

INTRAPROCEDURAL COMPLICATIONS
Bleeding

Bleeding during ESD often stains the submucosa causing a hematoma making subsequent dissection more difficult. Endocut current for dissection through the hematoma in the submucosa enables dissection without excessive charring and allows effective identification of the bleeding point. Massive hemorrhage during the procedure often obscures the view, and formation of clots in the lumen makes suction increasingly difficult. Change of position of the patient allows the bleeding vessel to be more accessible or placing the patient in a head down, or Trendelenburg position, with copious irrigation allows the blood flow into the proximal colon away from the endoscopic lens allowing quick and safe coagulation of the visible vessel. The evacuation of clots can be challenging and requires further suctioning often with the removal of the suction button to generate further power. In addition, a proctoscope or rigid sigmoidoscope can be inserted to evacuate any clots in the rectum quickly.

Perforation

Perforation is more likely if the knife is perpendicular to the muscular layer. In addition, errors in knife management can occur if there is undue tension in countertraction with the distal attachment, leading to the loss of endoscopic tip control. On occasion, the muscular fibers are split but perforation is not full thickness with no visible pericolic or perirectal fat. In these circumstances, it is prudent to continue with the dissection until the end of the procedure, and then evaluate the muscle layer carefully in order to identify areas that might require closure. In rare circumstances, the perforation is full thickness, and in this situation, the perforation should be closed with through the scope clips at a time when the polyp has been dissected away from the perforation site so that the clips do not interfere with subsequent submucosal dissection. In our experience, it is extremely rare for a procedure to be abandoned for such a complication.

Management of patients after procedure would depend on the institution guidelines and often can be managed as an outpatient if secure closure of the defect is achieved and appropriate prophylactic antibiotics are given. This would largely depend on the clinical status of the patient.

POSTOPERATIVE MANAGEMENT

In our practice, 90% of patients for colorectal ESD are treated as a day case (outpatient) procedure. In western practice, decisions regarding conscious sedation, propofol and general anesthesia are made after appropriate discussions with the patient and anesthesia colleagues. It is particularly advantageous for training, to perform procedures under general anesthesia because these are likely to be longer procedures; however, turning of the patient may be problematic if needed multiple times during the procedure. Therefore, appropriate planning and preoperative strategy as discussed earlier in this article are of paramount importance.

There is no evidence regarding utilization of antibiotics routinely during colorectal ESD.[17] However, this is used in our institution if patients have muscle parting or perforation requiring closure and also routinely for rectal ESD particularly for larger lesions involving dissection times greater than 2 hours.

In our institution, there is currently no restriction to postoperative intake and patients increase their diet from free fluids through to normal diet depending on their appetite and desires. It should be noted that 8.6% to 14.2% of patients may develop abdominal pain, fever, and disturbances in bowel habit with some abdominal tenderness as part of the postpolypectomy coagulation syndrome.[18] Risk factors include right colonic

Table 2
Japanese Society of Colon and Rectal Cancer Guidelines 2019 for treatment of colorectal cancer

Endoscopic Surveillance	Lymph Node Harvest and Surgical Resection
R0 resection	R1 resection
No vascular or lymphatic invasion	Vascular or lymphatic invasion
No tumor budding	Tumor budding
Depth of invasion <1 mm	Depth of invasion >1 mm

lesions, procedural times greater than 90 minutes, and lesion size greater than 40 mm. Often, this is a minor concern and can be easily managed in the outpatient setting. Rarely, patients are admitted for inpatient management and often cross-sectional imaging is undertaken to exclude perforation. We should note with caution that often small amounts of free fluid and locules of air can be seen adjacent to the dissected area. This is not an indication for further surgical intervention and close observation is often needed for conservative management. Collaboration with colorectal surgeons to manage these patients jointly is currently best practice.

OUTCOMES FOLLOWING ESD

An audit of intraoperative and postoperative complications and quality of colorectal submucosal dissection is important in order to have insight into your practice. This will enable us to benchmark our unit figures with comparisons against national and international standards from expert centers. In our institution, we aim for outcomes of less than 1% risk of perforation and postoperative bleeding requiring admission to hospital. En bloc and complete (R0) resection should aim to be greater than 90%. The literature suggests that the rate of postoperative complications vary significantly among institutions depending on their experience. The incidence of intraprocedural perforations is 2.7% to 5.7%, whereas the incidence for delayed perforations is relatively rare at 0.2% to 1.4%.[19–24] Delayed bleeding often varies between 1.5% and 8.1%[25–28] and risk factors include rectal and cecal lesions, large polyp size greater than 30 mm and those patients on anticoagulants.

Vertical margin positivity has been a contentious issue in many units. For patients that have incidental early colorectal cancer, many institutions use the surgical clearance of 1 mm being the minimum in the submucosa. This would mean that although there is a clear histologic margin, if this is less than 1 mm, it is deemed an involved margin (R1) resection. Unfortunately, this has consequences for the patient, and the advice that the colorectal multidisciplinary team often gives is that of formal colorectal surgical resection and lymph node harvest due to involved margins. In our practice, R1 is only stated if there is involved cancer at the resection margin. Other histologic high-risk features for lymph node metastasis include vascular and lymphatic invasion, tumor budding, invasive cancer greater than 1000 μm and poorly differentiated adenocarcinoma.[6,29–31] The Japanese guidelines[32] are summarized in **Table 2** and recommends which patients should proceed to lymph node harvest and formal surgical resection after histologic evaluation. This is also similar to the European guidelines.[3] In practice, detailed discussion regarding risk of lymph-node metastases needs to be conducted with the patient preoperatively and postoperatively to understand their risk strategy. The location of the colorectal cancer resected by ESD is important because complications associated with rectal resection are very different to those for proximal colonic surgery.

Isolated deep submucosal invasion without any of the other risk factors has a low risk of lymph node metastasis, and this should be discussed with patients before decision-making regarding further treatment. Utilization of early colorectal cancer specialist nurses and a specialist multidisciplinary meeting is best practice in order to manage such patients and support their decision-making.

SUMMARY

Colorectal ESD requires detailed multimodal assessment of polyps to make an accurate endoscopic diagnosis in order to identify lesions suitable for en bloc resection. Knowledge of colorectal anatomy with careful planning ensures that a successful strategy is adopted to minimize complications.

CLINICS CARE POINTS

- Rectal polyps should be resected en bloc by ESD to ensure vertical margin clearance in those with incidental cancer, thereby avoid over treatment with surgery if piecemeal EMR is undertaken. MRI should be performed preoperatively for all lesions as artifact will be present if done after ESD leading to overstaging.
- When planning for ESD, identify the colorectal anatomy to understand the intraperitoneal and retroperitoneal side.
- Mucosal incision and trimming of the oral side of the lesion and the gravity side should be planned early if not accessible with turiing the patient to increase success of completion.

DISCLOSURE

The author has nothing to disclose.

REFERENCES

1. Pimentel-Nunes P, Pioche M, Albeniz E, et al. Curriculum for endoscopic submucosal dissection training in Europe: European Society of Gastrointestinal Endoscopy (ESGE) Position Statement. Endoscopy 2019;51(10):980–92.
2. Tanaka, Kashida H, Saito Y, et al. Japan Gastroenterological Endoscopy Society guidelines for colorectal endoscopic submucosal dissection/endoscopic mucosal resection. Dig Endosc 2020;32(2):219–39.
3. Pimentel-Nunes P, Dinis-Ribeiro M, Ponchon T, et al. Endoscopic submucosal dissection: European Society of Gastrointestinal Endoscopy (ESGE) Guideline. Endoscopy 2015;47(9):829–54.
4. Emmanuel A, Lapa C, Ghosh A, et al. Multimodal Endoscopic Assessment Guides Treatment Decisions for Rectal Early Neoplastic Tumors. Dis Colon Rectum 2020;63(3):326–35.
5. Participants in the Paris Workshop. The Paris endoscopic classification of superficial neoplastic lesions: esophagus, stomach, and colon. Gastrointest Endosc 2003;58:s3–43.
6. Kitajima K, Fujimori T, Fujii S, et al. Correlations between lymph node metastasis and depth of submucosal invasion in submucosal invasive colorectal carcinoma: a Japanese collaborative study. J Gastroenterol 2004;39:534–43.
7. Kobayashi, Yamada M, Takamaru H, et al. Diagnostic yield of the Japan NBI Expert Team (JNET) classification for endoscopic diagnosis of superficial

colorectal neoplasms in a large-scale clinical practice database. United Eur Gastroenterol J 2019;7(7):914–23.

8. Kudo S, Tamura S, Nakajima T, et al. Diagnosis of colorectal tumorous lesions by magnifying endoscopy. Gastrointest Endosc 1996;44:8–14.

9. Kudo S, Wakamura K, Ikehara N, et al. Diagnosis of colorectal lesions with a novel endocytoscopic classification - a pilot study. Endoscopy 2011;43(10):869–75.

10. Haji A, Adams K, Bjarnason I, et al. High-frequency mini probe ultrasound before endoscopic resection of colorectal polyps–is it useful? Dis Colon Rectum 2014; 57(3):378–82.

11. Hassan C, Repici A, Sharma P, et al. Efficacy and safety of endoscopic resection of large colorectal polyps: a systematic review and meta-a- nalysis. Gut 2016;65: 806–20.

12. Senada PA, Kandel P, Bourke M, et al. S0138 Soft coagulation of the resection margin for the prevention of residual or recurrent adenoma after endoscopic mucosal resection of large sessile colonic polyps: a multi-center, randomized controlled trial. Am J Gastroenterol 2020;115:S68.

13. Emmanuel A, Williams S, Gulati S, et al. Incidence of microscopic residual adenoma after complete wide-field endoscopic resection of large colorectal lesions: evidence for a mechanism of recurrence. Gastrointest Endosc 2021;94(2): 368–75.

14. Emmanuel A, Lapa C, Ghosh A, et al. Risk factors for early and late adenoma recurrence after advanced colorectal endoscopic resection at an expert Western center. Gastrointest Endosc 2019;90(1):127–36.

15. Ban H, Sugimoto M, Otsuka T, et al. Usefulness of the clip-flap method of endoscopic submucosal dissection: A randomized controlled trial. World J Gastroenterol 2018;24(35):4077–85.

16. Kawaguchi K, Ikebuchi Y, Isomoto H, et al. Novel pre-incision clip and traction method for colorectal endoscopic submucosal dissection. Dig Endosc 2019; 31(6):e107–8.

17. Shichijo, Takeuchi Y, Shimodate Y, et al. Performance of perioperative antibiotics against post-endoscopic submucosal dissection coagulation syndrome: a multicenter randomized controlled trial. Astrointest Endosc 2022;95(2):349–59.

18. Jung Dahyun, Youn Young, Jahng Jaehoon, et al. Risk of electrocoagulation syndrome after endoscopic submucosal dissection in the colon and rectum. Endoscopy 2013;45:714–7.

19. Iwatsubo T, Takeuchi Y, Yamasaki Y, et al. Differences in clinical course of intraprocedural and delayed perforation caused by endoscopic submucosal dissection for colorectal neoplasms: a retrospective study. Dig Dis 2019;37:53–62.

20. Boda K, Oka S, Tanaka S, et al. Clinical outcomes of endoscopic submucosal dissection for colorectal tumors: a large multicenter retrospective study from the Hiroshima GI Endos- copy Research Group. Gastrointest Endosc 2018;87: 714–22.

21. Fujishiro M, Yahagi N, Kakushima N, et al. Outcomes of endoscopic sub- mucosal dissection for colorectal epithelial neoplasms in 200 consecutive cases. Clin Gastroenterol Hepatol 2007;5:678–83.

22. Isomoto H, Nishiyama H, Yamaguchi N, et al. Clinico- pathological factors associated with clinical outcomes of endo- scopic submucosal dissection for colorectal epithelial neoplasms. Endoscopy 2009;41:679–83.

23. Akintoye E, Kumar N, Aihara H, et al. Colorectal endoscopic submucosal dissection: a systematic review and meta-analysis. Endosc Int Open 2016;4:E1030–44.

24. Toyanaga T, Man IM, Ivanov D, et al. The results and limitations of endoscopic submucosal dissection for colorectal tumors. Acta Chir lugosl 2008;55:17–23.

25. Suzuki S, Chino A, Kishihara T, et al. Risk factors for bleeding after endoscopic submucosal dissection of colorectal neoplasms. World J Gastroenterol 2014; 20:1839–45.

26. Terasaki M, Tanaka S, Shigita K, et al. Risk factors for delayed bleeding after endoscopic submucosal dissection for colorectal neoplasms. Int J Colorectal Dis 2014;29:877–82.

27. Ogasawara N, Yoshimine T, Noda H, et al. Clinical risk factors for delayed bleeding after endoscopic submucosal dissection for colorectal tumors in Japanese patients. Eur J Gastroenterol Hepatol 2016;28:1407–14.

28. Seo M, Song EM, Cho JW, et al. A risk-scoring model for the prediction of delayed bleeding after colorec- tal endoscopic submucosal dissection. Gastrointest Endosc 2019;89(990–998):e992.

29. Hassan C, Zullo A, Risio M, et al. Histologic risk factors and clinical outcome in colorectal malignant polyp: a pooled-data analysis. Dis Colon Rectum 2005;48: 1588–96.

30. Netzer P, Forster C, Biral R, et al. Risk factor assessment of endoscopically removed malignant colorectal polyps. Gut 1998;43:669–74.

31. Kikuchi R, Takano M, Takagi K, et al. Management of early invasive colorectal cancer. Risk of recurrence and clinical guidelines. Dis Colon Rectum 1995;38: 1286–95.

32. Hashiguici Y, Muro K, Saito Y, et al. Japanese Society for Cancer of the Colon and Rectum (JSCCR) guidelines 2019 for the treatment of colorectal cancer. Int J Clin Oncol 2020;25(1):1–42.

Indications and Outcomes of Per Oral Endoscopic Myotomy from Mouth to Anus

Ashish Gandhi, MD, DNB[a,1], Jay Bapaye, MD[b,1],
Amol Bapaye, MD, (MS), FASGE, FJGES, FISG, FSGEI[a,*]

KEYWORDS

- Per oral endoscopic myotomy • POEM • G-POEM • D-POEM • Z-POEM
- Per rectal endoscopic myotomy • PREM • Third space endoscopy

KEY POINTS

- Submucosal endoscopy using a mucosal flap valve is a novel third space endoscopic technique that uses a submucosal tunneling approach to access deeper layers of the gastrointestinal (GI) tract.
- Per oral endoscopic myotomy (POEM) is the index procedure and has shown excellent clinical safety and efficacy for the treatment of achalasia cardia and its subtypes.
- Various modifications in the POEM technique have been described for other spastic disorders of the GI tract.
- G-POEM or endoscopic pyloromyotomy is an upcoming and potentially effective treatment for patients with refractory gastroparesis.
- More recently, diverticular myotomy for Zenker's and esophageal diverticula (Z-POEM and D-POEM), and per-rectal myotomy for Hirschsprung's disease (PREM) have been described and have shown impressive outcomes.
- Third space endoscopy procedures show potential in changing the way these spastic GI conditions can be treated in future.

INTRODUCTION

Third space endoscopy (TSE) or submucosal endoscopy using a mucosal flap valve (SEMF) was first described by Sumiyama and colleagues[1] as a potential peritoneal access route for natural orifice transoral endoscopic surgery (NOTES). The principle involves creation of a submucosal tunnel in the esophagus through a mucosal incision to

Disclosures: None.
[a] Shivanand Desai Center for Digestive Disorders, Deenanath Mangeshkar Hospital and Research Center, Pune 411004, Maharashtra, India; [b] Department of Internal Medicine, Rochester General Hospital, Rochester, New York, USA
[1] Both authors contributed equally to the article and are listed as joint first authors.
* Corresponding author.
E-mail address: amolbapaye@gmail.com

Gastrointest Endoscopy Clin N Am 33 (2023) 99–125
https://doi.org/10.1016/j.giec.2022.08.002
1052-5157/23/© 2022 Elsevier Inc. All rights reserved.

access the deeper muscle layers and peritoneal cavity, after which the mucosal incision is closed using clips (**Fig. 1**). The advantage of this technique is that because the mucosa and muscularis are breached at different locations, full-thickness perforation is prevented, and procedural safety is enhanced. In the same year, Pasricha and colleagues[2] showed the safety and feasibility of creating a tunnel and subsequent myotomy in the esophagus in porcine models and named it per oral endoscopic myotomy (POEM). POEM was envisioned to be implemented as a minimally invasive treatment for achalasia cardia (AC). Inoue and colleagues[3] reported the first human case series of POEM for patients of AC.

Since its original description, POEM has become an exceedingly popular and effective treatment for AC. Based on this popularity, endoscopists have implemented the SEMF principle for various other spastic disorders of the gastrointestinal (GI) tract. Gastric per oral endoscopic myotomy of the pylorus (G-POEM) has been described for refractory gastroparesis,[4] diverticular myotomy has been described for Zenker's and epiphrenic diverticula (Z-POEM and D-POEM, respectively),[5] and the technique has also been used for rectal myotomy of the spastic segment in patients with Hirschsprung's disease (per rectal endoscopic myotomy [PREM]).[6] This article describes the indications and outcomes of these various types of POEMs (or PREM) procedures from the mouth to the anus.

PER ORAL ENDOSCOPIC MYOTOMY
Indications

AC is a benign progressive motility disorder of the esophagus characterized by loss of esophageal body motility and nonrelaxation of the lower esophageal sphincter (LES) on wet swallows. It forms a part of a group of conditions collectively classified as spastic esophageal disorders (SEDs). The Chicago classification has classified

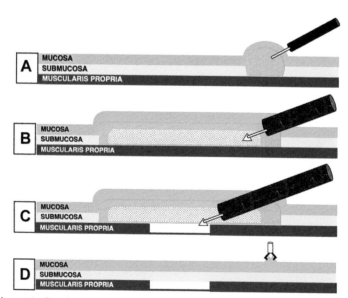

Fig. 1. Schematic showing principle of third space endoscopy: (*A*) layers of gastrointestinal tract represented with creation of submucosal cushion, (*B*) submucosal dissection and tunneling, (*C*) myotomy being performed distal to the site of mucosal incision, and (*D*) closure of mucosa creating sealing of submucosal tunnel thereby preventing bowel leak.

SEDs into AC with its three variant types–I, II, and III based on esophageal high-resolution manometry (HRM), and other SEDs–Jackhammer esophagus (JH), esophagogastric junction outflow obstruction (EGJOO), diffuse esophageal spasm (DES).[7]

Treatment of AC is palliative and is directed toward disruption of the spastic LES, with no therapy presently available to improve esophageal body motility. Surgical LES myotomy was described by Heller in 1913 and remained the mainstay of treatment for several decades until laparoscopic Heller myotomy (LHM) emerged and became the standard of care thereafter. Endoscopic approaches for treatment of AC also include endoscopic pneumatic balloon dilatation (PD) wherein a 30 to 40 mm diameter balloon is used to disrupt the LES, and endoscopic injection of botulinum toxin into the LES. Patients with advanced achalasia with a grossly dilated, nonmotile sigmoid esophagus and with no anticipated benefit by LES relaxation are recommended to undergo esophagectomy. POEM is the newest entrant in the variety of treatment options for AC and provides a minimally invasive option to perform myotomy of the LES (**Fig. 2**).

Indications, Patient Selection, and Contraindications for Per Oral Endoscopic Myotomy

POEM has been proposed as a minimally invasive technique for myotomy as a treatment of AC. It can be performed for all achalasia subtypes. POEM is preferred in patients with type III achalasia and SEDs, as these conditions require a personalized long myotomy.[8]

Common presentations of AC are dysphagia and regurgitation. Clinical evaluation involves calculation of the Eckardt score (ES) which includes four parameters: dysphagia, retrosternal pain, regurgitation, and weight loss; and has been shown to directly correlate with symptom severity. Diagnosis is by esophago-gastro-duodenoscopy (EGD), HRM, and sometimes barium swallow and/or a thoracic CT scan. EGD and/or HRM confirm AC, whereas barium swallow or computed tomography (CT) scan can rule out pseudo-achalasia caused by extrinsic compression by

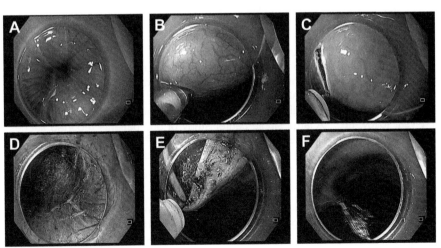

Fig. 2. POEM: (*A*) Tight LES, (*B*) Submucosal cushion, (*C*) mucosal incision, (*D*) submucosal dissection and tunneling, (*E*) full-thickness myotomy using triangular tip J knife, (*F*) mucosal incision closure using endoclips.

mediastinal mass lesions, and to determine the degree of sigmoidization in patients with sigmoid AC. Timed barium swallow is preferred to standard swallow, and the length of the vertical column of barium in the esophagus and the time for esophageal clearance of the barium are important considerations. Sigmoid AC is classified as S1 and S2 depending on degree of sigmoidization and on whether one or two esophageal lumens are visible on a single horizontal CT section (S1 and S2, respectively. Patients with S1 sigmoidization are likely to benefit by POEM (or any other myotomy) whereas S2 is less likely to benefit. Preoperative workup to evaluate fitness for general anesthesia is mandatory before POEM can be planned.

Although absolute contraindications for POEM are very few, several relative contraindications exist, wherein POEM can be technically challenging or potentially difficult to perform. Patients with severe coagulopathy, severe pulmonary disease, cirrhosis with portal hypertension, and conditions that cause severe, extensive fibrosis of the esophageal submucosa are absolute contraindications for POEM.[9] In general, patients unfit for general anesthesia due to comorbid conditions cannot be subjected to POEM. Severe stasis esophagitis and/or esophageal candidiasis are relative contraindications to performing POEM during that session. The esophageal mucosa in these patients is inflamed, friable, and bleeds during incision, is usually adherent to the muscle layer, which makes tunneling technically difficult. Furthermore, secure closure of such a mucosal incision is difficult because clips or sutures can cut through the friable tissues, subjecting the patient to the risk of mucosal dehiscence and mediastinitis. POEM in such situations is best postponed until mucosal inflammation heals. An important contraindication is extensive submucosal fibrosis wherein submucosal elevation cannot be obtained. In such cases, POEM may have to be aborted or deferred for safety concerns. Bing Hu has described a technique of open POEM for such cases with impressive safety and efficacy reported in a single-center case series of over 80 patients;[10] however, the overall acceptance of this technical variation at other centers have been limited.

Outcomes of per oral endoscopic myotomy

POEM has shown excellent short-, medium- and long-term clinical outcomes in various large series and meta-analyses. Outcomes are primarily reported based on improvement in ES.

Short- and Medium-Term Outcomes

Studies on POEM for AC have consistently reported high clinical success rates above 90% (**Table 1**).[11–25] A large multi-center retrospective study from Japan included 1346 patients and reported clinical success rates of 94.7% at 1-year follow-up.[11] Another single-center study from India reporting 400 patients showed 90.9% success rates at 1-year follow-up.[14] A large single-center study of 502 patients reported success rates of 91% at 2 year and 88.5% at 3 year follow-up.[18] Another large international multi-center study involving over 200 subjects reported 91% symptom relief at 2 year follow-up duration.[26]

Long-Term Outcomes

Long-term data on POEM is gradually emerging, with limited studies reporting long-term outcomes. A large single-center study evaluated 10-year sequential follow-up in 610 consecutive patients. The study reports impressive long-term outcomes as identified by Kaplan–Meier clinical success estimates at years 1, 2, 3, 4, 5, 6, and 7 as 98%, 96%, 96%, 94%, 92%, 91%, and 91%, respectively.[25] Other studies have reported similar outcomes. A multicenter retrospective cohort study involving 146

Table 1
Outcomes of per oral endoscopic myotomy in achalasia (select large studies)

Study	Patients (N)	Previous Therapy (%)	Mean/Median Follow-Up (months)	Pre-Eckardt Score	Post-Eckardt Score	Treatment Success (%)	Adverse Events (%)	GER (%)
Shiwaku et al.[10]	1346	31	12	6.1	1.1	95.1 at 6 m 94.7 at 1 y	3.7	14.8
Li et al.[11]	564	34.2	49	8	2	94.2 at 1 y 87.1 at 5 y	6.4	37.3
Kumbhari et al.[12]	282	28.6	12	7.8	1	94.3		23.2
Nabi et al.[13]	423	46	17	7	1.2	94 at 1 y 91 at 2 y	4.5	16.8
Shiwaku et al.[14]	100	47	3	5.9	0.8	99	10	28.5
Hungness et al.[15]	112	30	28	7	1	92	2.7	28
Ramchandani et al.[16]	220	41.3	13.4 (149)	7.1	1.25	94 at 6 m 92 at 1 y	6.4	21.6
Inoue et al.[17]	500	39	36	6	1	91 at 1 y 88.5 at 3 y	3.2	16.8 at 2 months, 21 at 3 y
Stavropoulos et al.[18]	100	27	13.3	7.8	0.2	98 at 3 months 96 at 1 y		32
Brewer Gutierrez et al.[19]	146	PD—19.9, Botulinum toxin injection—8.9, Heller's myotomy—8.9	55	7	1	95.2	5.5	Symptomatic reflux—32.1% Reflux esophagitis—16.8%
Wen-Gang Zhang et al.[20]	32	NR	88	7	2	88	22	Symptomatic reflux—38%

(continued on next page)

Table 1
(continued)

Study	Patients (N)	Previous Therapy (%)	Mean/Median Follow-Up (months)	Pre-Eckardt Score	Post-Eckardt Score	Treatment Success (%)	Adverse Events (%)	GER (%)
Teitelbaum et al.[21]	36	NR	65	6.4	1.7	83	NR	Reflux on pH studies (6 m)—38%; At 5 y: Erosive esophagitis—13%, Symptomatic reflux—26%
Werner et al.[22] (POEM vs LHM)	POEM—112, LHM—109	PD—27, Botulinum toxin injection—7, PD and BT—5	24	POEM - 6.8 ± 2 LHM—6.7 ± 2	POEM— 2 ± 1.9 LHM— 1.8 ± 1.7	POEM—83, LHM—81.7	POEM - 2.6, LHM—7.3	POEM group–3 months—57%, 24 months—44%
Ponds et al.[23] (POEM vs PD)	POEM—64, PD—66	None	24	POEM—med 8 (IQR 6–9), PD—med 7 (IQR 6–9)	POEM—1 (IQR 0–2) PD—1 (IQR 0–2)	POEM—92, PD—54	Serious procedure-related AE, PD—2, POEM - 0	Reflux esophagitis; POEM—41%, PD—7%
Modayil et al.[24]	610	47.9 – PD—17.7, BT—22.5, HM—13.6, POEM—2.8	30	Achalasia—7.6, non-achalasia—7.9	0.5, 1.2	97.6% (1 y), 96.2% (2 y), 95.9% (3 y), 93.8% (4 y), 91.9% (5 y), 91.2% (6 y), 91.2% (7 y)	Clinically significant AEs—3.4	Reflux on pH studies—57.1%, esophagitis on EGD—49.8%, GER symptoms—20.5% at 4 m; Normalization of pH at long term follow-up in 35% of initial positives

patients reported sustained clinical response in 95.2% at >48-month follow-up.[20] A single-center retrospective study of 32 patients reported 88% clinical success at median 88-month follow-up.[21] Two other studies have reported 87.1% and 83% long-term clinical success rates at 4 and 5 years, respectively.[12,22] Although some of these studies indicate that there may be a slight decline in clinical efficacy over the long term, most reported reductions are marginal, and can possibly be attributed to the continued impairment of esophageal body function rather than a recurrence of AC. Similar outcomes have been reported after LHM.

Per oral endoscopic myotomy for spastic esophageal disorders and type III achalasia cardia

POEM is the preferred treatment modality for the management of SEDs including type III AC. A recent systematic review and meta-analysis showed pooled clinical success rates of 89.6% (95% CI 83.5–93.1, 95% PI 83.4–93.7, I2 = 0%) for clinical success and adverse events (AEs) for all SED subtypes. Myotomy length (<10 cm or >10 cm) did not affect the clinical success rates. Furthermore, prior therapeutic intervention also did not affect the primary outcomes.[27] Another systematic review and meta-analysis showed a weighted pooled ratio (WPR) with a 95% confidence interval (CI) for clinical success of 87% (78, 93%), I^2 = 37%; the WPRs for clinical success for type III achalasia, DES, and JH were 92, 88, and 72%, respectively. WPR with 95% CI for AEs was 14% (9, 20%), I^2 = 0%.[28] An international, multicentric, retrospective study of 73 patients subjected to POEM for SEDs and followed up for mean of 234 days showed 93% clinical response and 11% AEs.[29]

Per Oral Endoscopic Myotomy for Pediatric Achalasia

POEM has proven to be a safe and effective modality to treat pediatric AC. A systematic review and meta-analysis of 12 studies included 146 pediatric patients with achalasia. Symptom resolution was seen in 93% patients. Significant reduction in mean ES by 6.88 points (95%CI, 6.28–7.48, P < .001) and LES pressure by 20.73 mm Hg (95% CI, 15.76–25.70, P < .001) was noted.[30] A single-center study from India evaluating 44 children with AC undergoing POEM reported excellent clinical success rates of 92.8%, 94.4%, 92.3%, and 83.3% at 1-, 2-, 3-, and 4-year follow-up, respectively. Intraoperative AEs were encountered in 25.6% and post-POEM gastro-esophageal reflux (GER) was documented by pH studies in 53.8%.[31]

A major limitation of data reporting outcomes of POEM for pediatric achalasia is that most studies have included patients up to 18 years of age. Most of the unique technical challenges while performing POEM for pediatric AC patients are encountered in a younger population, particularly infants and small-size children. Further subgroup analysis for this age group is therefore desirable.

Per Oral Endoscopic Myotomy for Recurrent Achalasia Cardia and Prior Treatment Failures

POEM has proved to be an effective salvage modality to treat these recurrences. A retrospective comparison of POEM for treatment naïve AC versus prior-treatment-failures showed no significant difference in technical and clinical success rates, complications, and operative times between the two groups.[32] An international multi-center study of 51 patients undergoing POEM for post-Heller's myotomy with recurrent AC showed excellent technical and clinical success rates of 100% and 94%, respectively. AEs were encountered in 13%.[33] A large Chinese single-center retrospective study of >1300 patients including 245 patients with prior treatment failure status showed 'prior treatment' as an independent predictor for clinical failure during follow-up (Hazard ratio 1.90, P = 0.002; Cox regression).[34] In another international multicenter case-controlled study of 181 patients comparing POEM for treatment naïve vs previous failed LHM, success rates, and AE were similar in both groups but post-LHM group showed poorer outcomes during follow-up (81 vs 94%, $p = 0.01$).[35] These results suggest that although POEM is safe and effective in treatment failures, the results may be inferior and may reflect disease progression in these patient groups. A study reporting pediatric achalasia patients revealed comparable results in both groups,[36] also suggesting that duration and natural disease progression could be additional factors responsible for successful outcomes. Endoluminal functional luminal imaging probe (EndoFLIP) has been evaluated as a predictor of response after POEM. A distensibility index (DI) < 7 has been shown to predict incomplete response.[37]

Per Oral Endoscopic Myotomy Compared with Other Treatment Modalities

POEM is the preferred therapy in patients with SEDs and type III AC. As reported in the earlier section, excellent outcomes have been consistently documented in several systematic reviews and metanalyses.[27,28] A retrospective multi-center study comparing POEM versus LHM for type III AC reported significantly superior clinical outcomes (98% vs 80.8%, $P < 0/01$), reduced procedural duration (102 min vs 264 min) and significantly few AEs (6% vs 27%, $P < 0.01$) for POEM as compared with LHM.[38]

For AC types I and II, outcomes of POEM and LHM are comparable. A systematic review and meta-analysis of 74 studies including 7792 patients compared POEM to LHM and reported predicted dysphagia improvement 93.5% for POEM and 91% for LHM at 12 months and 92.7% and 90%, at 24 months, respectively. Incidence of GER, however, was higher in patients undergoing POEM (odds ratio [OR] 1.69, 95% CI 1.33–2.14, $P < 0.0001$).[39]

In a multicenter prospective trial, Werner and colleagues[23] randomized 221 patients to POEM (112) or LHM plus Dor fundoplication (109), and reported comparable clinical success at 2-year follow-up (83.0% POEM and 81.7% LHM [difference, 1.4 percentage points; 95% CI, −8.7 to 11.4; $P = 0.007$ for noninferiority]). GER was more common in the POEM group as measured at 3 months (57% POEM vs 20% LHM, OR 5.74; 95% CI, 2.99 to 11.00) and at 2 years (44% vs 29%, OR 2.00; 95% CI, 1.03 to 3.85). Several other studies have also reported comparable short- and medium-term success rates. POEM achieved shorter operative times, reduced blood loss, and less pain compared with LHM.[38,40–47]

POEM and PD have been less frequently compared. A meta-analysis including 66 studies and >6000 patients compared POEM to PD. Superior clinical success rates were reported for POEM as compared with PD at 12, 24, and 36 months (92.9%, vs 76.9%, $P = 0.001$; 90.6% vs 74.8%, $P = 0.004$; and 88.4% vs 72.2%, $P = 0.006$, respectively). Pooled OR for GER was higher with POEM (symptomatic—2.95, $P = 0.02$ and endoscopic—6.98, $P = 0.001$) whereas esophageal perforation (0.3% vs 0.6%, $P = 0.8$) and significant bleeding (0.4% vs 0.7%, $P = 0.56$) were comparable in both groups.[48] A randomized study comparing PD to POEM in 133 patients showed significant superior clinical success with POEM as compared with PD (92 vs 54%, p < 0.01) despite no differences in the integrated relaxation pressures (IRP) or median barium column height in both groups. GER was significantly more frequent after POEM (41 vs 7%, $p = 0.002$).[24] Two other studies have reported 91.8% versus 68% ($p = 0.002$) and 92.3 vs 57.5% ($p < 0.0001$) clinical success after POEM and PD, respectively. Higher frequency of GER symptoms at 1-year follow-up was reported after POEM as compared with PD.[49,50]

A network meta-analysis of 19 studies including 5 randomized trials and 4407 patients comparing POEM to LHM and PD reported highest dysphagia remission rates after POEM as compared with LHM and PD (risk ratio [RR] = 1.21; 95% credible intervals [CIs] = 1.04–1.47 and RR = 1.40; 95% CIs = 1.14–1.79, respectively). However, higher postoperative GER was observed after POEM as compared with LHM and PD (RR = 1.75; 95% CIs = 1.35–2.03 and RR = 1.36; 95% CIs = 1.18–1.68, respectively). No major differences were seen between the LHM and PD arms.[51]

Gastro-esophageal reflux after per oral endoscopic myotomy

Incidence of post-POEM GER has been reported as high as 40-60% in recent literature.[11,13,22,23,25,39,51] GER is more frequent after POEM as compared with LHM or PD. An extensive meta-analysis of 74 studies (>7000 patients) compared POEM to LHM and reported higher risk of developing GER after POEM than after LHM on all measurable parameters–GER symptoms (OR 1.69, 95% CI 1.33–2.14, $P < 0.0001$), endoscopic evidence of erosive esophagitis (EE) (OR 9.31, 95% CI 4.71–18.85, $P < 0.0001$), and abnormal esophageal acid exposure (EAE) on pH testing (OR 4.30, 95% CI 2.96–6.27, $P < 0.0001$).[39] Another meta-analysis evaluating 17 and 28 studies with 1542 and 2581 patients of POEM and LHM reported higher abnormal EAE (pooled rate estimate 39% vs 16.8%) and esophagitis (29.4% vs 7.6%) for POEM and LHM, respectively.[52] The Werner study reported a significantly higher incidence of GER in the POEM group as compared with LHM (57% vs 20%; OR, 5.74; 95% CI, 2.99 to 11.00 at 3 months and 44% vs 29%; OR, 2.00; 95% CI, 1.03 to 3.85 at 24 months, respectively). However, incidence of severe grade C/D esophagitis was low in both groups.[23]

POEM experts have described technical modifications to minimize GER occurrence after POEM. Gastric length of myotomy should be limited to <2 cm (ideally observed and confirmed by double endoscope transillumination technique), and the myotomy should be performed in a manner that spares the sling fibers of the LES, especially while performing a posterior myotomy.[53,54] In the absence of double scope transillumination, other measures should be undertaken to ensure the optimal length and direction of myotomy. Tanaka and colleagues[55] have reported the consistent presence of two perforator vessels identified during posterior POEM that mark the boundary between the circular and sling muscle fibers. The second perforating vessels also form the optimal limit of dissection on the gastric side. Maintaining the myotomy direction to the right of these perforators minimizes risk to the sling fibers and may help prevent GER. These techniques collectively can be termed as anti-reflux measures during POEM.

Other factors that have been implicated for post-POEM GER include length of esophageal myotomy–a shorter myotomy could reduce GER; however, reports are conflicting.[56–58] Similarly, anterior versus posterior approach and selective circular versus full-thickness myotomy have failed to show consistently significant differences in post-POEM GER.[59,60] Teitelbaum and colleagues[61] have reported that a DI < 6 mm²/mm Hg was predictive of lower risk for GER.

A distinct peculiarity of post-POEM GER is that although most studies report high rates of abnormal EAE, endoscopic evidence of EE or symptomatic GER is significantly less frequent. Also, most GER is mild and easily treatable using proton pump inhibitors (PPI).[62,63] In the study by Kumbhari and colleagues,[13] although abnormal EAE was reported in 57.8%, EE was noted in only 23.2% and severe Grade C/D GER was seen in only 5.6%. In another multicenter Japanese study, GER was documented in 63% on pH but symptoms were observed in 14.8% and severe Grade C/D EE was seen in only 6.2%.[11] Repici and colleagues[52] reported GER in 39% on pH although EE, severe esophagitis, and symptoms were reported in 29.4%, 4.47%, and 19%, respectively. The Werner study confirmed that although GER was more frequent after POEM compared with LHM at 3 months, GER after LHM gradually increased so that the difference was less significant at 2 years. Furthermore, at 2 years, severe esophagitis was infrequent and was comparable in both groups (5 and 6%, respectively).[23] A single-center study comparing POEM with LHM reported significant EAE post-POEM (48.4% vs 13.6%, $P < 0.001$), although symptomatic GER was not significantly different in the two groups (28% vs 14.9%, $P = 0.38$).[40] A retrospective cohort study evaluating long-term outcomes of post-POEM GER in 68 patients reported >50% GER at 12-month follow-up; however, GER was mild and PPI responsive in >95% of patients and no GER-related AEs were noted at 5-year follow-up.[64] Similar outcomes have been reported in a study with long-term follow-up.[25] Therefore, although POEM does seem to predispose to GER, the majority of cases are mild, nonerosive, and responsive to PPI therapy.

Anti-reflux Procedures after Per Oral Endoscopic Myotomy. Anti-reflux procedures have been reported for treatment of refractory post-POEM GER. Second-stage transoral incisionless fundoplication (TIF) for symptomatic post-POEM GER was reported in 5 patients. All patients could discontinue PPI at a mean of 27 months of follow-up.[65,66] There have been few case reports of subsequent laparoscopic fundoplication following POEM.[62]

Inoue and colleagues[67] reported safety and feasibility of a novel endoscopic partial fundoplication performed in conjunction with POEM (POEM + F) as a potential minimally invasive option to prevent post-POEM GER. The procedure involves performing a standard anterior full-thickness POEM at 12 o'clock followed by entry into the peritoneal cavity by dissecting and opening the overlying serosa over the gastric myotomy. The gastric fundus is folded and fixed to the distal end of the myotomy using endoclips and endoloop to create a partial wrap. At 3-month follow-up, an intact wrap was shown in 19/21 patients. Results of POEM + F were also evaluated at 1-year follow-up in a single-arm study published from the authors' group. Wrap integrity was confirmed in 82.6% and GER was identified in 11.1% patients at median 1-year follow-up, much lower than that reported for most POEM studies.[68] Longer-term outcomes are under evaluation.

Currently, there is a debate about whether ARP should be offered prophylactically at every POEM or whether it should be reserved for those who develop refractory GER following POEM. This presently remains an unanswered question. Toshimori and colleagues[69] have described an endoscopic fundoplication (POEF) performed as a second stage following a posterior POEM. Accurate pre-POEM identification of patients who are at risk of developing GER in the post-POEM period could help provide insights into these decisions.

In conclusion, POEM has shown excellent outcomes in all achalasia subtypes and SEDs. It is effective for naïve as well as recurrent AC after failed initial therapy. Outcomes of POEM are comparable to LHM and are superior to PD. Post-POEM GER occurs in a significant number of patients, although most of it is mild, nonerosive, and responsive to PPI therapy. ARPs for post-POEM GER have been described and are currently under evaluation.

GASTRIC PER ORAL ENDOSCOPIC MYOTOMY

Gastroparesis is a motility disorder defined as a clinical syndrome and objective evidence of delayed gastric emptying in the absence of mechanical obstruction. Characteristic features of gastroparesis include early satiety, postprandial nausea, vomiting, bloating, and abdominal pain.[70,71] Gastroparesis has shown to have a significant impact on morbidity and mortality, especially in diabetics making it crucial to manage this condition appropriately.[71] Dietary modifications such as consuming small frequent low residue meals are not efficacious in all patients. Pharmacotherapy in the form of metoclopramide has been recommended for gastroparesis; however, data on its long-term efficacy are limited and are limited by its black box warning due to the risk of tardive dyskinesia.[72] Endoscopic management for gastroparesis has been studied more recently. Two randomized controlled trials showed that intra-pyloric botulinum toxin injection improved gastric emptying. However, symptom benefit was not evident. Therefore, intra-pyloric botulinum toxin injection is not recommended for the management of gastroparesis.[73] Endoscopic transpyloric stenting showed short-term efficacy but was limited by frequent stent migration up to 48%. The procedure therefore, has been considered as a temporizing measure to treat hospitalized patients, or to identify patients who may respond to durable pylorus-directed therapies.[74] Surgical or laparoscopic pyloroplasty is effective, however these procedures are invasive and can be associated with significant morbidity.[75]

This inspired Kawai and colleagues[76] to envision endoscopic myotomy of the pyloric sphincter based on the principles of SEMF which was subsequently performed and reported by Khashab and colleagues[4] G-POEM involves submucosal tunneling at the pylorus followed by a full-thickness short (2–3 cm) myotomy of the pyloric ring (**Fig. 3**).[8]

Currently, G-POEM has been performed and reported for medically refractory gastroparesis of all etiologies.

Outcomes of gastric per oral endoscopic myotomy

Technical Success
Data on G-POEM is still growing and is currently limited to observational studies and one randomized, sham-controlled trial (**Table 2**).[77–90] G-POEM is a complex procedure based on surgical principles and the mean procedure time for G-POEM ranges from 33 to 119 min indicative of its variable learning curve.[91] Procedure time has reduced as procedural proficiency has improved and was reported to be 43 min (34–56.5) in a 2022 multicenter study.[89] Technical success rates reported for G-POEM are high. A meta-analysis of ten studies of 292 patients from multiple

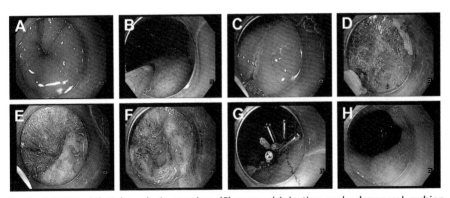

Fig. 3. G-POEM: (*A*) tight pyloric opening, (*B*) mucosal injection and submucosal cushion approximately 5 cm proximal to pyloric ring on posterior gastric wall, (*C*) mucosal incision, (*D*) submucosal dissection and tunneling perpendicular to circular muscle fibers, (*E*) duodenal mucosa visualized rising vertically beyond the pyloric ring, (*F*) short full-thickness pyloromyotomy, (*G*) mucosal incision closed using endoclips, and (*H*) opened-up pylorus.

Table 2
Outcomes for gastric per oral endoscopic myotomy

Study	Patients (N)	Technical Success (%)	Procedure Time (min)	Clinical Success (%)	Adverse Events	Follow-up (months)
Shlomovitz et al.[79]	7	100	90–120	6/7 (86)	1 bleeding (clips)	6.5 ± 2.1
Mekaroonkamol et al.[80]	3	100	74 (55–93)	3/3 (100)	None	3
Rodriguez et al.[81]	47	100	41.2 ± 28.5	31/47—(66)	1 death (cardiac disease, unrelated to procedure)	3
Dacha et al.[82]	16	100	49.7 ± 22.1	13/16 (81)	None	6
Gonzalez et al.,[83] 2017	29	100	47 (32–118)	3 m—23/29 (79%); 6 m—20/29 (69%)	1 bleeding (clips), 1 abscess (conservatively managed)	10 ± 6.4
Khashab et al.,[84] 2018	30	100	72 (35–223)	26/30 (86)	1 capnoperitoneum, 1 ulcer	5.5
Gonzalez et al.[85]	12	100	51 (32–105)	10/12 (85)	2 capnoperitoneum	5
Kahaleh et al.[86]	33	100	77.6 (37–255)	28/33 (85)	1 bleeding (clips), 1 ulcer	11.5
Xu et al.[87]	16	100	45.25 ± 12.96	13/16 (81.25)	NR	14.5
Mekaroonkamol et al.[88]	30	100	NR	23/30 (76.7)	NR	18
Malik et al.[89]	13	100	119 ± 23	GCSI and GES revealed statistically insignificant improvements; 11/13 patients reported feeling somewhat better on questionnaire	1 pulmonary embolism	6
Abdefatah et al.[90]	97	100	50 ± 13	73/97 (81.1%)	2 mild, 2 moderate—1 tension capnoperitoneum (needle decompression), 1 bleeding ulcer (endoscopic treatment)	36

Vosoughi et al.[91]	80	100	43 (34–56.5)	45/80 (56)		3 Capnoperitoneum (needle decompression), 1 mucosotomy, 1 thermal mucosal injury (clips)	12
Martinek et al.[92]	21	95.23 (20/21), 1 G-POEM unable to be completed due to severe SM fibrosis	76 ± 41	At 6 months—14/20 (70) vs 4/19 (22) in sham group. Patients from sham group when crossed over to G-POEM—9/12 (75)	2 serious AE related to procedure in G-POEM group—1 pyloric ulcer (required hospitalization managed conservatively), 1 mucosal injury (managed conservatively)	6

centers in 3 countries reported a 100% technical success rate.[91] These studies included patients who had undergone prior treatments including botulinum toxin injections (28.1%), gastric electrical stimulator (12.6%), transpyloric stenting (1.4%) and dilation (0.3%), and laparoscopic pyloric surgery (1.4%) which did not affect technical success. Similarly, a study on 80 patients reported a 100% technical success after patients had undergone botulinum toxin injection (35%) or transpyloric stenting (20%).[89]

Clinical Success

Clinical success with G-POEM has been reported in the form of symptomatic improvement, objective improvement in gastric emptying, and overall quality of life.

Symptoms. Symptomatic improvement has been assessed with standardized subjective criteria namely Gastric Cardinal Symptom Index (GCSI) comprising three symptoms: (1) post-prandial fullness/early satiety, (2) nausea/vomiting, and (3) bloating.[92] A randomized sham-controlled trial reported a 71% clinical success rate in the G-POEM group and 22% in the sham group. GCSI scores were reduced by 2.4 (95% CI 2–2.8) in the G-POEM group compared with 0.7 (95% CI 0–1.2) in the sham group.[90]

Uemura and colleagues[93] compared pre and post-G-POEM GCSI scores in patients across 10 studies and 281 patients in their meta-analysis of observational studies. All studies showed a decreased GCSI score, and the pooled mean difference was a statistically significant reduction of 1.76 points (95% CI 1.43, 2.08, $p = 0.0002$). This was consistent with findings reported by other reviews evaluating the effect of G-POEM on GCSI.[91,94] An international prospective trial reported a reduction in GCSI by 1.2 ± 1.3, $p < 0.001$ at 12 months, and a clinical success rate of 56.3% (95% CI 44.8–66.7).[89] Studies reported GCSI scores at different times in the follow-up period; however, an improvement in these scores was seen at 3, 6, 12, and 18 months.[93]

Abdominal pain is not assessed in the GCSI but can be a common symptom of gastroparesis. A study showed improvement in abdominal pain in 56% to 73% of patients following G-POEM when followed up for a mean of 11.5 months.[86]

Gastric Emptying Studies. Objective evaluation of gastric emptying using a 4-hour gastric emptying scintigraphy (GES) was also a marker of clinical success of G-POEM in several studies. Some variability has been reported in GES results with improvement seen in 70-100% of the study population.[87] One randomized sham-controlled trial showed a significant decrease in 4-h gastric retention in the G-POEM group compared with no change in the sham group. There was no correlation between GCSI and gastric retention at 3 months ($r = 0.15$, 95% CI –0.18 to 0.42).[90]

Ten observational studies individually showed an improvement in GES. When pooled together, they revealed a 26.28% (95% CI 19.74–32.83, $p < 0.0001$) reduction in gastric retention at 4 h following G-POEM.[93] Mohan and colleagues[95] reported an 85.1% pooled clinical success rate based on improvement in 4-h GES. This study also showed comparable improvement in 4-h GES with G-POEM (85.1%) and surgery (84%), ($p = 0.91$).

Other Outcomes. Endoscopic functional luminal imaging probe (EndoFLIP) measurements have revealed increased length, cross-sectional area (CSA), and distensibility of the pylorus in patients following G-POEM.[90] However, only increased CSA has been associated with better clinical outcomes.[87] Studies have also shown improvement in quality-of-life (assessed by SF36 questionnaires) in 70-78% of patients. In addition, emergency room visits, gastroparesis-related hospitalization rate, and anti-emetic use significantly reduced following G-POEM as compared with controls.[86]

Patient Selection for Gastric Per Oral Endoscopic Myotomy

Gastroparesis is a complex clinical disorder and both impaired gastric dysmotility and pylorospasm play a variable role in its pathophysiology.[96] Impaired gastric motility is likely the predominant mechanism in diabetic gastroparesis, whereas pylorospasm may be an important factor in postoperative (after vagal injury or vagotomy) gastroparesis. Therefore, analyzing outcomes for G-POEM based on etiology of gastroparesis becomes crucial. Data regarding G-POEM are still emerging and are quite varied across studies. Predictors of poor outcomes after G-POEM identified are diabetes,[79,81] female gender,[81] higher BMI, history of psychiatric or pain medication use.[88] However, Mekaroonkamol and colleagues[86] reported similar benefits with G-POEM in diabetics and nondiabetics. Moreover, among diabetics, the baseline HbA1c levels did not influence outcomes. Longer duration of gastroparesis before G-POEM may have inferior outcomes at 12 months; however, this has not shown to influence outcomes at 1 month or 6 months. Vosoughi and colleagues[89] in their multi-center prospective study of 80 patients reported comparable clinical success with G-POEM at 12 months regardless of the demographics, etiology, and duration of gastroparesis. Investigators identified that a baseline GCSI score greater than 2.6 (OR = 3.23, $p = 0.04$) and a baseline gastric retention >20% at 4 hours (OR = 3.65, $p = 0.03$) was an independent predictor of clinical success at 12 months. Benefits of G-POEM were shown to be evident at 1-month post-procedure. Patients who had clinical improvement at 1-month post-procedure were significantly more likely (OR 8.75 [95% CI 2.9–26.38], $p < 0.001$) to have a sustained benefit at 12 months. A scoring system has been developed to predict clinical response to G-POEM based on symptom subsets among the GCSI and results of GES study (**Table 3**). It was validated in 46 patients and showed 93.3% sensitivity, 56.3% specificity, 80% PPV, 81.8% NPV, and 80.4% accuracy. Patients with a score >/2 were more likely to be responders at 3 years than those with a score < 2 (80% and 18%, respectively, $p = 0.0004$).[97]

Gastric Per Oral Endoscopic Myotomy versus Other Treatment Modalities

In medically refractory gastroparesis, G-POEM can be compared with gastric electrical stimulators and surgery. G-POEM has shown a 60% lower risk of clinical recurrence along with a higher 24-month clinical response rate (76.6% vs 53.7%).[86,98] G-POEM (4.3%) had fewer AEs than electric stimulators (26.1%), $p = 0.1$, and was effective across all types of gastroparesis whereas electric stimulators had limited

Table 3 Gastric per oral endoscopic myotomy patient selection predictive model scoring system	
Criterion	**Score**
Nausea subscale < 2	+ 1
Satiety subscale >/4	+ 1
Bloating subscale > 3.5	+ 1
Retention at 4 hours > 50% on GES	+ 1

Data from Labonde A, Lades G, Debourdeau A, et al. Gastric peroral endoscopic myotomy in refractory gastroparesis: long-term outcomes and predictive score to improve patient selection. Gastrointest Endosc. 2022;96(3):500-508.e2.

benefit in patients with idiopathic gastroparesis.[98] G-POEM has shown comparable clinical success to surgical pyloroplasty based on GCSI scores (75.8% vs 77.3%, $p = 0.81$) and improvement in 4-h gastric emptying studies (85.1% vs 84%, $p = 0.91$).[95,99]

Adverse Events

G-POEM has been reported to have a low rate of AE at approximately 6-11%.[89,91,95] The most common AEs following G-POEM are bleeding (32%), abdominal pain (30%), and capnoperitoneum (24%). In one randomized sham-controlled study, seven AE were reported in the G-POEM group compared with three in the sham group. Of these seven, three were related to the G-POEM procedure, gastric ulcer ($n = 1$), mucosal injury ($n = 1$), and delayed dumping syndrome ($n = 1$).[90] Bleeding can usually be managed with proton pump inhibitor therapy and/or endoscopic therapy. Capnoperitoneum is often managed conservatively and resolves spontaneously and rarely needle decompression can be used to treat severe cases.[86] Two deaths have been reported in G-POEM-related studies; however, none of them were related to the procedure.[93]

Data on G-POEM has grown over the last few years as it continues to get incorporated in clinical practice. G-POEM has shown robust efficacy in gastroparesis of all etiologies. Results with G-POEM are comparable to surgical pyloroplasty and are superior to gastric electrical stimulators with an excellent short- and long-term safety profile. Appropriate patient selection is crucial to improve clinical success rates and the development and validation of predictive models is essential.

DIVERTICULAR PER ORAL ENDOSCOPIC MYOTOMY

Diverticular or D-POEM is an inclusive term for endoscopic myotomy performed for esophageal diverticula (ED). It has been reported for Zenker's diverticula, epiphrenic diverticula, and mid esophageal diverticula.

Zenker's Per Oral Endoscopic Myotomy or submucosal tunneling endoscopic septum division

Zenker's diverticulum (ZD) is a rare clinical condition characterized by sac-like herniation of the mucosal and submucosal layers originating from the pharyngoesophageal junction due to a defect in the cricopharyngeus muscle. Traditionally ZD are treated by surgical resection of the diverticulum with cricopharyngeal myotomy; however, morbidity and mortality rates have been reported to be 30% and 3%, respectively.[100–102] Flexible endoscopic cystotomy (FES) soon became the preferred treatment modality which was attributable to its preferable safety profile, shorter procedure time and length of hospital stay.[103] FES however carried the limitation of recurrence rates much higher than surgery (11%) possibly due to incomplete division of the septum.[103,104] This led to the conceptualization of submucosal tunneling endoscopic septum division (STESD or Z-POEM).[5] This technique allowed for a longer septotomy length which is a prognostic marker of septotomy success.[105]

Literature on outcomes after Z-POEM is still emerging (**Table 4**).[106–109] An international multicenter study of 75 patients undergoing Z-POEM for mean ZD size 31.3 $\pm$ 1.6 mm reported 97.3% technical and 92% clinical success rates. AEs were low at 6.7% which included bleeding (1) and perforation (4). Length of hospital stay was mean 1.8 $\pm$ 0.2 days. Patients were followed up for a mean 291.5 days (interquartile range [IQR] 103.5–436) and one recurrence was noted. Dysphagia scores reduced from mean 1.96 to 0.25 ($P < 0.0001$).[106] Another study of 22 patients with symptomatic ZD (mean size 30 mm [IQR, 24–40]) undergoing Z-POEM reported

Table 4
Diverticular per oral endoscopic myotomy (diverticular per oral endoscopic myotomy and Z-per oral endoscopic myotomy)

Study	Procedure Details	Patients (N)	Clinical Success	Adverse Events	Follow-up (Median)
Yang et al.[109]	Z-POEM	75	92%	6.7%	291.5 d (IQR 103.5–436)
Budnicka et al.[110]	Z-POEM	22	90.9%	13.6%	266 d (IQR 213–306)
Sanaei et al.[111]	Z-POEM	32	96.7%	12.5%	166 d (IQR 39–566)
Kahaleh et al.[112]	Z-POEM vs Septotomy	Septotomy—49, Z-POEM—52	Septotomy—84%, Z-POEM—92%	Septotomy—30.6%, Z-POEM—9.6%	Mean, Septotomy—7.9 m, Z-POEM—3.4 m
Yang et al.[114]	D-POEM, esophageal diverticula	11 (ZD—7, Mid esophagus—1, EED—3)	100%	0%	145 d (IQR 126–273)
Nabi et al.[115]	D-POEM, EED	13	84.6%	7.69% (1 AE requiring surgery)	25 m
Zeng et al.[116]	D-POEM	10 (ZD—2, mid-esophagus—5, EED—3)	90%	0%	11 m (IQR 10.25–17.25)
Maydeo et al.[117]	D-POEM	25 (ZD—20, EED—5)	86%	0%	12 m

100% technical and 90.9% clinical success rates. At a mean follow-up duration of 266 days, no recurrences were seen. AEs included mild (2) and severe (1) subcutaneous emphysema.[107]

A recent study of 32 patients looked at outcomes of Z-POEM after failed prior interventions such as surgery (10), rigid (9) and flexible endoscopy (13), Z-POEM (3), and Botulinum toxin injection (1). Overall technical success rate was 93.8%. Two technical failures occurred due to presence of extensive fibrosis preventing the creating of a submucosal tunnel. The clinical success rate after excluding technical failures was 96.7%. Ten patients followed up for at least 12 months and did not have symptom recurrence. AE rate was 12.5% (two inadvertent mucosotomies and two leaks), none of which were severe or fatal.[108]

A multicenter retrospective study compared outcomes of Z-POEM with FES in 101 patients and reported comparable dysphagia relief in both arms although AEs were significantly lower in the Z-POEM group (9.6% vs 30.6%, $p = 0.02$).[110]

Diverticular Per Oral Endoscopic Myotomy

Diverticular per oral endoscopic myotomy (D-POEM) is similar to Z-POEM and has been performed for epiphrenic and mid-esophageal diverticula. Esophageal epiphrenic diverticula (EED) are rare pulsion-type outpouchings at the lower end the esophagus, most commonly occurring in association with AC. Data on outcomes for D-POEM are scarce and include studies with small sample sizes due to the low incidence of EEDs (see **Table 4**).[111–114] Yang and colleagues[111] studied 11 patients undergoing D-POEM for ZD, mid-esophageal and epiphrenic diverticula. Technical success was achieved in 10/11 (91%) and clinical success was reported in 10/10 (100%) patients with mean dysphagia score decreasing from 2.1 to 0.1 ($p < 0.001$). No AEs were reported. A retrospective study of 13 patients who underwent D-POEM for EED reported a technical success rate of 12/13 (92.3%). At 25-month(-median) follow-up, clinical success was achieved in 84.6% cases. Mean integrated relaxation pressures reduced significantly after D-POEM (25.80 ± 13.24 vs 9.40 ± 3.10, $p = 0.001$). There was one AE requiring surgical intervention.[112] A study by Zeng and colleagues[113] reported patients with ZD (2), mid-esophageal diverticulum (5) and EED (3) who underwent D-POEM. Technical success rate was 100%, clinical success achieved in 9/10, symptomatic score reduced from 2.5 to 1 ($p = 0.007$) during a median follow-up of 11 (IQR 10.25–17.25) months. A single-center study reported outcomes of 20 ZDs and 5 EEDs treated by Z-POEM or D-POEM and reported 86% clinical response at 12-month follow-up.[114]

Nevertheless, additional safety data are needed before D-POEM becomes standard of care for all patients with esophageal diverticula. It must be kept in mind that ED is more commonly seen in the elderly, who may harbor significant additional comorbidities. FES is technically easier and quicker compared with D-POEM and therefore the benefits of a more invasive procedure should be carefully weighed against the potential consequences.

PER-RECTAL ENDOSCOPIC MYOTOMY

Hirschsprung's disease (HD) is a congenital disorder characterized by the absence of intrinsic ganglion cells in the submucosal and myenteric plexuses of the hindgut. Single or multistage surgical or laparoscopic pull-through procedures have been the standard of care for HD for several decades. However, there is considerable morbidity associated with these surgeries, especially anal incontinence, fecal soiling, enterocolitis, and poor quality of life.[115,116]

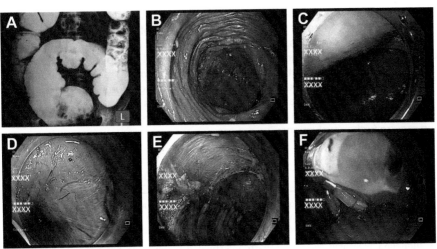

Fig. 4. PREM: (*A*) barium enema showing dilated proximal colon with spastic distal segment in a case of HD, (*B*) endoscopic view of dilated proximal colon, (*C*) submucosal injection and cushion, (*D*) submucosal tunneling in oral direction following horizontal mucosal incision just proximal to anal verge, (*E*) full-thickness myotomy in aboral direction, (*F*) mucosal incision closure using endoclips.

PREM was conceptualized based on the principle of POEM wherein a myotomy of the spastic bowel segment leads to relief of the functional obstruction.[6] Optimal preoperative mapping of the aganglionic segment is mandatory before planning PREM and can be performed using suction EMR biopsies that include the deep submucosal layer in the biopsy specimen.[117,118] The PREM procedure involves creating a retrograde submucosal tunnel starting at the anorectal junction extending proximally of a predetermined length based on the pre-PREM mapping biopsies, and performing a full-thickness myotomy, which must necessarily include the internal anal sphincter **(Fig. 4)**.[6,119]

Data on PREM has been limited to case reports and case series. To date, it has been performed for infantile, pediatric, and adult HD.[6,117,120] A case series on nine patients of median age 4 years (range, 1–24) undergoing PREM for HD reported technical success of 100%. Mean aganglionic segment length was 6.3 ($\pm$4.4) cm. No periprocedural AE's or new-onset incontinence was observed. Patients were followed up for a median 17 months (IQR 11–35) and stool frequency improved from pre-PREM 1 in 4.4 ($\pm$1.5) days to post-PREM 1 in 1.2 ($\pm$0.4) days (P = 0.0004). Laxative usage reduced from pre-PREM mean 5.4 UL ($\pm$4.9, range 2–18) to post-PREM mean 0.4 UL ($\pm$0.7, range 0–2) (P = 0.0002). Laxative could be discontinued in six patients, whereas a dose reduction of > 50% was seen in the remaining three.[119] A recent case report showed safety and efficacy of PREM after failed surgical myectomy (Lynn procedure) for a 9-year-old with HD.[121] Further studies on this topic are necessary to establish the role of PREM in the management of HD.

SUMMARY

In conclusion, the SEMF technique has provided access to the muscle layer of the bowel wall and can be used to perform a minimally invasive endoscopic myotomy of spastic segments in the GI tract. The concept has been used from the esophagus to the anus in the form of various procedures which have been described and named accordingly. Esophageal POEM is the index procedure in this group and has proved to be an effective procedure for the treatment of AC. It is useful for all AC subtypes and is effective to treat recurrences. Although post-POEM GER remains a concern, the majority of cases are mild, nonerosive and responsive to PPI therapy. G-POEM is an upcoming and potentially effective treatment for patients with refractory gastroparesis. Optimal patient selection remains the current challenge for G-POEM. Z-POEM, D-POEM, and PREM have shown impressive outcomes for patients with ZD, EED, and HD, respectively, although these procedures are relatively new, less studied, and require further evaluation.

CLINICS CARE POINTS

- Submucosal endoscopy using a mucosal flap valve technique provides safe access to the muscle layer of the bowel wall and can be used to perform a minimally invasive endoscopic submucosal tunneling myotomy of spastic segments in the GI tract.

- Tunneling myotomy for spastic gastrointestinal (GI) segments has been described for achalasia cardia (AC) (per oral endoscopic myotomy [POEM]), refractory gastroparesis (G-POEM), Zenker's and esophageal diverticula (Z-POEM and D-POEM, respectively), and Hirschsprung's disease (per-rectal endoscopic myotomy [PREM]).

- POEM is a safe and effective procedure for the treatment of AC. It is useful for all AC subtypes and for treating recurrent AC. Outcomes of POEM are comparable to LHM for AC types I and II and superior to PD. POEM is superior to all other modalities for type III AC and spastic esophageal disorders.

- Gastro-esophageal reflux frequently occurs after POEM, but is mostly mild, nonerosive, and responsive to PPI therapy.

- G-POEM is an upcoming and potentially effective treatment for carefully selected patients with refractory gastroparesis. Optimal patient selection remains the current challenge.

- Z-POEM, D-POEM, and PREM have shown impressive outcomes for patients with Zenker's diverticulum, esophageal epiphrenic diverticula, and Hirschsprung's disease, respectively. They have been newly described and require further evaluation in larger studies.

REFERENCES

1. Sumiyama K, Gostout CJ, Rajan E, et al. Submucosal endoscopy with mucosal flap safety valve. Gastrointest Endosc 2007;65(4):688–94.
2. Pasricha PJ, Hawari R, Ahmed I, et al. Submucosal endoscopic esophageal myotomy: a novel experimental approach for the treatment of achalasia. Endoscopy 2007;39(9):761–4.
3. Inoue H, Minami H, Kobayashi Y, et al. Peroral endoscopic myotomy (POEM) for esophageal achalasia. Endoscopy 2010;42(4):265–71.
4. Khashab MA, Stein E, Clarke JO, et al. Gastric peroral endoscopic myotomy for refractory gastroparesis: first human endoscopic pyloromyotomy (with video). Gastrointest Endosc 2013;78(5):764–8.
5. Li QL, Chen WF, Zhang XC, et al. Submucosal Tunneling endoscopic septum division: a novel technique for treating zenker's diverticulum. Gastroenterology 2016;151(6):1071–4.
6. Bapaye A, Wagholikar G, Jog S, et al. Per rectal endoscopic myotomy for the treatment of adult Hirschsprung's disease: First human case (with video). Dig Endosc 2016;28(6):680–4.

7. Pandolfino JE, Kwiatek MA, Nealis T, et al. Achalasia: a new clinically relevant classification by high-resolution manometry. Gastroenterology 2008;135(5): 1526–33.

8. Bapaye A, Korrapati SK, Dharamsi S, et al. Third Space Endoscopy: Lessons Learnt From a Decade of Submucosal Endoscopy. J Clin Gastroenterol 2020; 54(2):114–29.

9. Stavropoulos SN, Modayil R, Friedel D. Extended indications and contraindications for peroral endoscopic myotomy. Tech Gastrointest Endosc 2013;15(3): 149–52.

10. Liu W, Zeng XH, Yuan XL, et al. Open peroral endoscopic myotomy for the treatment of achalasia: a case series of 82 cases. Dis Esophagus 2019. https://doi.org/10.1093/dote/doz052.

11. Shiwaku H, Inoue H, Onimaru M, et al. Multicenter collaborative retrospective evaluation of peroral endoscopic myotomy for esophageal achalasia: analysis of data from more than 1300 patients at eight facilities in Japan. Surg Endosc 2019. https://doi.org/10.1007/s00464-019-06833-8.

12. Li QL, Wu QN, Zhang XC, et al. Outcomes of per-oral endoscopic myotomy for treatment of esophageal achalasia with a median follow-up of 49 months. Gastrointest Endosc 2018;87(6):1405–1412 e3.

13. Kumbhari V, Familiari P, Bjerregaard NC, et al. Gastroesophageal reflux after peroral endoscopic myotomy: a multicenter case-control study. Endoscopy 2017;49(7):634–42.

14. Nabi Z, Ramchandani M, Chavan R, et al. Per-oral endoscopic myotomy for achalasia cardia: outcomes in over 400 consecutive patients. Endosc Int Open 2017;5(5):E331–9.

15. Shiwaku H, Inoue H, Sasaki T, et al. A prospective analysis of GERD after POEM on anterior myotomy. Surg Endosc 2016;30(6):2496–504.

16. Hungness ES, Sternbach JM, Teitelbaum EN, et al. Per-oral Endoscopic Myotomy (POEM) after the learning curve: durable long-term results with a low complication rate. Ann Surg 2016;264(3):508–17.

17. Ramchandani M, Nageshwar Reddy D, Darisetty S, et al. Peroral endoscopic myotomy for achalasia cardia: Treatment analysis and follow-up of over 200 consecutive patients at a single center. Dig Endosc 2016;28(1):19–26.

18. Inoue H, Sato H, Ikeda H, et al. Per-oral endoscopic myotomy: a series of 500 patients. J Am Coll Surg 2015;221(2):256–64.

19. Stavropoulos SN, Modayil RJ, Friedel D, et al. The international per oral endoscopic myotomy survey (IPOEMS): a snapshot of the global POEM experience. Surg Endosc 2013;27(9):3322–38.

20. Brewer Gutierrez OI, Moran RA, Familiari P, et al. Long-term outcomes of per-oral endoscopic myotomy in achalasia patients with a minimum follow-up of 4 years: a multicenter study. Endosc Int Open 2020;8(5):E650–5.

21. Zhang W-G, Chai N-L, Zhai Y-Q, et al. Long-term outcomes of peroral endoscopic myotomy in achalasia patients with a minimum follow-up of 7 years. Chin Med J 2020;133(8):996–8.

22. Teitelbaum EN, Dunst CM, Reavis KM, et al. Clinical outcomes five years after POEM for treatment of primary esophageal motility disorders. Surg Endosc 2018;32(1):421–7.

23. Werner YB, Hakanson B, Martinek J, et al. Endoscopic or surgical myotomy in patients with idiopathic achalasia. N Engl J Med 2019;381(23):2219–29. https://doi.org/10.1056/NEJMoa1905380.

24. Ponds FA, Fockens P, Lei A, et al. Effect of peroral endoscopic myotomy vs pneumatic dilation on symptom severity and treatment outcomes among treatment-naive patients with achalasia: a randomized clinical trial. JAMA 2019;322(2):134–44.

25. Modayil RJ, Zhang X, Rothberg B, et al. Peroral endoscopic myotomy: 10-year outcomes from a large, single-center U.S. series with high follow-up completion and comprehensive analysis of long-term efficacy, safety, objective GERD, and endoscopic functional luminal assessment. Gastrointest Endosc 2021;94(5):930–42.

26. Ngamruengphong S, Inoue H, Chiu P, et al. Long-term outcomes of per-oral endoscopic myotomy in achalasia patients with a minimum follow-up of 2 years: an international multicenter study. Gastrointest Endosc 2016. https://doi.org/10.1016/j.gie.2016.09.017.

27. Chandan S, Mohan BP, Chandan OC, et al. Clinical efficacy of per-oral endoscopic myotomy (POEM) for spastic esophageal disorders: a systematic review and meta-analysis. Surg Endosc 2020;34(2):707–18.

28. Khan MA, Kumbhari V, Ngamruengphong S, et al. Is POEM the Answer for Management of Spastic Esophageal Disorders? A Systematic Review and Meta-Analysis. Dig Dis Sci 2017;62(1):35–44.

29. Khashab MA, Messallam AA, Onimaru M, et al. International multicenter experience with peroral endoscopic myotomy for the treatment of spastic esophageal disorders refractory to medical therapy (with video). Gastrointest Endosc 2015;81(5):1170–7.

30. Lee Y, Brar K, Doumouras AG, et al. Peroral endoscopic myotomy (POEM) for the treatment of pediatric achalasia: a systematic review and meta-analysis. Surg Endosc 2019;33(6):1710–20.

31. Nabi Z, Ramchandani M, Chavan R, et al. Outcome of peroral endoscopic myotomy in children with achalasia. Surg Endosc 2019;33(11):3656–64.

32. Yeniova AO, Yoo IK, Jeong E, et al. Comparison of peroral endoscopic myotomy between de-novo achalasia and achalasia with prior treatment. Surg Endosc 2021;35(1):200–8.

33. Tyberg A, Sharaiha RZ, Familiari P, et al. Peroral endoscopic myotomy as salvation technique post-Heller: International experience. Dig Endosc 2018;30(1):52–6.

34. Liu ZQ, Li QL, Chen WF, et al. The effect of prior treatment on clinical outcomes in patients with achalasia undergoing peroral endoscopic myotomy. Endoscopy 2019;51(4):307–16.

35. Ngamruengphong S, Inoue H, Ujiki MB, et al. Efficacy and Safety of Peroral Endoscopic Myotomy for Treatment of Achalasia After Failed Heller Myotomy. Clin Gastroenterol Hepatol 2017;15(10):1531–1537 e3.

36. Nabi Z, Ramchandani M, Darisetty S, et al. Impact of prior treatment on long-term outcome of peroral endoscopic myotomy in pediatric achalasia. J Pediatr Surg 2019. https://doi.org/10.1016/j.jpedsurg.2019.07.010.

37. Yoo IK, Choi SA, Kim WH, et al. Assessment of Clinical Outcomes after Peroral Endoscopic Myotomy via Esophageal Distensibility Measurements with the Endoluminal Functional Lumen Imaging Probe. Gut Liver 2019;13(1):32–9.

38. Kumbhari V, Tieu AH, Onimaru M, et al. Peroral endoscopic myotomy (POEM) vs laparoscopic Heller myotomy (LHM) for the treatment of Type III achalasia in 75 patients: a multicenter comparative study. Endosc Int Open 2015;3(3):E195–201.

39. Schlottmann F, Luckett DJ, Fine J, et al. Laparoscopic heller myotomy versus peroral endoscopic myotomy (POEM) for achalasia: a systematic review and meta-analysis. Ann Surg 2018;267(3):451–60.

40. Sanaka MR, Thota PN, Parikh MP, et al. Peroral endoscopic myotomy leads to higher rates of abnormal esophageal acid exposure than laparoscopic Heller myotomy in achalasia. Surg Endosc 2019;33(7):2284–92.

41. Hanna AN, Datta J, Ginzberg S, et al. Laparoscopic heller myotomy vs per oral endoscopic myotomy: patient-reported outcomes at a single institution. J Am Coll Surg 2018;226(4):465–472 e1.

42. Ramirez M, Zubieta C, Ciotola F, et al. Per oral endoscopic myotomy vs laparoscopic Heller myotomy, does gastric extension length matter? Surg Endosc 2018;32(1):282–8.

43. Chan SM, Wu JC, Teoh AY, et al. Comparison of early outcomes and quality of life after laparoscopic Heller's cardiomyotomy to peroral endoscopic myotomy for treatment of achalasia. Dig Endosc 2016;28(1):27–32.

44. Kumagai K, Tsai JA, Thorell A, et al. Per-oral endoscopic myotomy for achalasia. Are results comparable to laparoscopic Heller myotomy? Scand J Gastroenterol 2015;50(5):505–12.

45. Bhayani NH, Kurian AA, Dunst CM, et al. A comparative study on comprehensive, objective outcomes of laparoscopic Heller myotomy with per-oral endoscopic myotomy (POEM) for achalasia. Ann Surg 2014;259(6):1098–103.

46. Hungness ES, Teitelbaum EN, Santos BF, et al. Comparison of perioperative outcomes between peroral esophageal myotomy (POEM) and laparoscopic Heller myotomy. J Gastrointest Surg 2013;17(2):228–35.

47. Ujiki MB, Yetasook AK, Zapf M, et al. Peroral endoscopic myotomy: a short-term comparison with the standard laparoscopic approach. Surgery 2013;154(4): 893–7 [discussion: 897-900].

48. Ofosu A, Mohan BP, Ichkhanian Y, et al. Peroral endoscopic myotomy (POEM) vs pneumatic dilation (PD) in treatment of achalasia: A meta-analysis of studies with >/= 12-month follow-up. Endosc Int Open 2021;9(7):E1097–107.

49. Kim GH, Jung KW, Jung HY, et al. Superior clinical outcomes of peroral endoscopic myotomy compared with balloon dilation in all achalasia subtypes. J Gastroenterol Hepatol 2019;34(4):659–65.

50. Zheng Z, Zhao C, Su S, et al. Peroral endoscopic myotomy versus pneumatic dilation - result from a retrospective study with 1-year follow-up. Z Gastroenterol 2019;57(3):304–11. Perorale endoskopische Myotomie im Vergleich zu Ballondilatation - Ergebnisse einer retrospektiven Studie mit einjahrigem Follow-up.

51. Aiolfi A, Bona D, Riva CG, et al. Systematic review and bayesian network meta-analysis comparing laparoscopic heller myotomy, pneumatic dilatation, and peroral endoscopic myotomy for esophageal achalasia. J Laparoendosc Adv Surg Tech A 2019. https://doi.org/10.1089/lap.2019.0432.

52. Repici A, Fuccio L, Maselli R, et al. GERD after per-oral endoscopic myotomy as compared with Heller's myotomy with fundoplication: a systematic review with meta-analysis. Gastrointest Endosc 2018;87(4):934–943 e18.

53. Inoue H, Shiwaku H, Iwakiri K, et al. Clinical practice guidelines for peroral endoscopic myotomy. Dig Endosc 2018;30(5):563–79.

54. Zaninotto G, Bennett C, Boeckxstaens G, et al. The 2018 ISDE achalasia guidelines. Dis Esophagus 2018;31(9). https://doi.org/10.1093/dote/doy071.

55. Tanaka S, Kawara F, Toyonaga T, et al. Two penetrating vessels as a novel indicator of the appropriate distal end of peroral endoscopic myotomy. Dig Endosc 2018;30(2):206–11.

56. Shiwaku H, Inoue H, Sato H, et al. Peroral endoscopic myotomy for achalasia: a prospective multicenter study in Japan. Gastrointest Endosc 2020;91(5):1037–1044 e2.

57. Chandan S, Facciorusso A, Khan SR, et al. Short versus standard esophageal myotomy in achalasia patients: a systematic review and meta-analysis of comparative studies. Endosc Int Open 2021;9(8):E1246–54.

58. Nabi Z, Ramchandani M, Sayyed M, et al. Comparison of short versus long esophageal myotomy in cases with idiopathic achalasia: a randomized controlled trial. J Neurogastroenterol Motil 2021;27(1):63–70.

59. Ichkhanian Y, Abimansour JP, Pioche M, et al. Outcomes of anterior versus posterior peroral endoscopic myotomy 2 years post-procedure: prospective follow-up results from a randomized clinical trial. Endoscopy 2021;53(5):462–8.

60. Li C, Gong A, Zhang J, et al. Clinical outcomes and safety of partial full-thickness myotomy versus circular muscle myotomy in peroral endoscopic myotomy for achalasia patients. Gastroenterol Res Pract 2017;2017:2676513.

61. Teitelbaum EN, Soper NJ, Pandolfino JE, et al. Esophagogastric junction distensibility measurements during Heller myotomy and POEM for achalasia predict postoperative symptomatic outcomes. Surg Endosc 2015;29(3):522–8.

62. Inoue H, Shiwaku H, Kobayashi Y, et al. Statement for gastroesophageal reflux disease after peroral endoscopic myotomy from an international multicenter experience. Esophagus 2020;17(1):3–10.

63. Bapaye A, Gandhi AR, Bapaye J. Gastroesophageal reflux after peroral endoscopic myotomy: myth or reality? J Dig Endosc 2021;12(12):202–13.

64. Hernández-Mondragón OV, Solórzano-Pineda OM, González-Martínez M, et al. Gastroesophageal reflux disease after peroral endoscopic myotomy: Short-term, medium-term, and long-term resultsGastroesophageal reflux disease after peroral endoscopic myotomy (POEM). Revista de Gastroenterología de México (English Edition 2020;85(1):4–11.

65. Tyberg A, Choi A, Gaidhane M, et al. Transoral incisional fundoplication for reflux after peroral endoscopic myotomy: a crucial addition to our arsenal. Endosc Int Open 2018;6(5):E549–52.

66. Kumta NA, Kedia P, Sethi A, et al. Transoral incisionless fundoplication for treatment of refractory GERD after peroral endoscopic myotomy. Gastrointest Endosc 2015;81(1):224–5.

67. Inoue H, Ueno A, Shimamura Y, et al. Peroral endoscopic myotomy and fundoplication: a novel NOTES procedure. Endoscopy 2019;51(2):161–4.

68. Bapaye A, Dashatwar P, Dharamsi S, et al. Single-session endoscopic fundoplication after peroral endoscopic myotomy (POEM+F) for prevention of post gastroesophageal reflux - 1-year follow-up study. Endoscopy 2020. https://doi.org/10.1055/a-1332-5911.

69. Toshimori A, Inoue H, Shimamura Y, et al. Peroral endoscopic fundoplication: a brand-new intervention for GERD. VideoGIE 2020;5(6):244–6.

70. Camilleri M, Parkman HP, Shafi MA, et al, American College of G. Clinical guideline: management of gastroparesis. Am J Gastroenterol 2013;108(1):18–38.

71. Camilleri M, Bharucha AE, Farrugia G. Epidemiology, mechanisms, and management of diabetic gastroparesis. Clin Gastroenterol Hepatol 2011;9(1):5–12 [quiz; e7].

72. Rao AS, Camilleri M. Review article: metoclopramide and tardive dyskinesia. Aliment Pharmacol Ther 2010;31(1):11–9.

73. Bai Y, Xu MJ, Yang X, et al. A systematic review on intrapyloric botulinum toxin injection for gastroparesis. Digestion 2010;81(1):27–34.

74. Brewer Gutierrez OI, Khashab MA. Stent placement for the treatment of gastroparesis. Gastrointest Endosc Clin N Am 2019;29(1):107–15.

75. Hibbard ML, Dunst CM, Swanstrom LL. Laparoscopic and endoscopic pyloroplasty for gastroparesis results in sustained symptom improvement. J Gastrointest Surg 2011;15(9):1513–9.

76. Kawai M, Peretta S, Burckhardt O, et al. Endoscopic pyloromyotomy: a new concept of minimally invasive surgery for pyloric stenosis. Endoscopy 2012; 44(2):169–73.

77. Shlomovitz E, Pescarus R, Cassera MA, et al. Early human experience with peroral endoscopic pyloromyotomy (POP). Surg Endosc 2015;29(3):543–51.

78. Mekaroonkamol P, Li LY, Dacha S, et al. Gastric peroral endoscopic pyloromyotomy (G-POEM) as a salvage therapy for refractory gastroparesis: a case series of different subtypes. Neurogastroenterol Motil 2016;28(8):1272–7.

79. Rodriguez JH, Haskins IN, Strong AT, et al. Per oral endoscopic pyloromyotomy for refractory gastroparesis: initial results from a single institution. Surg Endosc 2017. https://doi.org/10.1007/s00464-017-5619-5.

80. Dacha S, Mekaroonkamol P, Li L, et al. Outcomes and quality-of-life assessment after gastric per-oral endoscopic pyloromyotomy (with video). Gastrointest Endosc 2017;86(2):282–9.

81. Gonzalez JM, Benezech A, Vitton V, et al. G-POEM with antro-pyloromyotomy for the treatment of refractory gastroparesis: mid-term follow-up and factors predicting outcome. Aliment Pharmacol Ther 2017;46(3):364–70.

82. Khashab MA, Ngamruengphong S, Carr-Locke D, et al. Gastric per-oral endoscopic myotomy for refractory gastroparesis: results from the first multicenter study on endoscopic pyloromyotomy (with video). Gastrointest Endosc 2017; 85(1):123–8.

83. Gonzalez JM, Lestelle V, Benezech A, et al. Gastric per-oral endoscopic myotomy with antropyloromyotomy in the treatment of refractory gastroparesis: clinical experience with follow-up and scintigraphic evaluation (with video). Gastrointest Endosc 2017;85(1):132–9.

84. Kahaleh M, Gonzalez JM, Xu MM, et al. Gastric peroral endoscopic myotomy for the treatment of refractory gastroparesis: a multicenter international experience. Endoscopy 2018. https://doi.org/10.1055/a-0596-7199.

85. Xu J, Chen T, Elkholy S, et al. Gastric peroral endoscopic myotomy (G-POEM) as a treatment for refractory gastroparesis: long-term outcomes. Can J Gastroenterol Hepatol 2018;2018:6409698.

86. Mekaroonkamol P, Shah R, Cai Q. Outcomes of per oral endoscopic pyloromyotomy in gastroparesis worldwide. World J Gastroenterol 2019;25(8):909–22. https://doi.org/10.3748/wjg.v25.i8.909.

87. Malik Z, Kataria R, Modayil R, et al. Gastric per oral endoscopic myotomy (G-POEM) for the treatment of refractory gastroparesis: early experience. Dig Dis Sci 2018;63(9):2405–12.

88. Abdelfatah MM, Noll A, Kapil N, et al. Long-term outcome of gastric per-oral endoscopic pyloromyotomy in treatment of gastroparesis. Clin Gastroenterol Hepatol 2021;19(4):816–24.

89. Vosoughi K, Ichkhanian Y, Benias P, et al. Gastric per-oral endoscopic myotomy (G-POEM) for refractory gastroparesis: results from an international prospective trial. Gut 2022;71(1):25–33.

90. Martinek J, Hustak R, Mares J, et al. Endoscopic pyloromyotomy for the treatment of severe and refractory gastroparesis: a pilot, randomised, sham-controlled trial. Gut 2022. https://doi.org/10.1136/gutjnl-2022-326904.

91. Spadaccini M, Maselli R, Chandrasekar VT, et al. Gastric peroral endoscopic pyloromyotomy for refractory gastroparesis: a systematic review of early outcomes with pooled analysis. Gastrointest Endosc 2020;91(4):746–52.e5.

92. Revicki DA, Rentz AM, Dubois D, et al. Gastroparesis Cardinal Symptom Index (GCSI): development and validation of a patient reported assessment of severity of gastroparesis symptoms. Qual Life Res 2004;13(4):833–44.

93. Uemura KL, Chaves D, Bernardo WM, et al. Peroral endoscopic pyloromyotomy for gastroparesis: a systematic review and meta-analysis. Endosc Int open 2020;8(7):E911–23.

94. Aghaie Meybodi M, Qumseya BJ, Shakoor D, et al. Efficacy and feasibility of G-POEM in management of patients with refractory gastroparesis: a systematic review and meta-analysis. Endosc Int Open 2019;7(3):E322–9.

95. Mohan BP, Chandan S, Jha LK, et al. Clinical efficacy of gastric per-oral endoscopic myotomy (G-POEM) in the treatment of refractory gastroparesis and predictors of outcomes: a systematic review and meta-analysis using surgical pyloroplasty as a comparator group. Surg Endosc 2020;34(8):3352–67.

96. Camilleri M, Sanders KM. Gastroparesis. Gastroenterology 2022;162(1):68–87.e1.

97. Labonde A, Lades G, Debourdeau A, et al. Gastric peroral endoscopic myotomy in refractory gastroparesis: long-term outcomes and predictive score to improve patient selection. Gastrointest Endosc. doi:10.1016/j.gie.2022.04.002

98. Shen S, Luo H, Vachaparambil C, et al. Gastric peroral endoscopic pyloromyotomy versus gastric electrical stimulation in the treatment of refractory gastroparesis: a propensity score-matched analysis of long term outcomes. Endoscopy 2020;52(5):349–58.

99. Landreneau JP, Strong AT, El-Hayek K, et al. Laparoscopic pyloroplasty versus endoscopic per-oral pyloromyotomy for the treatment of gastroparesis. Surg Endosc 2019;33(3):773–81.

100. Bizzotto A, Iacopini F, Landi R, et al. Zenker's diverticulum: exploring treatment options. Acta Otorhinolaryngol Ital 2013;33(4):219–29.

101. Chang CY, Payyapilli RJ, Scher RL. Endoscopic staple diverticulostomy for Zenker's diverticulum: review of literature and experience in 159 consecutive cases. Laryngoscope 2003;113(6):957–65.

102. Bonafede JP, Lavertu P, Wood BG, et al. Surgical outcome in 87 patients with Zenker's diverticulum. Laryngoscope 1997;107(6):720–5.

103. Albers DV, Kondo A, Bernardo WM, et al. Endoscopic versus surgical approach in the treatment of Zenker's diverticulum: systematic review and meta-analysis. Endosc Int Open 2016;4(6):E678–86.

104. Ishaq S, Sultan H, Siau K, et al. New and emerging techniques for endoscopic treatment of Zenker's diverticulum: State-of-the-art review. Dig Endosc 2018;30(4):449–60.

105. Costamagna G, Iacopini F, Bizzotto A, et al. Prognostic variables for the clinical success of flexible endoscopic septotomy of Zenker's diverticulum. Gastrointest Endosc 2016;83(4):765–73.

106. Yang J, Novak S, Ujiki M, et al. An international study on the use of peroral endoscopic myotomy in the management of Zenker's diverticulum. Gastrointest Endosc 2019. https://doi.org/10.1016/j.gie.2019.04.249.

107. Budnicka A, Januszewicz W, Białek AB, et al. Peroral endoscopic myotomy in the management of zenker's diverticulum: a retrospective multicenter study. J Clin Med 2021;10(2):187.

108. Sanaei O, Ichkhanian Y, Mondragon OVH, et al. Impact of prior treatment on feasibility and outcomes of Zenker's peroral endoscopic myotomy (Z-POEM). Endoscopy 2021;53(7):722–6.

109. Martinek J, Svecova H, Vackova Z, et al. Per-oral endoscopic myotomy (POEM): mid-term efficacy and safety. Surg Endosc 2018;32(3):1293–302.

110. Kahaleh M, Mahpour NY, Tyberg A, et al. Per oral endoscopic myotomy for zenker's diverticulum: a novel and superior technique compared with septotomy? J Clin Gastroenterol 2022;56(3):224–7.

111. Yang J, Zeng X, Yuan X, et al. An international study on the use of peroral endoscopic myotomy (POEM) in the management of esophageal diverticula: the first multicenter D-POEM experience. Endoscopy 2019;51(4):346–9.

112. Nabi Z, Chavan R, Asif S, et al. Per-oral Endoscopic Myotomy with Division of Septum (D-POEM) in Epiphrenic Esophageal Diverticula: Outcomes at a Median Follow-Up of Two Years. Dysphagia 2021. https://doi.org/10.1007/s00455-021-10339-8.

113. Zeng X, Bai S, Zhang Y, et al. Peroral endoscopic myotomy for the treatment of esophageal diverticulum: an experience in China. Surg Endosc 2021;35(5):1990–6.

114. Maydeo A, Patil GK, Dalal A. Operative technical tricks and 12-month outcomes of diverticular peroral endoscopic myotomy (D-POEM) in patients with symptomatic esophageal diverticula. Endoscopy 2019;51(12):1136–40.

115. Sharma S, Gupta DK. Hirschsprung's disease presenting beyond infancy: surgical options and postoperative outcome. Pediatr Surg Int 2012;28(1):5–8.

116. Pini Prato A, Gentilino V, Giunta C, et al. Hirschsprung's disease: 13 years' experience in 112 patients from a single institution. Pediatr Surg Int 2008;24(2):175–82.

117. Bapaye A, Bharadwaj T, Mahadik M, et al. Per-rectal endoscopic myotomy (PREM) for pediatric Hirschsprung's disease. Endoscopy 2018;50(6):E644–5.

118. Nabi Z, Chavan R, Shava U, et al. A novel endoscopic technique to obtain rectal biopsy specimens in children with suspected Hirschsprung's disease. VideoGIE 2018;3(5):157–8.

119. Bapaye A, Dashatwar P, Biradar V, et al. A novel third space endoscopic procedure, per-rectal endoscopic myotomy, for Hirschsprung's disease: Medium and long-term outcomes. Endoscopy 2020. https://doi.org/10.1055/a-1332-6902.

120. Bapaye A, Mahadik M, Kumar Korrapati S, et al. Per rectal endoscopic myotomy (PREM) for infantile hirschsprung's disease. Endoscopy 2018;50(04):OP209V.

121. Bandres D, Prada C, Soto J, et al. Per-anal endoscopic myotomy as rescue therapy for hirschsprung disease after unsuccessful surgical myectomy. ACG Case Rep J 2022;9(4):e00755.

Peroral Endoscopic Myotomy Technique, from Mouth to Anus

Roberta Maselli, MD, PhD[a,b], Marco Spadaccini, MD[a,b,*],
Gaia Pellegatta, MD[b], Alessandro Repici, MD[a,b]

KEYWORDS

- Third-space endoscopy • Submucosal tunneling • Endoscopic myotomy
- Vessel hemostasis • Clip closure

KEY POINTS

- From its introduction, peroral endoscopic myotomy (POEM) concept, intended as the ability to perform endoscopic myotomy, has been extended from the management of achalasia to several different dysmotility disorders along the entire gastrointestinal (GI) tract.
- Access to muscularis propria of the GI tract requires a preparation step with expansion of the submucosal layer and subsequent tunneling with creation of the third space.
- Despite several anatomic and technical variations, all POEM procedures are based on a very similar approach that entails, in most of the cases, general anesthesia and very similar setting of devices and electrosurgical modalities.
- Available data confirm that endoscopic myotomy performed in different clinical situations is an extremely safe procedure associated with outcomes at least equivalent to myotomy performed under surgical techniques.

INTRODUCTION

Peroral endoscopic myotomy (POEM) is a novel minimally invasive technique that has been established as an alternative treatment of esophageal achalasia more than 10 years ago.[1–3]

As originally described, POEM was an endoluminal procedure aimed at dissection of esophageal muscle fibers after extensive submucosal tunneling. After Inoue's first attempt of POEM for achalasia, indications of POEM expanded to include different subclasses of achalasia such as type I, type II, type III, failed prior treatments for achalasia, other dysmotility esophageal disorders, management of esophageal diverticula such as Zenker or epiphrenic diverticula (ED), gastroparesis, and treatment of selected cases of Hirschsprung disease.[4–8]

[a] Department of Biomedical Sciences, Pieve Emanuele, Humanitas University, Rozzano, Italy;
[b] Humanitas Clinical and Research Center -IRCCS-, Endoscopy Unit, Rozzano, Italy
* Corresponding author.
E-mail address: marco.spadaccini@humanitas.it

Gastrointest Endoscopy Clin N Am 33 (2023) 127–142
https://doi.org/10.1016/j.giec.2022.09.008
1052-5157/23/© 2022 Elsevier Inc. All rights reserved.

giendo.theclinics.com

It is important to remark that all variations of POEM procedures, regardless of the underlying disease, are challenging endoscopic surgical procedures that require advanced endoscopic skills. The authors believe that physicians approaching these procedures should prepare themselves and the entire team with an appropriate laboratory training and should perform the initial cases under proctoring of experts in POEM.

ACHALASIA AND ESOPHAGEAL DYSMOTILITY DISORDERS

POEM for achalasia represents the first natural orifice endoscopic surgical technique for "scarless" myotomy and has been the index technique over which all other POEM-like procedures have been modeled and rearranged.

Equipment

The key equipment for POEM include a high-definition standard upper gastrointestinal (GI) scope with water jet and carbon dioxide (CO_2) insufflator; an array of different transparent caps; and the latest generation, high-frequency electrosurgical units with intelligent systems for delivering current modalities with the ability to adapt response to tissue impedance and vessels coagulation. The distal attachment cap, whether straight or tapered, should be fixed with a highly adhesive, water-resistant tape to firmly attach the cap to the end of the scope, in order to minimize the risk of intraprocedural cap dislodgment.

Currently, 2 varieties of knives are used for most of the POEM procedures: the triangle tip (TT) knife (Olympus Medical, Tokyo, Japan) introduced by Inoue and the HybridKnife (ERBE, Tübingen, Germany) introduced by the Shanghai group. The HybridKnife is the only currently available knife that allows for pressure-controlled injection of fluid into the submucosa. In challenging situations, due to fibrosis, a narrow space for myotomy, or difficulty with orientation, an insulted tip (IT) knife has been also used, as the insulated tip may help in preventing injury to the mucosa of the esophageal side or to avoid direct contact with vessels located outside the distal esophageal wall or the gastroesophageal junction (GEJ) during the myotomy. The last device required for POEM procedures is a coagulation grasper to provide preventive coagulation of broad vessels and to control active bleeding that cannot be controlled with the knife.[9]

With regard to the most commonly used current settings, most of the studies report Endocut-Q for the mucosal incision, Swift Coag and Spray Coag for tunneling, and a combination of both for the myotomy. For the coagrasper, the recommended modality is Soft Coag, which allows for gentle coagulation with deep penetration, without carbonization, resulting in minimal adhesion of the device to the tissue.[9]

A wide range of different disposable and nondisposable, rotatable and nonrotatable clips have been reported with POEM procedures, and presently there is no evidence that one specific type is superior to the others.[10]

Preprocedure Preparation

The preoperative evaluation of patients with achalasia should include a barium swallow and manometry. Endoscopy should be performed to confirm diagnosis, evaluate the anatomic status of esophagus, and exclude other conditions such as cancer. High-resolution manometry is instrumental to provide a tailored approach based on the subtype of achalasia.[11,12]

Before POEM, patients should be prepared with clear fluids diet for at least 1 day. In our practice, we perform endoscopy at least 4 hours before the procedure to clear the esophagus from food or other debris and assess for candida esophagitis. Intravenous administration of a broad-spectrum antibiotic is recommended just before starting the procedure. Anticoagulants and antiplatelet medication are to be withheld before the intervention in accordance with relevant guidelines on operative and endoscopic procedures.

General anesthesia is required for when performing POEM. And although initially all procedures were carried out in the operating theater, nowadays many centers have moved POEM into the endoscopy suite without finding substantial changes in terms of safety for the patients, while improving operational time and patient turnover.[13]

For operative planning, appropriate scope orientation within the esophageal lumen is fundamental with the anterior point of the esophagus identified at the 12 o'clock position and the posterior point at the 6 o'clock position. Additional orientation on esophageal anatomy and preparation of intervention is determined by using imprints of recognizable extrinsic structures such as the aorta or spine when visible and pooling of instilled water along the posterior wall.[14]

Peroral Endoscopic Myotomy Steps

The POEM technique, originally described for achalasia, consists of 4 sequential steps: mucosotomy to get access to submucosal space; submucosal dissection and tunneling; myotomy proper; and finally closure of the mucosal defect.[15]

Mucosotomy

For the mucosal incision, an injection of a mixture of saline, epinephrine, and indigo carmine or methylene blue is performed to raise a submucosal bleb on top of where the mucosal incision will be performed. Since the standard technique of POEM includes 8 to 10 cm of myotomy, the mucosotomy should be started about 12 cm above the located GEJ. The incision is traditionally done longitudinally with careful dissecting of the lateral submucosal fibers at the edges of the linear incision to allow the gastroscope to be advanced into the third space (submucosa).

The main and most obvious advantage of a longitudinal mucosotomy is easy clip closure. Potential downsides may include difficult entry into the tunnel and a higher risk of insufflation-related adverse events.[16] Zhai and colleagues first reported the utility of a transverse mucosal incision[17] in order to facilitate access to submucosa and reduce the incidence of insufflation-related adverse events. According to this study, POEM with a transverse entry incision is associated with a significantly decrease in the operation time and reduction of the incidence of pneumatosis-related complications. A quite obvious downside of transverse incision is difficulty in the closure with clips. Subsequently, Ma and colleagues[18] described an inverted "T"-shaped incision for entry into the tunnel claiming easier scope entry, low incidence of gas-related events, and fewer clips required for closure. Presently, there is no randomized controlled trial demonstrating superiority of these modifications of the mucosotomy technique over the longitudinal incision.

Submucosal tunneling

After creation of the entry site, the scope is carefully advanced within the submucosa to create a longitudinal tunnel along the esophageal axis (**Fig. 1**). During this step, it is very important to preserve the mucosa, as it will be the only remaining barrier between the mediastinal space and esophageal lumen once myotomy has been completed. The technique of submucosal tunneling is identical to submucosal dissection during endoscopic submucosal dissection. Inside the tunnel, small blood vessels should be coagulated using the tip of the knife and forced coagulation current, whereas

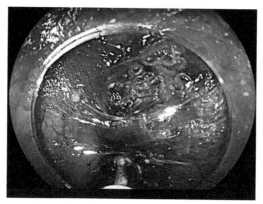

Fig. 1. POEM: submucosal tunneling during POEM for achalasia.

prophylactic hemostasis of larger vessels should be treated with coagraspers (**Fig. 2**). In the case of active bleeding, the irrigation with the water jet is of paramount importance to precisely identify the location of the bleed and proceed with coagulation using the tip of the knife or the coagrasper based on entity of bleeding and size of the vessel.[19]

The submucosal tunnel has to be extended a few centimeters below the GEJ, which is usually identified by multiple anatomic landmarks including visualization of the longitudinal muscle bundles, large-caliber, perforating vessels in the cardia representing branches of the left gastric artery, observation of aberrant longitudinal muscle bundle, progressive narrowing of the submucosal space, and resistance of advancing the endoscope thought GEJ, followed by expansion of the space in the gastric cardia. The presence of spiral or comma-shaped small vessels into the submucosa is an additional indicator.[20,21] Depth of insertion is also easily determined by the centimeter marks on the endoscope, and confirmation of extension of the submucosal tunnel to the cardia can be obtained with inspection of the cardia with a retroflexed scope in the gastric lumen, looking for markedly raised and blue-stained mucosa.

There is unanimous consensus among experts that overextension of the tunnel on the gastric side may result in an excessive myotomy, which may hypothetically predispose the patients to an increased risk of complications and development of post-POEM reflux.[22]

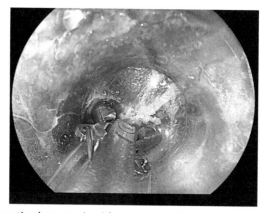

Fig. 2. POEM: preventive hemostasis with coagrasper during tunneling.

Myotomy

A selective myotomy is started 2 cm distal to the mucosotomy and should be extended 2 cm below the GEJ. Initially, the knife carefully dissects the muscle with spray or swift Coag until the proper dissection plane is found between the longitudinal muscle layer and the circular muscle layer. Once this plane is found, dissection is continued trying to preserve the longitudinal layer (**Fig. 3**). Even though a selective myotomy of the inner circular layer is targeted, most of the cases end up with full myotomy in the distal part of the esophagus and across the GEJ. Unintended full myotomy often occurs because of the pressure of the cap against the longitudinal outer muscle layer (which is very thin and fragile) in the narrow space of distal esophagus. Several experts have described this approach as progressive full-thickness myotomy: selective circular in upper portion and full thickness in distal part of the tunnel. In several studies, full-thickness myotomy seems to significantly reduce procedural time without increasing the risk of adverse events or reflux.[23]

The orientation of myotomy, originally reported on the anterior side, constitutes one of the most common variations in the technique. POEM via the posterior route (5 o'clock) has been described with the intent to facilitate the procedure and reduce the risk of adverse events. In several randomized trials comparing the outcomes of POEM when performed via an anterior or posterior approach, clinical success and adverse events rate have been found to be very similar.[24–27]

In several situations, myotomy by conventional routes (anterior or posterior) may not be feasible due to anatomic challenges or prior surgical or endoscopic attempts. In these cases, endoscopic myotomy can be performed successfully via a greater curvature approach, that is, 8 o'clock.[28]

The length of myotomy of the initial study by Inoue was approximately 8 cm (6 cm in the esophagus and 2 cm on gastric side). Subsequent studies described more or less similar length of myotomies. Although the length of gastric myotomy has been considered instrumental to the clinical success after surgical myotomy,[29] the same may not be true for esophageal myotomy. Recent studies have challenged the original dogma of long esophageal myotomy, introducing the concept of a short myotomy, which normally extends for approximately 5 cm in total. According to several studies and recent meta-analysis, short and longer myotomies reported similar outcomes with respect to clinical and technical success, length of hospital stay, and adverse events. However, abnormal esophageal acid exposure was less frequent and the procedure duration significantly shorter in the short myotomy group.[30,31]

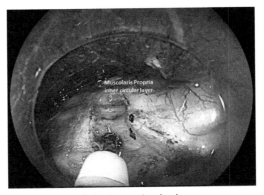

Fig. 3. POEM: selective myotomy of the inner circular layer.

Closure of the mucosotomy

After successful completion of the myotomy, careful inspection of the submucosal tunnel should be performed ensuring that any active bleeding is stopped before closure. The esophageal mucosa is then inspected for prompt diagnosis of incidental tear. Closure of the initial mucosal incision is usually performed with endoscopic clips, even though the use of endoscopic suturing devices has been reported.[32]

Special Situations

The presence of massive submucosal fibrosis (SMF) may pose several challenges to the POEM procedure. Indeed, severe fibrosis in the submucosal layer has been found to be the most important reason for technical failure during POEM.[33] In such situations, modified techniques may overcome the technical barriers. A modification technique of POEM (open-POEM) has been reported in 82 patients with achalasia.[34] With this approach, a mucosal incision is created 6 to 10 cm above the GEJ and extended at least 2 cm beyond the GEJ. Afterward, submucosal dissection and selective circular myotomy are performed without creating a submucosal tunnel.

Also, the double tunnel (DT) approach has been proposed[35] in patients with extensive SMF, which is typically associated with long disease duration, sigmoid esophagus, mucosal edema or extensive inflammation, and prior interventions. For the technique of DT-POEM, the mucosal incision and submucosal tunneling are similar to the standard fashion. When severe SMF is found and is not allowing proper distal extension of the submucosal tunnel, a second tunnel is created along the anterior or posterior esophageal wall depending on the initial site of tunneling. The site of the second submucosal injection is usually selected at least 1 to 2 cm distal to the initial incision along the alternate route (anterior or posterior). Subsequent procedure is completed using the standard technique of POEM. The mucosal incisions of both the tunnels are closed using a standard approach with clips.

Postprocedural Care

A soft diet can be started on day 2 postoperatively and continued for 10 to 14 days before starting a regular diet. Most of the investigators suggest the use of postprocedural antibiotics up to 7 days; however, their impact is still debated.[36] Proton pump inhibitors should be prescribed for a minimum of 14 days.

ZENKER DIVERTICULUM

Zenker diverticulum (ZD) is a pulsion-type diverticulum of the pharyngoesophageal junction, consisting of a posteriorly directed pouch between the cricopharyngeal muscle and inferior pharyngeal constrictor muscle.[37–39] Killian-Jamieson diverticulum is a mucosal protrusion distal to the cricopharyngeal muscle through an area of anatomic weakness, the Killian dehiscence. It is commonly asymptomatic but can also present dysphagic symptoms similar to ZD. However, this kind of diverticulum is usually distinguished from Zenker because of its location.

Traditionally, ZD has been treated surgically; however, the unneglectable risk of adverse events and mortality has made endotherapy the preferred approach since early 2000s. Initially the developed endoscopic approach,[40–42] also called flexible endoscopic septal division, has been associated with a significant risk of incomplete septotomy, especially in cases of a pouch with a septum shorter than 20 to 30 mm. The application of the third-space concept with protected access to the target muscle has been proposed with the intent to provide a more complete myotomy, without increasing the risks of adverse events.[6,43]

The preprocedural workup for patients with ZD is based on upper endoscopy and barium esophagogram. Dysphagia scores (ie, Dakkak and Bennet[44]) are used to grade symptoms severity and to assess treatment efficacy. The procedure is performed under general anesthesia with endotracheal intubation (ETI), having the patient in the left lateral decubitus position. No prophylactic antibiotic therapy is required. A standard gastroscope (2.8 mm working channel) with water jet and a transparent distal attachment is used. CO2 is required for insufflation.

Zenker Peroral Endoscopic Myotomy

This technique was described first by Zhou's group in 2016.[5] Once the septum is identified, a submucosal injection is performed 1 to 2 cm proximal to the septum using 5 to 10 mL of a blue-stained (indigo carmine or methylene blue) saline-based solution. A 1.5-cm longitudinal mucosotomy is subsequently performed with a standard endoscopic submucosal dissection knife using EndoCut current. The edges of the mucosal incision are undermined with coagulation current (forced or spray coagulation) to achieve access into the submucosal space with the aid of the cap.

A submucosal tunnel is then created in the direction of the septum maintaining the mucosal layer at 12 o'clock. The progression is facilitated by repeated injection of blue-dyed saline to bulk the submucosal space. Once the muscular septum is reached, tunneling is extended along both sides of the septum, ending 1 to 2 cm distal to the bottom of the diverticulum, in order to have an adequate endoscopic access of the entire muscular septum. During the dissection, any blood vessel encountered (or accidentally injured) is to be carefully coagulated with the tip of the knife. More rarely, in case of bigger vessels the use of hemostatic forceps with soft coagulation current may be required.

The cricopharyngeal muscle fibers of the septum are completely dissected using EndoCut current, down till the bottom of the diverticulum. We do suggest to extend the myotomy about 1 to 2 cm further to ensure completeness of myotomy and minimize risks of recurrence (**Fig. 4**). The esophageal mucosa is then inspected for any evidence of mucosal injury, and the mucosal incision site is finally sealed with up to 3 clips.

Peroral Endoscopic Septotomy

A variation of the "standard" Z-POEM was developed to overcome the technical challenges of this procedure.[45] Scoping at the boundaries between the pharynx and the upper esophageal sphincter, muscular spasms as well as anatomic limitations may reduce the ability to properly open and close the mucosal incision and access the submucosal space.

Hence, in order to allow more direct access to the septal muscle fibers, peroral endoscopic septotomy is performed by incising the mucosa directly on top of the septum, along its long axis (**Fig. 5**). Then submucosal dissection along both sides and the subsequent steps of standard Z-POEM are performed. Anatomic landmarks for myotomy extension are similar to Z-POEM. In our practice we try to extend myotomy until the muscularis propria of the esophagus becomes thin and easily distinguishable into the third space.

This approach may also allow to complete the treatment under deep sedation rather than general anesthesia with endotracheal intubation in order to avoid the risks of ETI and reduce the procedural time.[46]

Postprocedural Care

After the procedure, patients are kept fasting for 8 hours and then may have a trial of clear fluids. In the absence of symptoms or signs of early adverse events, patients may

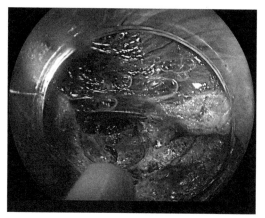

Fig. 4. Z-POEM: complete myotomy of the cricopharyngeal muscle.

be discharged home and are allowed to resume oral feeding with a soft diet the day after. Proton pump inhibitors should be prescribed for a minimum of 14 days.

EPIPHRENIC DIVERTICULA

ED are pulsion-type diverticula of the distal esophagus often associated with esophageal motility disorders, partially explaining the pathophysiology of this uncommon condition.[47] Traditional surgical options have high morbidity and mortality, whereas endoscopic septal division may properly manage the underlying motility dysfunction.[48] Hence the D-POEM procedure has been recently proposed.[49]

The diagnostic workup should include an upper endoscopy and a barium esophagogram in order to exclude alternative/associated conditions (ie, cancer) and complications (ie, fistulae). High-resolution esophageal manometry should be also performed during the initial assessment to precisely identify the underlying motility disorder. However, negotiating the access through the LES may be difficult by blind intubation during manometry.[50]

Patients are treated in left lateral position under general anesthesia and endotracheal intubation. A standard endoscope with water jet, fitted with a clear cap is used. As per all other third-space procedures, CO_2 insufflation system is mandatory. A broad-spectrum antibiotic given intravenously is recommended just before starting the procedure.[49,51–53]

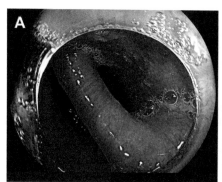
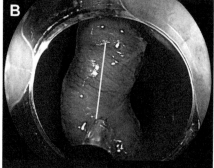

Fig. 5. Peroral Endoscopic Septotomy. (*A*) Zenker Diverticulum, endoscopic view. (*B*) Mucosal submucosal injection and mucosal incision.

As per standard POEM, patients should be instructed to follow a clear liquid diet for 2 days before the procedure to reduce the risk of retained food. In many cases, after the initial endoscopic examination, cleaning of the esophageal lumen and the diverticulum may be required using saline

Following the POEM principles, a mucosal bleb is created a few centimeters proximal to the diverticular septum by injecting 10 to 20 mL of a blue-stained saline-based solution. Then a 1-cm longitudinal mucosal incision, serving as the tunnel entry, is created with an endoscopic submucosal dissection knife using EndoCut mode. The submucosal fibers are dissected with coagulation current toward the septum with the aid of the clear cap, creating the submucosal tunnel. The tunnel is extended along both sides of the septum until it is entirely exposed. In this situation extra caution is recommended either during tunneling or during myotomy due to close contact with most of the relevant anatomic structures of the mediastinum including the heart and great vessels. The esophageal side tunnel is extended at the level of the GEJ to ensure complete myotomy and to deal with the underlying condition. The septotomy is then performed using the EndoCut current. Under direct endoscopic view, the muscle fibers of the septum are completely dissected down to the bottom of the diverticulum. The myotomy is then extended at least 2 cm beyond the GEJ. The mucosotomy is finally sealed starting from the most distal end of the incision to facilitate approximation.[49,51–53]

Patients are routinely admitted overnight for observation and kept nil per os (NPO) until the following day when a liquid diet can be started. The postprocedural management of standard POEM is routinely followed.

Gastroparesis

Gastroparesis is a chronic disorder characterized by delayed gastric emptying in the absence of a mechanical obstruction. The main types are idiopathic, postsurgical, and diabetes related. Regardless of the type, very limited treatment options are available, mainly comprising medications or surgical approaches. Diagnosis is confirmed based on evocative symptoms and delayed gastric emptying by gastric emptying scintigraphy.

The first gastric peroral pyloromyotomy (G-POEM) was reported in humans in 2013 by Khashab and colleagues,[7] and since then many specialized centers globally have reported data on the technical outcomes and mid- to long-term results of G-POEM showing excellent safety outcomes.

In general, G-POEM has shown good early-term and satisfactory mid- and long-term outcomes. Recently the G-POEM has also been described in pediatric patients.[54]

Typically, patients remained on a clear liquid diet for 72 hours before the procedure and (NPO) from midnight on the day of the procedure to ensure adequate gastric clearance on the procedure day. Antibiotic prophylaxis, typically with third-generation cephalosporins, is commonly administered.

The procedure is performed by an expert physician with the patient under general anesthesia and endotracheal intubation, in the supine position. Some centers place the patient on the left lateral position, to reduce the loop of the endoscope in the stomach. As far as the accessories are concerned, the use of different knifes has been described, depending on operator preference: TT-knife (Olympus), HybridKnife (ERBE, Tübingen, Germany), HookKnife (Olympus), and IT-Knife (Olympus).[55]

From a technical point of view, the procedure can be divided into 4 main steps:

Step 1: after submucosal injection of a blue-stained solution (saline solution or glycerol mixture), a longitudinal mucosal 15-mm incision is made 4 to 5 cm from the pylorus. (EndoCut I, effect 2, VIO-200D or 300D; ERBE, Tübingen, Germany). The incision is generally performed on the greater gastric curvature, about 5 to 6 cm proximal to pylorus with the endoscope in a neutral position (**Fig. 6**). Some operators prefer the lesser curvature and rarely the anterior or posterior wall.

Step 2: entering from this point, a submucosal tunnel is made using an electrosurgical knife reaching the pylorus. Submucosal vessels are carefully coagulated using the tip of the knife or coagulation forceps with soft coagulation.

Step 3: after the identification of the pylorus (usually it has a white arch appearance), it is dissected distally to proximally (from the duodenal to the gastric side) until the serosa (visible as a pink membrane) has been reached in case of a full-thickness myotomy. The length of the myotomy should be between 2 cm and 3.5 cm, proximally including 2 cm from the antral muscularis propria (EndoCut I, effect 2). Either single or double direct myotomy on the ring can be performed.

Step 4: the tunnel entry is firmly closed; closure has been described using standard clips, over-the-scope clips, cyanoacrylate, or more recently endo-suturing, according to availability and expertise.[56]

Throughout the procedure, the abdomen of the patients is carefully evaluated for any abnormal distension and/or emphysema. P_{CO_2} and peak pressure on the ventilator as well are closely monitored as an early indicator of capnoperitoneum. At the end of the procedure, if no significant abdominal distension or subcutaneous emphysema is noted, patients are extubated and moved to a recovery unit.

Complications of the procedure are mainly the abovementioned pneumoperitoneum (minor complication), intra- and postprocedural bleeding, perforation of the mucosa overlying the tunnel (mucosotomy), and, rarely, gastric ulcers and pyloric stenosis (6.8%).[57]

Postprocedure Care

In most of the centers the procedure is done with admitted patients, but recent evidences of a same-day discharge have been reported.[58] Patients are allowed to resume a liquid diet on the day after the operation (in most of the center after an upper GI radiography to rule out any complication) and begin a solid diet on the third to the seventh day, depending by local protocols.

Proton pump inhibitor therapy is initiated after the procedure and continued for 1 to 2 months.[59,60]

Patients are usually followed-up after 4 weeks with a repeat gastric emptying study. Clinical and endoscopic evaluations can be performed every 6 months, depending on patients' symptoms and local protocols.

HIRSCHSPRUNG DISEASE

The per-rectal endoscopic myotomy (PREM) is a minimally invasive procedure first described in 2016 by Bapaye and colleagues[8] for the treatment of Hirschsprung disease (HD), a congenital disorder characterized by the loss of intrinsic ganglion cells in the bowel submucosal and myenteric plexuses.[61] The rationale behind PREM is to perform tailored myotomy of the distal hypertonic colonic segments using a third-space endoscopic technique.

The PREM approach has been reported both in adults and pediatric patients.[8,61–63]

Preoperative Evaluation

The preoperative evaluation procedure includes a contrast enema and an anorectal manometry. A sigmoidoscopy with serial deep muco-submucosal biopsies should also be performed in order to confirm the diagnosis of HD and to measure the

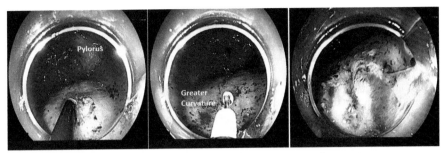

Fig. 6. G-POEM: mucosal incision performed on the greater gastric curvature.

aganglionic segment and tailor the myotomy length. Deep biopsies should be carried out with the specific cap-assisted endoscopic mucosal resection technique from the dilated segment up to 2 cm above the dentate line.[64]

Patients should be on a clear liquid and low-residue diet and receive bowel preparation with polyethylene glycol solution for 2 days before the procedure.

Per-rectal Endoscopic Myotomy

An intravenous third-generation cephalosporin and metronidazole is administered on the day of the intervention. As with the other third-space endoscopic procedures, the PREM should also be performed under general anesthesia with an endotracheal intubation with patients placed in a prone position.

Subsequent to the creation of a submucosal bleb, using a saline solution and methylene blue, the mucosal incision should be performed 1 cm beyond the anorectal junction along the posterior rectal wall. After the careful disruption of the submucosal fibers, it is possible to introduce the endoscope into the submucosa and create the tunnel, dissecting close to the muscle layer and perpendicular to the circular muscular fibers. The submucosal tunnel should be extended for 1 to 2 cm proximal to the transition zone, whose position is established during the preoperative sigmoidoscopy.

In the first description of PREM, Bapaye and colleagues[8] suggested to use fluoroscopy to confirm crossing of the sacral promontory and the tunnel adequacy.

Full-thickness myotomy is then performed starting from the proximal apex of the submucosal tunnel to the distal rectum. The fibers of the internal anal sphincter are divided from the circular muscle fibers that undergo myotomy; the external anal sphincter must be preserved from the myotomy.

At the end of the procedure, the closure of the mucosal incision is achieved with endoscopic clips.

Postprocedural Care

Twelve hours after PREM, an oral diet can be initiated, and the patients should be discharged after the first bowel movement. Low doses of lactulose should be prescribed for 14 days.

CLINICS CARE POINTS

- All patients undergoing POEM should have preprocedural imaging with esophagram, manometry, and upper endoscopy to confirm diagnosis, rule out other pathology, and define anatomy.

- The 4 steps of POEM, mucosotomy, tunneling, myotomy, and mucosal closure, are invariable regardless of the anatomic location of the procedure. Care should be taken at each step to ensure that no adverse events have occurred. Hemostasis should be confirmed before tunnel closure. The mucosa should be inspected at the completion of the procedure to ensure no defects.

- It is important to prophylactically coagulate vessels during all steps of the procedure, particularly during dissection of the tunnel, in order to prevent severe bleeding. The device used, with either the electrosurgical knife or coagulation graspers, should be determined based on vessel size and source.

- Attention should be paid to the degree of SMF when starting the tunnel. If an adequate tunnel cannot be created, a second tunnel should be attempted in order to prevent mucosal damage.

- If capnoperitoneum or capnothorax occur, needle decompression should be performed.

DISCLOSURES

Repici A: Boston Scientific consulting fee, research grant, speaker fee, ERBE consulting fee, research grant, speaker fee, Fujifilm consulting fee, research grant, speaker fee, Olympus consulting fee. Maselli R: Consulting fee Erbe and Boston Scientific. Spadaccini M and Pellegatta G have no conflicts of interest to disclose.

REFERENCES

1. Pasricha PJ, Hawari R, Ahmed I, et al. Submucosal endoscopic esophageal myotomy: a novel experimental approach for the treatment of achalasia. Endoscopy 2007;39:761–4. https://doi.org/10.1055/s-2007-966764.
2. Inoue H, Minami H, Satodate H, et al. First clinical experience of submucosal endoscopic esophageal myotomy for esophageal achalasia with no skin incision. Gastrointest Endosc 2009;69:AB122.
3. Werner YB, Hakanson B, Martinek J, et al. Endoscopic or surgical myotomy in patients with idiopathic achalasia. N Engl J Med 2019;381:2219–29.
4. Ichkhanian Y, Sanaei O, Canakis A, et al. Esophageal peroral endoscopic myotomy (POEM) for treatment of esophagogastric junction outflow obstruction: results from the first prospective trial. Endosc Int Open 2020;8(9):E1137–43. https://doi.org/10.1055/a-1198-4643.
5. Li QL, Chen WF, Zhang XC, et al. Submucosal Tunneling Endoscopic Septum Division: A Novel Technique for Treating Zenker's Diverticulum. Gastroenterology 2016;151:1071–4.
6. Brewer Gutierrez OI, Ichkhanian Y, Spadaccini M, et al. Zenker's Diverticulum Per-Oral Endoscopic Myotomy Techniques: Changing Paradigms. Gastroenterology 2019;156(8):2134–5.
7. Khashab MA, Stein E, Clarke JO, et al. Gastric peroral endoscopic myotomy for refractory gastroparesis: first human endoscopic pyloromyotomy (with video). Gastrointest Endosc 2013;78:764–8.
8. Bapaye A, Wagholikar G, Jog S, et al. Per rectal endoscopic myotomy for the treatment of adult Hirschsprung's disease: first human case (with video). Dig Endosc 2016;28:680–4.
9. Stavropoulos SN, Desilets DJ, Fuchs K-H, et al. Per-oral endoscopic myotomy white paper summary. Gastrointest Endosc 2014;80(1):1–15.

10. Inoue H, Tianle KM, Ikeda H, et al. Peroral endoscopic myotomy for esophageal achalasia: technique, indication, and outcomes. Thorac Surg Clin 2011;21(4): 519–25.

11. Yadlapati R, Kahrilas PJ, Fox MR, et al. Esophageal motility disorders on high-resolution manometry: Chicago classification version 4.0(a). Neu- Rogastroen-terol Motil 2021;33:e14058.

12. Campagna RAJ, Carlson DA, Hungness ES, et al. Intraoperative assessment of esophageal motility using FLIP during myotomy for achalasia. Surg Endosc 2019. https://doi.org/10.1007/s00464-019-07028-x.

13. Yang D, Pannu D, Zhang Q, et al. Evaluation of anesthesia management, feasi-bility and efficacy of peroral endoscopic myotomy (POEM) for achalasia per-formed in the endoscopy unit. Endosc Int Open 2015;3:E289–95. https://doi.org/10.1055/s-0034-1391965.

14. Stavropoulos SN. Per Oral Endoscopic Myotomy, Equipment and Technique: A Step-by-Step Explanation. Video J Encyclopedia GI Endosc 2013;1(1):96–100.

15. Khashab MA, Kumbhari V, Kalloo AN, et al. Peroral endoscopic myotomy: a 4-step approach to a challenging procedure. Gastrointest Endosc 2014;79:997–8.

16. Chai NL, Li HK, Linghu EQ, et al. Consensus on the digestive endoscopic tunnel technique. World J Gastroenterol 2019;25(7):744–76.

17. Zhai Y, Linghu E, Li H, et al. Comparison of peroral endoscopic myotomy with transverse entry incision versus longitudinal entry incision for achalasia Nan Fang Yi Ke Da Xue Xue Bao 2013;33:1399–402.

18. Ma XB, Linghu EQ, Li HK, et al. [Factors affecting the safety and efficacy of peroral endoscopic myotomy for achalasia], 36. Nan Fang Yi Ke Da Xue Xue Bao; 2016. p. 892–7.

19. Bechara R, Onimaru M, Ikeda, et al. Per-oral endoscopic myotomy, 1000 cases later: pearls, pitfalls, and practical considerations. Gastrointest Endosc 2016; 84(2):330–8.

20. Minami H, Inoue H, Haji A, et al. Per-oral endoscopic myotomy: emerging indica-tions and evolving techniques. Dig Endosc 2015;27:175–81.

21. Stavropoulos SN, Modayil RJ, Friedel D, et al. The International Per Oral Endo-scopic Myotomy Survey (IPOEMS): a snapshot of the global POEM experience. Surg Endosc 2013;27:3322–38.

22. Grimes KL, Bechara R, Shimamura Y, et al. Gastric myotomy length affects severity but not rate of post-procedure reflux: 3-year follow-up of a prospective randomized controlled trial of double-scope per-oral endoscopic myotomy (POEM) for esophageal achalasia. Surg Endosc 2020;34(7):2963–8.

23. Li QL, Chen WF, Zhou PH, et al. Peroral endoscopic myotomy for the treatment of achalasia: a clinical comparative study of endoscopic full-thickness and circular muscle myotomy. J Am Coll Surg 2013;217:442–51.

24. Ramchandani M, Nabi Z, Reddy DN, et al. Outcomes of anterior myotomy versus posterior myotomy during POEM: a randomized pilot study. Endosc Int Open 2018;6:E190–8. https://doi.org/10.1055/s-0043-121877.

25. Tan Y, Lv L, Wang X, et al. Efficacy of anterior versus posterior per-oral endo-scopic myotomy for treating achalasia: a randomized, prospective study. Gastro-intest Endosc 2018;88:46–54. https://doi.org/10.1016/j.gie.2018.03.009.

26. Khashab MA, Sanaei O, Rivory J, et al. Peroral endoscopic myotomy: anterior versus posterior approach: a randomized single-blinded clinical trial. Gastroint-est Endosc 2020;91:288–297e7.

27. Ichkhanian Y, Abimansour JP, Pioche M, et al. Outcomes of anterior versus posterior peroral endoscopic myotomy 2 years post-procedure: prospective follow-up results from a randomized clinical trial. Endoscopy 2021;53:462–8.

28. Onimaru M, Inoue H, Ikeda H, et al. Greater curvature myotomy is a safe and effective modified technique in per-oral endoscopic myotomy (with videos). Gastrointest Endosc 2015;81:1370–7.

29. Oelschlager BK, Chang L, Pellegrini CA. Improved outcome after extended gastric myotomy for achalasia. Arch Surg 2003;138:490–5, discussion 495–497.

30. Nabi Z, Talukdar R, Mandavdhare H, et al. Short versus long esophageal myotomy during peroral endoscopic myotomy: A systematic review and meta-analysis of comparative trials. Saudi J Gastroenterol 2022;28(4):261–7.

31. Vaezi MF, Pandolfino JE, Yadlapati RH, et al. ACG clinical guidelines: diagnosis and management of achalasia. Am J Gastroenterol 2020;115:1393–411.

32. Kumbhari V, Azola A, Saxena P, et al. Closure methods in submucosal endoscopy. Gastrointest Endosc 2014;80:894–5.

33. Wu QN, Xu XY, Zhang XC, et al. Submucosal fibrosis in achalasia patients is a rare cause of aborted peroral endoscopic myotomy procedures. Endoscopy 2017;49:736–44.

34. Liu W, Zeng XH, Yuan XL, et al. Open peroral endoscopic myotomy for the treatment of achalasia: a case series of 82 cases. Dis Esophagus 2019;32(10):1–7.

35. Nabi Z, Ramchandani M, Chavan R, et al. Double tunnel technique reduces technical failure during POEM in cases with severe submucosal fibrosis. Endosc Int Open 2021;16:9.

36. Maselli R, Oliva A, Badalamenti M, et al. Single-dose versus short-course prophylactic antibiotics for peroral endoscopic myotomy: a randomized controlled trial. Gastrointest Endosc 2021;94(5):922–9. https://doi.org/10.1016/j.gie.2021.05.045.

37. Zenker FA, von Ziemssen H. Krankheiten des oesophagus. In: von Ziemssen H, ed. Handbuch der Speciellen. Pathologie and Therapie 1877;7(Suppl) Leipzig: FCW Vogel.

38. Shaw DW, Cook IJ, Jamieson GG, et al. Influence of surgery on deglutitive upper oesophageal sphincter mechanics in Zenker's diverticulum. Gut 1996;38:806–11.

39. Cook IJ, Gabb M, Panagopoulos V, et al. Pharyngeal (Zenker's) diverticulum is a disorder of upper esophageal sphincter opening. Gastroenterology 1992;103: 1229–35.

40. Ishioka S, Sakai P, Maluf Filho F, et al. Endoscopic incision of Zenker's diverticula. Endoscopy 1995;27:433–7.

41. Costamagna G, Iacopini F, Tringali A, et al. Flexible endoscopic Zenker's diverticulotomy: cap-assisted technique vs. diverticuloscope-assisted technique. Endoscopy 2007;39:146–52.

42. Repici A, Cappello A, Spadaccini M, et al. Cap-Assisted Endoscopic Septotomy of Zenker's Diverticulum: Early and Long-Term Outcomes. Am J Gastroenterol 2021;116(9):1853–8. https://doi.org/10.14309/ajg.0000000000001356.

43. Maselli R, Spadaccini M, Cappello A, et al. Flexible endoscopic treatment for Zenker's diverticulum: from the lumen to the third space. Ann Gastroenterol 2021;34(2):149–54. https://doi.org/10.20524/aog.2021.0575.

44. Dakkak M, Bennett JR. A new dysphagia score with objective validation. J Clin Gastroenterol 1992;14:99–100.

45. Repici A, Spadaccini M, Belletrutti PJ, et al. Peroral endoscopic septotomy for short-septum Zenker's diverticulum. Endoscopy 2020;52(7):563–8. https://doi.org/10.1055/a-1127-3304.

46. Spadaccini M, Maselli R, Chandrasekar VT, et al. Submucosal tunnelling techniques for Zenker's diverticulum: a systematic review of early outcomes with pooled analysis. Eur J Gastroenterol Hepatol 2021;33(1S Suppl 1):e78–83. https://doi.org/10.1097/MEG.0000000000002318.

47. Soares R, Herbella FA, Prachand VN, et al. Epiphrenic diverticulum of the esophagus. From pathophysiology to treatment. J Gastrointest Surg 2010;14:2009 –15.

48. Tapias LF, Morse CR, Mathisen DJ, et al. Surgical management of esophageal epiphrenic diverticula: a transthoracic approach over four decades. Ann Thorac Surg 2017;104:1123–30.

49. Yang J, Zeng X, Yuan X, et al. An international study on the use of peroral endoscopic myotomy (POEM) in the management of esophageal diverticula: the frst multicenter D-POEM experience. Endoscopy 2019;51:346–9.

50. Nadaleto BF, Herbella FAM, Patti MG. Treatment of Achalasia and Epiphrenic Diverticulum. World J Surg 2022;46(7):1547–53. https://doi.org/10.1007/s00268-022-06476-2.

51. Samanta J, Mandavdhare HS, Kumar N, et al. Per oral endoscopic myotomy for the management of large esophageal diverticula (D-POEM): safe and efective modality for complete septotomy. Dysphagia 2022;37(1):84–92.

52. Zeng X, Bai S, Zhang Y, et al. Peroral endoscopic myotomy for the treatment of esophageal diverticulum: an experience in China. Surg Endosc 2021;35(5): 1990–6.

53. Maydeo A, Patil GK, Dalal A. Operative technical tricks and 12-month outcomes of diverticular peroral endoscopic myotomy (D-POEM) in patients with symptomatic esophageal diverticula. Endoscopy 2019;51:1136–40.

54. Zhang H, Liu Z, Ma L, et al. Gastric Peroral Endoscopic Pyloromyotomy for Infants with Congenital Hypertrophic Pyloric Stenosis. Am J Gastroenterol 2022.

55. Verga MC, Mazza S, Azzolini F, et al. Gastric per-oral endoscopic myotomy: Indications, technique, results and comparison with surgical approach. World J Gastrointest Surg 2022;14(1):12–23.

56. Hustak R, Vackova Z, Krajciova J, et al. Endoscopic clips versus overstitch suturing system device for mucosotomy closure after peroral endoscopic pyloromyotomy (G-POEM): a prospective single-center study. Surg Endosc 2022.

57. Spadaccini M, Maselli R, Chandrasekar VT, et al. Gastric peroral endoscopic pyloromyotomy for refractory gastroparesis: a systematic review of early outcomes with pooled analysis. Gastrointest Endosc 2020;91:746–52, e5.

58. Shah R, Chen H, Calderon LF, et al. Safety and feasibility of same day discharge after per oral endoscopic pyloromyotomy in refractory gastroparesis: a pilot study. Chin Med J (Engl) 2022.

59. Labonde A, Lades G, Debourdeau A, et al. Gastric peroral endoscopic myotomy in refractory gastroparesis: long-term outcomes and predictive score to improve patient selection. Gastrointest Endosc 2022;96(3):500–8.e2.

60. Hernández Mondragón OV, Contreras LFG, Velasco GB, et al. Gastrointest Gastric peroral endoscopic myotomy outcomes after 4 years of follow-up in a large cohort of patients with refractory gastroparesis (with video). Endosc 2022;96(3):487–99.

61. Martucciello G. Hirschsprung's disease, one of the most difficult diagnoses in pediatric surgery: a review of the problems from clinical practice to the bench. Eur J Pediatr Surg 2008;18(3):140–9.

62. Bapaye A, Bharadwaj T, Mahadik M, et al. Correction: Per-rectal endoscopic myotomy (PREM) for pediatric Hirschsprung's disease. Endoscopy 2018;50(6):C9. https://doi.org/10.1055/a-0666-6232.

63. Bapaye A, Dashatwar P, Biradar V, et al. Initial experience with per-rectal endoscopic myotomy for Hirschsprung's disease: medium and long term outcomes of the first case series of a novel third-space endoscopy procedure. Endoscopy 2021;53(12):1256–60. https://doi.org/10.1055/a-1332-6902.
64. Nabi Z, Chavan R, Shava U, et al. A novel endoscopic technique to obtain rectal biopsy specimens in children with suspected Hirschsprung's disease. VideoGIE 2018;3:157.

Submucosal Tunneling Techniques for Tumor Resection

Zi-Han Geng, MD[a,b], Ping-Hong Zhou, MD, PhD[a,b],
Ming-Yan Cai, MD, PhD[a,b],*

KEYWORDS

- Third space endoscopy • Endoscopic submucosal tunnel dissection (ESTD)
- Submucosal tunneling endoscopic resection (STER) • Submucosal tumors (SMTs)
- Extraluminal tumors

KEY POINTS

- Endoscopic submucosal tunnel dissection is an innovative technique for large superficial esophageal squamous cell neoplasms.
- Submucosal tunneling endoscopic resection (STER) is a safe and effective treatment modality for gastrointestinal (GI) submucosal tumors (SMTs), preferably originating from the muscularis propria layer.
- STER for extraluminal tumors is a feasible, safe, and effective endoscopic technique to achieve a curative resection for SMTs with a predominant extraluminal growth pattern or extra-GI tumors.

INTRODUCTION

The first space represented the natural lumen of the gastrointestinal (GI) tract. Conventional endoscopic procedures are considered as the first space endoscopy. In the last two decades, endoscopic pioneers described natural orifice transluminal endoscopic surgery (NOTES) which allowed entry into the peritoneal cavity (the second space) for surgical interventions.[1] Given the major concern with NOTES that is the secure closure of the entry point into the peritoneal cavity, the third space with mucosal flap safety valve was applied.[2] Submucosal space, as the third space, is a potential space located between the mucosa and muscularis propria (MP) layer of the GI wall, and can be opened up and used as a working tunnel. Because the intact mucosal flap prevented any peritoneal leakage, the endoscopist could use the tunnel to perform

a Endoscopy Center and Endoscopy Research Institute, Zhongshan Hospital, Fudan University, Shanghai, China; b Shanghai Collaborative Innovation Center of Endoscopy, Shanghai, China
* Corresponding author. Endoscopy Center and Endoscopy Research Institute, Zhongshan Hospital, Fudan University, 180 FengLin Road, Shanghai 200032, P. R. China.
E-mail address: cai.mingyan@qq.com

Gastrointest Endoscopy Clin N Am 33 (2023) 143–154
https://doi.org/10.1016/j.giec.2022.07.002
1052-5157/23/© 2022 Elsevier Inc. All rights reserved.

interventions in the MP layer or breech it to enter the mediastinum or peritoneal cavity without full thickness perforation. Therefore, the era of clinical third space endoscopy started. The third space endoscopy opened up horizons for endoscopic interventions, such as achalasia, mucosal lesions, submucosal tumors (SMTs), extraluminal tumors, gastroparesis, and Zenker diverticulum. In this review article, the authors aimed to discuss the indications, techniques, clinical management, and adverse events of submucosal tunneling techniques for tumor resection.

Indications

Through the tunnel, endoscopic diagnosis and treatment can be performed for mucosal lesions, SMTs, and even tumors outside the GI tract. The application of submucosal tunneling techniques covers the following,[1] mucosal lesions, such as esophageal or rectal large or circular early-stage cancer[3–6];[2] GI SMTs; and[3] tumors outside the GI tract, such as benign tumor excision in the mediastinum[7] or abdominal cavity[8] (**Fig. 1**).

Circumferential endoscopic resection for esophageal mucosal lesions has been considered to be noninvasive, with a low complication rate and good short-term clinical efficacy.[9–11] Next, endoscopic submucosal tunnel dissection (ESTD), as an innovative technique, was introduced to treat large superficial esophageal squamous cell neoplasms.[12,13] ESTD has been rapidly spread and widely used around the world, especially in the endoscopic treatment of large or circular early esophageal cancer. Single-tunnel or multi-tunnel procedures are optional for lesions of different sizes. Compared with endoscopic submucosal dissection (ESD), ESTD had a shorter operation time, faster dissection, higher complete resection rate, and lower complication rate.[14] A consensus reported that ESTD is indicated for lesions not invading deeper than SM_1 and without clinical evidence of lymph node metastasis, and at least one-third of the circumference and ≥ 20 mm in diameter.[13] The Japan Gastroenterological Endoscopy Society has developed endoscopic dissection guidelines for esophageal cancer and suggested that endoscopic resection is weakly recommended for superficial squamous cell carcinomas with a major axis length ≤ 50 mm and involving the entire circumference of the esophagus, upon implementing preventive measures for stenosis.[15]

Submucosal tunneling endoscopic resection (STER) was first described by Xu and colleagues.[16] This technique is a paradigm shift in endoscopy, which is considered as a solution for the endoscopic removal of SMTs. This technique was first introduced for

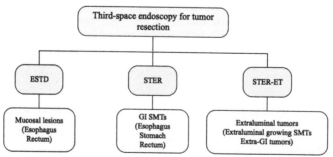

Fig. 1. Third-space endoscopy procedures for tumor resection. ESTD, endoscopic submucosal tunnel dissection; GI, gastrointestinal; SMTs, submucosal tumors; STER, submucosal tunneling endoscopic resection; STER-ET, submucosal tunnel endoscopic resection for extraluminal tumors.

esophageal SMTs and then extended to the gastric and the rectal tumors. It has been reported that SMTs less than 3.0 cm in diameter from the esophagus and cardia might be the appropriate application for STER.[17,18] Size may determine whether a lesion will be amenable to STER. Giant SMTs are difficult to retrieve after the endoscopic resection.[19] Besides, giant SMTs may have effects on en bloc resection and adverse events.[17,20–22] It was suggested that the implementation of STER for SMTs with a long diameter ≤5.0 cm and a transverse diameter ≤3.5 cm could facilitate a high en bloc resection rate.[23] However, some endoscopists considered that even when the tumor size was larger than 3.5 cm, STER still seems to be a feasible and effective method for SMTs in the upper GI tract.[24] It was believed that both endoscopic submucosal excavation (ESE) and STER had satisfactory therapeutic results for SMTs less than 10 mm, and STER was a preferable choice for SMTs more than 10 mm, especially when the perforation is likely to happen.[25] Therefore, the upper limit of the tumor diameter for a successful STER remains controversial. An alternative approach is to generate a second window, either in the area of the tumor or through a distal mucosal incision to facilitate en bloc extraction for large tumors.

Irregular morphology of SMTs was an independent risk factor for failure of en bloc resection.[26] Chen identified that STER for large tumors with irregular shapes in the deep MP layer is feasible but associated with a relatively high likelihood of piecemeal resection and complications.[23] In addition, in order to create the submucosal space, relatively straight and tubular structures are suitable locations for STER, such as the esophagus and cardia.[27] However, STER is also applicable in the stomach and rectum without an increase in adverse events.[27,28] The size, morphology, and location of the tumor that are fit for endoscopic resection has no fixed criteria but rather depends on the comfort level of the operator.

It is essential that SMTs with ulcers are not recommended for STER as the integrity of the mucosa cannot be maintained. Besides, STER should not be used if there is any evidence of metastasis, vascular invasion, or abundance of vascular supply in SMTs.[22,24,29] In addition to the above factors of SMTs, our study indicated that the direction of the gastroscope also contributed to determining endoscopic methods. The direction of the gastroscope where SMTs were observed directly could help endoscopists estimate the maneuverable space and directions of endoscopic instruments. Based on our clinical observations and experiences, we summarized the propriety of STER and non-tunnel techniques for SMTs in different aspects[30] (**Table 1**).

Besides mucosal lesions and SMTs, STER can also be used for extraluminal tumors (STER-ET) including extraluminal growing SMTs and extra-GI tumors.[7,8,31–34] It has been reported that STER appeared to be a feasible, safe, and effective endoscopic technique to achieve a curative resection for SMTs with a predominant extraluminal growth pattern or extra-GI tumors at the level of cardia or the proximal part of the lesser curvature of the stomach.[32] Mediastinal tumors, such as mediastinal cysts and superficial pancreatic tumors were removed with transesophageal and transgastric endoscopy, respectively.[7,8] This technique may revolutionize the treatment outcomes with a less invasiveness, and reduce the risk of postoperative adverse events. In the future, prospective studies are required to gauge the efficacy and safety of this novel technique compared with conventional methods.

Principles of Endoscopic Resection by Tunneling Technique

Preoperative evaluation with endoscopy, computed tomography (CT) scan, or endoscopic ultrasonography (EUS) is essential to evaluate the location, morphology, and layer of SMTs, and the relation with extra-luminal structures. Sometimes, EUS-guided fine needle aspiration is obtained according to the indication to prove the

Table 1
The propriety of STER and non-tunnel techniques for SMTs in different aspects

Factors	STER	Non-tunnel	Suggestions
Mucosa			
Smooth	Yes	Yes	STER
Ulcerative	No	Yes	Non-tunnel
Direction of the gastroscope			
Both	Yes	Yes	STER
Reverse	No	Yes	Non-tunnel
Enter	Yes	Yes	STER
Layer			
Muscularis mucosa and submucosa	Yes	Yes	Non-tunnel
Muscularis propria	Yes	Yes	STER

Abbreviation: STER, submucosal tunneling endoscopic resection
Adapted from Geng ZH, Zhu Y, Chen WF, et al. A scoring system to support surgical decision-making for cardial submucosal tumors [published correction appears in Endosc Int Open. 2022 May 24;10(4):C5]. *Endosc Int Open.* 2022;10(4):E468-E478. Published 2022 Apr 14.

histologic diagnosis. The patients were under general anesthesia with endotracheal intubation. Prophylactic intravenous antibiotics were administered routinely 30 min before the procedure, and CO_2 was used during the procedure to reduce gas-related complications.

A standard single-channel therapeutic scope is used during the procedure with an auxiliary water channel is used. A transparent cap is attached to the front of the scope. Water-jet-assisted knives are preferred to create the submucosal tunnel. Other accessories included hot biopsy forceps, a polypectomy snare, and hemostatic clips are also needed.

Procedures for ESTD included[5]:[1] Make the circumferential markings at least 5 mm outside the margin of the lesion by argon plasma coagulation (APC) or an electric knife after the lesion evaluation, revealing the anal and oral margins[2]; make two transversal or cambered incisions in the anal and oral mucosa after sufficient submucosal injection[3]; inject and dissect between the submucosal and muscular layers to create a submucosal tunnel from the oral incision to the anal incision[4]; resect the remaining bilateral mucosa at 5 mm outside the marking points to completely dissect the whole lesion[5]; use APC or hot biopsy forceps to prevent delayed bleeding with fibrin glue sprayed on the ulcer when necessary. A fully covered retrievable metal stent was suggested for lesions over 3/4 of the whole circle to prevent postoperative stricture.[35] Besides, oral steroid prophylaxis appeared to be more commonly used as a safe and effective treatment in preventing stricture and improving patients' quality of life.[36]

The main steps of STER procedures contained[37]:[1] Inject a mixture solution of normal saline and indigo carmine into the submucosa 3 to 5 cm proximal to the lesion and make a mucosal incision as the tunnel entry[2]; inject and dissect between the submucosal and muscular layers to create a tunnel to the lesion. The tunnel should be expanded 2 cm past the distal margin of the SMT to ensure appropriate working space[24,3] gradually dissect the tumor as deep as the bottom around the lesion with an insulated tip knife[4]; take the tumor out with a snare[5]; use APC or hot biopsy forceps to prevent delayed bleeding[6]; close the mucosal entry with metal clips (**Fig. 2**).

There were some differences in STER in different locations of the GI tract. For example, SMTs at the esophagus, cardia, or the fundus close to the cardia can

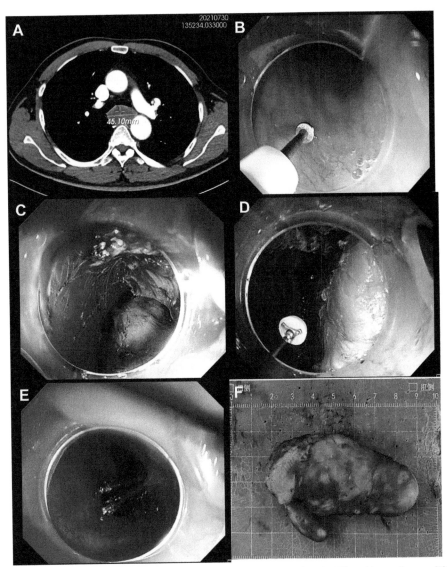

Fig. 2. STER for a giant esophageal leiomyoma. (*A*) CT showed an SMT in mid-esophagus. (*B*) A water-jet assisted knife was used to create a mucosal opening of the tunnel. (*C*) The tumor was dissected in the tunnel. (*D*) An insulated-tip knife was used to dissect the mediastinal side. (*E*) The mucosal entry was sealed by clips after tumor retrieval. (*F*) The retrieved specimen was measured 8.5 cm × 4.5 cm.

typically be excised with STER. By comparison, it was challenging to create a tunnel in the stomach due to the wide lumen, unfixed position, and thick mucosa. Thus, SMTs that were located in the front/posterior side of the gastric body/antrum or the great curvature can be dissected in a direct view. In addition, it was also difficult to create the tunnel in the rectum because of the redundant mucosa and tortuous lumen.

As for STER-ET, submucosal injection and tunnel establishment were the same as STER. Then, the full-thickness myotomy was performed above the estimated location of the extraluminal tumor, and connective tissue surrounding the tumor was dissected to ensure the tumor capsule intact. After that, the tumor was extracted with either a retrieval basket or a snare. Finally, the mucosal entry was closed with metal clips after an inspection of the submucosal tunnel for any evidence of bleeding sites.

After the endoscopic surgery, a nasogastric/anal tube was placed to decompress and monitor delayed bleeding of the wound. Besides, we observed postoperative symptoms of fever, hematemesis or melena, dyspnea, chest pain, and signs of pneumothorax. If the patient had persistent fever, hematemesis, melena, or pain, emergent endoscopy and CT would be performed. In addition, proton pump inhibitors (PPIs) and antibiotics were applied.

Clinical Management After Endoscopic Resection

Based on the pathologic results of surgical specimens, the subsequent clinical management was formulated. Leiomyoma is the most common GI SMTs, followed by stromal tumor, fibroma, and lipoma.[38,39] Gastrointestinal stromal tumor (GIST), leiomyosarcoma, and liposarcoma accompany the possibility of malignancies. It is important to differentiate these pathologies, as relatively aggressive intervention or surveillance are recommended for SMTs with malignant potentials.[40,41]

Patients should be examined with endoscopy for the evaluation of the wound healing and local recurrence at 3 to 6 months after the resection. Subsequently, the frequency of endoscopy should be adjusted according to the risk of recurrence and the timing and conditions of treatment, especially for patients whose pathology tends to be malignant such as GIST, leiomyosarcoma, and liposarcoma.[42]

For patients who suffered relapses, endoscopy and EUS were performed to check for recurrent tumors, and the abdominal US and CT were conducted to examine the distant metastasis.

Outcomes and Adverse Event

The efficacy and safety of submucosal tunneling techniques for tumor resection have been shown in multiple small to large studies (**Table 2**). The effectiveness of surgery was mainly reflected in the en bloc resection rate, complete resection rate, and recurrence rate. Although the complication rate was used to evaluate its safety. The en bloc resection was defined as the excision of the tumor in one piece without fragmentation, and based on the en bloc resection, the complete resection was defined as the excision without apparent residual tumors assessed macroscopically by the endoscopist at the resection site and with negative margins (both lateral and basal resection margins) on the pathologic examination.

A meta-analysis found that the en bloc resection rate of SMTs in the upper, middle, lower esophagus, and the cardia were more than 94%.[43] The large size and irregular shape of SMTs may preclude en bloc resection.[20,23,44] Therefore, en bloc resection rates were better for smaller tumors, typically less than 2 cm and the large size usually resulted in piecemeal resection and lowered the en bloc resection rate.[45,46] Patients with SMTs who were treated with STER were free from local recurrence and metastasis at follow-up.[43,47]

The overall incidence of complications with STER ranged from 5% to 25%,[48,49] including air leakage, mucosal injury, bleeding, perforation, and postoperative infection. Among these complications, gas-related adverse events were the most common, and the majority did not require an intervention.[50] It is suggested that SMTs with large size and irregular shape, SMTs arising from the deep MP layer, resection of synchronous lesions, air usage for insufflation, and long operation time were risk factors of complications.[23,29,50]

Table 2
Efficacy and safety of submucosal tunneling techniques for tumor resection

Study	Patients Number	Location	Mean Size (cm)	En-Bloc Resection (%)	Complications (%)	Recurrence (%)
ESTD for mucosal lesions						
Zhu et al.[55]	124	Esophagus: 124	22.2 cm²	100	43.5	0
Li et al.[3]	15	Esophagus: 15	4.2	86.7	46.7	0
Liu et al.[57]	6	Cardia: 6	2.1	100	0	0
Linghu et al.[12]	11	Esophagus: 11	4.8	100	54.5	0
STER for GI SMTs						
Ye et al.[29]	85	Esophagus: 60, Cardia: 16, Stomach: 9	1.9	100	9.4	0
Wang et al.[24]	80	Esophagus: 67, Cardia: 16	2.3	97.6	8.8	0
Chen et al.[50]	290	Esophagus: 199, Cardia: 68, Stomach: 23	2.1	89.3	23.4	NA
Mao et al.[58]	56	Esophagus: 18, Stomach: 38	1.8	100	15.3	0
Li et al.[21]	74	Esophagus: 74	1.9	98.6	5.4	2.7
Wu et al.[59]	242	Esophagus: 242	2.2	98.3	4.5	0
Wang et al.[60]	24	Esophagus: 24	4.7	100	0	0
Hu et al.[61]	12	Rectum: 12	1.4	100	16.7	0
STER-ET for extraluminal tumors						
Cai et al.[32]	8	Tumor impression on GI wall, Cardia: 1, LCUGB: 6, No apparent mucosal bulge: 1	2.8	100	0	0
Ma et al.[7]	10	Mediastinum: 10	3.3	60.0	0	0

Abbreviations: ESTD, endoscopic submucosal tunnel dissection; GI, gastrointestinal; LCUGB, lesser curvature of the upper gastric body; SMTs, submucosal tumors; STER, submucosal tunneling endoscopic resection; STER-ET, submucosal tunnel endoscopic resection for extraluminal tumors.

Air leakage mainly included subcutaneous emphysema, pneumomediastinum, pneumothorax, and pneumoperitoneum. Most gas-related adverse events were managed conservatively.[43] In addition, perforation can be conservatively treated by complete endoscopic closure with metal clips. Delayed perforation is rare; however, it can result in serious conditions that often require emergent surgery. Therefore, recognizing delayed perforation is very important when patients who have previously undergone endoscopic resection for SMTs show signs of peritoneal irritation.

In terms of bleeding, it is classified into immediate and delayed bleeding. Immediate bleeding can be successfully treated in most cases through coagulation of the bleeding vessels or placement of metallic clips. Delayed bleeding may be associated with the size and location of SMTs, presence of ulcers, longer operation time, and the use of antithrombotic agents.[51,52] In addition, the mucosal injury may occur but tend to be small (<1 cm) and it can be closed with hemostatic clips.[53,54]

In addition, postoperative esophageal stenosis is of most concern for large mucosal defects after ESTD. The incidence of esophageal stricture after ESTD for large mucosal lesions was about 50%.[3,12,55] Therefore, preventive intervention should be implemented such as endoscopic pneumatic dilation (EPD), steroids, and fully covered self-expandable metal stents (FCSEMs).[56]

SUMMARY

The submucosal tunneling technique is an effective and safe method for the resection of GI mucosal lesions, SMTs, and extra-GI tumors. The en bloc resection rate was comparable to other endoscopic techniques. Furthermore, it has several advantages such as maintaining mucosal integrity, reducing the risk of postoperative GI leak and secondary infection, rapid recovery, and short hospital stay. In addition, accurate diagnosis, selection of patients, and proper appreciation of technical aspects are essential to perform this technique. In the next decade, technological advances in the submucosal tunneling technique are expected.

CLINICS CARE POINTS

- Endoscopic submucosal tunnel dissection is an efficient technique for large superficial esophageal squamous cell neoplasms. Attention should be paid to the prophylactic measures and treatments of postoperative stricture.
- Submucosal tunneling endoscopic resection (STER) is a safe and an effective treatment modality for gastrointestinal (GI) submucosal tumors (SMTs), preferably originating from the muscularis propria layer. STER for extraluminal tumors is a feasible, safe and effective endoscopic technique to achieve a curative resection for SMTs with a predominant extraluminal growth pattern or extra-GI tumors.

GRANT SUPPORT

This study was supported by Innovation Funds of Zhongshan Hospital (2021ZSCX29).

DISCLOSURE

The authors have nothing to disclose.

REFERENCES

1. Kalloo AN, Singh VK, Jagannath SB, et al. Flexible transgastric peritoneoscopy: a novel approach to diagnostic and therapeutic interventions in the peritoneal cavity. Gastrointest Endosc 2004;60(1):114–7.
2. Sumiyama K, Gostout CJ, Rajan E, et al. Submucosal endoscopy with mucosal flap safety valve. Gastrointest Endosc 2007;65(4):688–94.
3. Li L, Wang W, Yue H, et al. Endoscopic submucosal multi-tunnel dissection for large early esophageal cancer lesions. Acta Gastroenterol Belg 2019;82(3): 355–8.
4. Gan T, Yang JL, Zhu LL, et al. Endoscopic submucosal multi-tunnel dissection for circumferential superficial esophageal neoplastic lesions (with videos). Gastrointest Endosc 2016;84(1):143–6.
5. Zhai YQ, Li HK, Linghu EQ. Endoscopic submucosal tunnel dissection for large superficial esophageal squamous cell neoplasms. World J Gastroenterol 2016; 22(1):435–45.
6. Li P, Ma B, Gong S, et al. Endoscopic submucosal tunnel dissection for superficial esophageal neoplastic lesions: a meta-analysis. Surg Endosc 2020;34(3): 1214–23.
7. Ma LY, Liu ZQ, Yao L, et al. Transesophageal endoscopic resection of mediastinal cysts (with video). Gastrointest Endosc 2022;95(4):642–9.e2.
8. Ma L-Y, Liu Z-Q, Chen W-F, et al. Transgastric Endoscopic Resection of a Superficial Pancreatic Tumor: The First Report in Human Beings. Official J Am Coll Gastroenterol ACG 2022;117(3):373–4.
9. Lopes CV, Hela M, Pesenti C, et al. Circumferential endoscopic resection of Barrett's esophagus with high-grade dysplasia or early adenocarcinoma. Surg Endosc 2007;21(5):820–4.
10. Giovannini M, Bories E, Pesenti C, et al. Circumferential endoscopic mucosal resection in Barrett's esophagus with high-grade intraepithelial neoplasia or mucosal cancer. Preliminary results in 21 patients. Endoscopy 2004;36(9):782–7.
11. Chennat J, Konda VJ, Ross AS, et al. Complete Barrett's eradication endoscopic mucosal resection: an effective treatment modality for high-grade dysplasia and intramucosal carcinoma–an American single-center experience. Am J Gastroenterol 2009;104(11):2684–92.
12. Linghu E, Feng X, Wang X, et al. Endoscopic submucosal tunnel dissection for large esophageal neoplastic lesions. Endoscopy 2013;45(1):60–2.
13. Chai NL, Li HK, Linghu EQ, et al. Consensus on the digestive endoscopic tunnel technique. World J Gastroenterol 2019;25(7):744–76.
14. Deprez PH, Moons LMG, O'Toole D, et al. Endoscopic management of subepithelial lesions including neuroendocrine neoplasms: European Society of Gastrointestinal Endoscopy (ESGE) Guideline. Endoscopy 2022;54(4):412–29.
15. Ishihara R, Arima M, Iizuka T, et al. Endoscopic submucosal dissection/endoscopic mucosal resection guidelines for esophageal cancer. Dig Endosc 2020; 32(4):452–93.
16. Xu MD, Cai MY, Zhou PH, et al. Submucosal tunneling endoscopic resection: a new technique for treating upper GI submucosal tumors originating from the muscularis propria layer (with videos). Gastrointest Endosc 2012;75(1):195–9.
17. Inoue H, Ikeda H, Hosoya T, et al. Submucosal endoscopic tumor resection for subepithelial tumors in the esophagus and cardia. Endoscopy 2012;44(3): 225–30.

18. Li Q-L, Yao L-Q, Zhou P-H, et al. Submucosal tumors of the esophagogastric junction originating from the muscularis propria layer: a large study of endoscopic submucosal dissection (with video). Gastrointest Endosc 2012;75(6): 1153–8.

19. Liu BR, Song JT. Submucosal Tunneling Endoscopic Resection (STER) and Other Novel Applications of Submucosal Tunneling in Humans. Gastrointest Endosc Clin N Am 2016;26(2):271–82.

20. Chen T, Lin ZW, Zhang YQ, et al. Submucosal Tunneling Endoscopic Resection vs Thoracoscopic Enucleation for Large Submucosal Tumors in the Esophagus and the Esophagogastric Junction. J Am Coll Surg 2017;225(6):806–16.

21. Li QY, Meng Y, Xu YY, et al. Comparison of endoscopic submucosal tunneling dissection and thoracoscopic enucleation for the treatment of esophageal submucosal tumors. Gastrointest Endosc 2017;86(3):485–91.

22. Liu BR, Song JT, Kong LJ, et al. Tunneling endoscopic muscularis dissection for subepithelial tumors originating from the muscularis propria of the esophagus and gastric cardia. Surg Endosc 2013;27(11):4354–9.

23. Chen T, Zhou PH, Chu Y, et al. Long-term Outcomes of Submucosal Tunneling Endoscopic Resection for Upper Gastrointestinal Submucosal Tumors. Ann Surg 2017;265(2):363–9.

24. Wang H, Tan Y, Zhou Y, et al. Submucosal tunneling endoscopic resection for upper gastrointestinal submucosal tumors originating from the muscularis propria layer. Eur J Gastroenterol Hepatol 2015;27(7):776–80.

25. Lu J, Jiao T, Zheng M, et al. Endoscopic resection of submucosal tumors in muscularis propria: the choice between direct excavation and tunneling resection. Surg Endosc 2014;28(12):3401–7.

26. Tan Y, Zhou B, Zhang S, et al. Submucosal Tunneling Endoscopic Resection for Gastric Submucosal Tumors: a Comparison Between Cardia and Non-cardia Location. J Gastrointest Surg 2019;23(11):2129–35.

27. Rajan E, Kee W, Song LM. Endoscopic Full Thickness Resection. Gastroenterology 2018;154(7):1925–37.e2.

28. Li QL, Chen WF, Zhang C, et al. Clinical impact of submucosal tunneling endoscopic resection for the treatment of gastric submucosal tumors originating from the muscularis propria layer (with video). Surg Endosc 2015;29(12):3640–6.

29. Ye LP, Zhang Y, Mao XL, et al. Submucosal tunneling endoscopic resection for small upper gastrointestinal subepithelial tumors originating from the muscularis propria layer. Surg Endosc 2014;28(2):524–30.

30. Geng Z-H, Zhu Y, Chen W-F, et al. A scoring system to support surgical decision-making for cardial submucosal tumors. Endosc Int Open 2022;10(04):E468–78.

31. Turner BG, Gee DW, Cizginer S, et al. Endoscopic transesophageal mediastinal lymph node dissection and en bloc resection by using mediastinal and thoracic approaches (with video). Gastrointest Endosc 2010;72(4):831–5.

32. Cai MY, Zhu BQ, Xu MD, et al. Submucosal tunnel endoscopic resection for extraluminal tumors: a novel endoscopic method for en bloc resection of predominant extraluminal growing subepithelial tumors or extra-gastrointestinal tumors (with videos). Gastrointest Endosc 2018;88(1):160–7.

33. Liu X, Chen T, Cheng J, et al. Endoscopic transmural route for dissection of gastric submucosal tumors with extraluminal growth: experience in two cases. Gut 2021;70(11):2052–4.

34. Gao P, Li Q, Hu J, et al. Transoesophageal endoscopic removal of a benign mediastinal tumour: a new field for endotherapy? Gut 2020;69(10):1727–9.

35. Wen J, Lu Z, Yang Y, et al. Preventing stricture formation by covered esophageal stent placement after endoscopic submucosal dissection for early esophageal cancer. Dig Dis Sci 2014;59(3):658–63.
36. Pih GY, Kim DH, Gong EJ, et al. Preventing esophageal strictures with steroids after endoscopic submucosal dissection in superficial esophageal neoplasm. J Dig Dis 2019;20(11):609–16.
37. Cai M, Chen J, Zhou P, et al. The rise of tunnel endoscopic surgery: a case report and literature review. Case Rep Gastrointest Med 2012;2012:847640.
38. Ponsaing LG, Kiss K, Hansen MB. Classification of submucosal tumors in the gastrointestinal tract. World J Gastroenterol 2007;13(24):3311–5.
39. Tsai SJ, Lin CC, Chang CW, et al. Benign esophageal lesions: endoscopic and pathologic features. World J Gastroenterol 2015;21(4):1091–8.
40. Demetri GD, von Mehren M, Antonescu CR, et al. NCCN Task Force report: update on the management of patients with gastrointestinal stromal tumors. J Natl Compr Canc Netw 2010;8(Suppl 2):S1–41 [quiz:S2-S4].
41. Kulke MH, Anthony LB, Bushnell DL, et al. NANETS treatment guidelines: well-differentiated neuroendocrine tumors of the stomach and pancreas. Pancreas 2010;39(6):735–52.
42. Nishida T, Blay JY, Hirota S, et al. The standard diagnosis, treatment, and follow-up of gastrointestinal stromal tumors based on guidelines. Gastric Cancer 2016; 19(1):3–14.
43. Lv XH, Wang CH, Xie Y. Efficacy and safety of submucosal tunneling endoscopic resection for upper gastrointestinal submucosal tumors: a systematic review and meta-analysis. Surg Endosc 2017;31(1):49–63.
44. Li Z, Gao Y, Chai N, et al. Effect of submucosal tunneling endoscopic resection for submucosal tumors at esophagogastric junction and risk factors for failure of en bloc resection. Surg Endosc 2018;32(3):1326–35.
45. Rahman SA, Walker RC, Lloyd MA, et al. Machine learning to predict early recurrence after oesophageal cancer surgery. Br J Surg 2020;107(8):1042–52.
46. Aslanian HR, Sethi A, Bhutani MS, et al. ASGE guideline for endoscopic full-thickness resection and submucosal tunnel endoscopic resection. VideoGIE 2019;4(8):343–50.
47. Zhang M, Wu S, Xu H. Comparison Between Submucosal Tunneling Endoscopic Resection (STER) and Other Resection Modules for Esophageal Muscularis Propria Tumors: A Retrospective Study. Med Sci Monit 2019;25:4560–8.
48. Du C, Linghu E. Submucosal Tunneling Endoscopic Resection for the Treatment of Gastrointestinal Submucosal Tumors Originating from the Muscularis Propria Layer. J Gastrointest Surg 2017;21(12):2100–9.
49. Du C, Chai NL, Ling-Hu EQ, et al. Submucosal tunneling endoscopic resection: An effective and safe therapy for upper gastrointestinal submucosal tumors originating from the muscularis propria layer. World J Gastroenterol 2019;25(2): 245–57.
50. Chen T, Zhang C, Yao LQ, et al. Management of the complications of submucosal tunneling endoscopic resection for upper gastrointestinal submucosal tumors. Endoscopy 2016;48(2):149–55.
51. So S, Ahn JY, Kim N, et al. Comparison of the effects of antithrombotic therapy on delayed bleeding after gastric endoscopic resection: a propensity score-matched case-control study. Gastrointest Endosc 2019;89(2):277–85, e2.
52. Mukai S, Cho S, Kotachi T, et al. Analysis of delayed bleeding after endoscopic submucosal dissection for gastric epithelial neoplasms. Gastroenterol Res Pract 2012;2012:875323.

53. Lu J, Jiao T, Li Y, et al. Heading toward the right direction–solution package for endoscopic submucosal tunneling resection in the stomach. PLoS One 2015; 10(3):e0119870.

54. Lu J, Zheng M, Jiao T, et al. Transcardiac tunneling technique for endoscopic submucosal dissection of gastric fundus tumors arising from the muscularis propria. Endoscopy 2014;46(10):888–92.

55. Zhu LL, Wu JC, Wang YP, et al. Endoscopic Submucosal Single- or Multi-tunnel Dissection for Near-Circumferential and Circumferential Superficial Esophageal Neoplastic Lesions. Gastroenterol Res Pract 2019;2019:2943232.

56. Oliveira JF, Moura EG, Bernardo WM, et al. Prevention of esophageal stricture after endoscopic submucosal dissection: a systematic review and meta-analysis. Surg Endosc 2016;30(7):2779–91.

57. Liu L, Guo HM, Miao F, et al. Endoscopic Esophageal Submucosal Tunnel Dissection for Cystic Lesions Originating from the Muscularis Propria of the Gastric Cardia. J Oncol 2020;2020:5259717.

58. Mao XL, Ye LP, Zheng HH, et al. Submucosal tunneling endoscopic resection using methylene-blue guidance for cardial subepithelial tumors originating from the muscularis propria layer. Dis Esophagus 2017;30(4):1–7.

59. Wu BH, Shi RY, Zhang HY, et al. Feasibility and Safety of Mark-Guided Submucosal Tunneling Endoscopic Resection for Treatment of Esophageal Submucosal Tumors Originating from the Muscularis Propria: A Single-Center Retrospective Study. Can J Gastroenterol Hepatol 2021;2021:9916927.

60. Wang GX, Yu G, Xiang YL, et al. Submucosal tunneling endoscopic resection for large symptomatic submucosal tumors of the esophagus: A clinical analysis of 24 cases. Turk J Gastroenterol 2020;31(1):42–8.

61. Hu JW, Zhang C, Chen T, et al. Submucosal tunneling endoscopic resection for the treatment of rectal submucosal tumors originating from the muscular propria layer. J Cancer Res Ther 2014;10(Suppl):281–6.

Nontunneling Full Thickness Techniques for Neoplasia

Grace E. Kim, MD[a],*, Shivangi Kothari, MD[b], Uzma D. Siddiqui, MD[c]

KEYWORDS

- Endoscopic full-thickness resection • Full thickness resection device
- Locally advanced cancer

KEY POINTS

- Endoscopic full-thickness resection (EFTR) is an increasingly used technique that can be considered as a highly successful alternative curative treatment of locally invasive gastrointestinal cancers or scarred benign lesions.
- There are 2 approaches to a nontunneling EFTR: nonexposed and exposed. The nonexposed technique typically uses over-the-scope clip for lumen closure before resection, whereas the exposed technique uses clips, sutures, or endoloops after performing ESD.
- Limitations of using the full-thickness resection device (FTRD) include size less than 2 to 3 cm and technical issues related to device passage.
- Rare complications have been associated with FTRD at the appendiceal orifice include fistula and appendicitis.

INTRODUCTION

Colorectal cancer is the third most common cancer worldwide and the fourth leading cause of cancer-related deaths in the world,[1] second in the United States.[2] T1 lesions are tumors that invade the submucosal layer with lower risks of lymph node invasion, whereas T2 tumors invade the muscularis propria.[3] T1 is further subclassified into T1a (invading $<1000\ \mu m$) and T1b carcinomas (invading deeper than $1000\ \mu m$), where the latter is usually treated surgically due to higher risk of lymph node invasion. The current guidelines recommend endoscopic removal of suspected malignant lesions unless there is a deeper submucosal invasion or the lesion has high-risk histologic features for which they should be referred to surgery.[3–5] High-risk features include poor

[a] Section of Gastroenterology, Hepatology, and Nutrition, University of Chicago, 15841 South Maryland Avenue MC4076, Chicago, IL 60637, USA; [b] Division of Gastroenterology/Hepatology, University of Rochester Medical Center & Strong Memorial Hospital, 2601 Elmwood Avenue, Box 646, Rochester, NY 14642, USA; [c] Section of Gastroenterology, Hepatology, and Nutrition, Center for Endoscopic Research and Therapeutics and Advanced Endoscopy Training, University of Chicago, 35700 South Maryland Avenue MC 8043, Chicago, IL 60637, USA
* Corresponding author.
E-mail address: grace.kim@uchospitals.edu

Gastrointest Endoscopy Clin N Am 33 (2023) 155–168
https://doi.org/10.1016/j.giec.2022.09.002
1052-5157/23/© 2022 Elsevier Inc. All rights reserved.

differentiation, invasion into the deep submucosa or muscularis propria, and lympho-vascular involvement.

Although many polypoid lesions in the gastrointestinal (GI) tract can be removed endoscopically using advanced techniques such as endoscopic mucosal resection (EMR) or endoscopic submucosal dissection (ESD), these techniques are limited in that they only resect down to the submucosal layer. Lesions that infiltrate deeper than the superficial aspect of the submucosal layer may have a nonlifting sign, which makes EMR and ESD technically difficult. Prior resections also often cause scarring that prevents adequate lift between the submucosal and muscularis propria layer.[6] EMR and ESD can lead to higher complication rates and incomplete resections when attempted on lesions located at difficult locations such as the appendiceal orifice.[7]

Endoscopic full-thickness resection (EFTR) is an emerging technique that enables these challenging lesions to be still managed endoscopically with high success rates and low adverse events. Because EFTR includes the muscularis propria, EFTR can be used as a curative treatment of early cancers that invade deeper into the submucosa.[8,9] Not only that, but having a transmural resection enables better assessment of the depth of infiltration into the submucosal layer and lymphatic spread, which can help risk stratify for management planning.

There are different techniques to accomplish EFTR, either resecting the lesion first then closing the defect (ie, exposed or open EFTR),[10,11] which can be done using a submucosal tunnel to gain access to the lesion (submucosal tunnel endoscopic resection) or with a nontunneling technique. The more commonly used method for EFTR is a nontunneling, nonexposed technique where a pseudopolyp of the lesion is created with serosa-to-serosa apposition by first placing a closure device such as an over-the-scope clip (OTSC; Ovesco Endoscopy AG, Tübingen, Germany[12]) or a Padlock clip (Steris, Mentor, OH, USA)[13] and then resecting the lesion with a snare over it (ie, nonexposed or closed EFTR).[14] The 2 types of OTSCs currently available in the United States are the Padlock clip and the Ovesco OTSC (**Fig. 1**). The Food and Drug Administration (FDA) has also approved a full-thickness resection device (FTRD) system (Ovesco Endoscopy AG, Tübingen, Germany), which facilitates EFTR (**Fig. 2**). This will be the focus of our review and will be discussed in more depth in a later section.

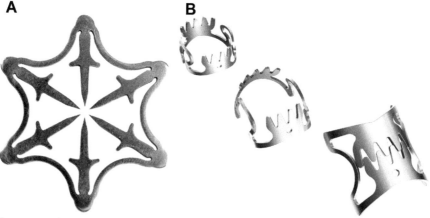

Fig. 1. Over the scope clips. (*A*) Padlock clip (*Courtesy* of STERIS, Mentor, OH) and (*B*) OTSC. (*Courtesy of* Ovesco Endoscopy, Cary, NC).

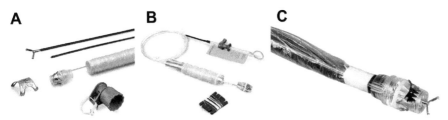

Fig. 2. Full-thickness resection device. (**A**) FTRD system with FTRD grasper. (**B**) FTRD system. (**C**) FTRD system fully mounted on endoscope. (*Courtesy of* Ovesco Endoscopy AG, Tübingen, Germany.)

INDICATIONS

EFTR is a reasonable approach in difficult lesions such as those with significant fibrosis and scarring that have a "nonlifting" sign, subepithelial tumors especially those arising deeper in the muscularis propria such as GI stromal tumor (GIST) or early malignancy (T1 with submucosal infiltration), and those in difficult locations such as appendiceal orifice or lesions involving a diverticulum.[14,15] Other indications include recurrent or incompletely resected T1 carcinoma, adenomas in a coagulopathic patient, and suspected Hirschsprung disease for diagnostic resection.[16]

The National Comprehensive Cancer Network guidelines recommend surgical resection of GIST greater than 20 mm in diameter as well as those less than 20 mm with high-risk sonographic features seen on endoscopic ultrasound such as irregular borders, ulcerations, and heterogeneity.[17] With the advent of EFTRs, GIST lesions originating from the muscularis propria have been increasingly managed via EFTRs with high success rates and safety profile.[18]

EFTR is a less invasive management option for those who otherwise would have needed a more aggressive surgical intervention. Although some advocates have suggested lesions up to 3 cm may be removed using EFTR, this technique is generally recommended for GI tract lesions 2 cm or lesser with studies showing higher success rates with this size lesion.[6,15]

Box 1 lists indications for EFTR.

Box 1
Indications for endoscopic full-thickness resection

Upper GI Lesions
- GISTs
- Neuroendocrine tumors
- T1 carcinoma
- Incomplete or recurrent T1 carcinoma
- Lesions with significant fibrosis or scarring (with "non lifting sign")
- Difficult locations (ie, gastroesophageal junction)

Lower GI lesions
- T1 carcinoma
- Incomplete or recurrent T1 carcinoma
- Lesions with significant fibrosis or scarring (with "non lifting sign")
- Lesions in difficult locations (ie, appendiceal orifice, near or involving diverticulum)
- Hirschsprung disease

VARIOUS ENDOSCOPIC FULL-THICKNESS RESECTION TECHNIQUES

There are 2 ways to perform EFTR: nonexposed and exposed. FTRD is the most commonly used method to perform nonexposed EFTRs; **Fig. 2** [19]; and **Fig. 3** illustrate the EFTR technique using FTRD of a small descending colon T1 adenocarcinoma. FTRD is an over-the-scope device system using a cap that is mounted over a colonoscope. The cap is longer at 23 mm (vs a conventional OTSC system with a cap that is 6 mm in depth) and includes a preloaded 13 mm snare at the tip as well as a modified OTSC that is 14 mm wide. The outer diameter of the cap is 21 mm. The modified FTRD for gastroduodenal EFTRs is slightly smaller (19.5 mm diameter).[20] **Fig. 4** shows the modified FTRD for gastroduodenal EFTR.

Ideally, when using FTRDs for nonexposed EFTRs, it is helpful to prepare 2 endoscopes in advance, one with the FTRD mounted. First, one starts with the regular endoscope to mark the lesion via argon plasma coagulation or clips. On withdrawal, it is important to irrigate and clean the surroundings. Then one switches to the endoscope with the mounted FTRD system, and the central part of the lesion is grabbed with forceps or a grasper such as an over-the-scope Ovesco Twin Grasper or Anchor (Ovesco Endoscopy AG, Tübingen, Germany; **Fig. 5**). The tissue is pulled slowly into the cap while the endoscope is advanced slowly; it is pulled until the marked margins are visible in the cap. It is recommended to use the grasping device to bring the lesion into the cap, and it is acceptable to use gentle suction. Aggressive suctioning is not advised because there is potential for structures adjacent to the GI tract to come into the cap. Immediately afterward, the snare is closed and cautery applied resulting in resection of the lesion. The resected lesion is usually retrieved via cap suction, and the regular endoscope then is used to inspect the resection site.

There are several ways to troubleshoot FTRDs. If the clip does not deploy, one can straighten out the scope and turn the handle to reattempt clip deployment. However, if it still does not work, then the scope needs to be removed. If the clip is deployed but snare does not close appropriately or does not cut, the high-frequency unit should be checked and the snare shaft should be straightened. If this does not fix it, the endoscope needs to be removed, and the lesion can be cut with the additional snare above the FTRD clip. If the clip does not get deployed but the lesion is cut, it is likely that a perforation may have occurred. This can be converted into exposed EFTR and push the resected lesion out of the cap to grasp the resection margins with a twin grasper and close the defect with FTRD clips.

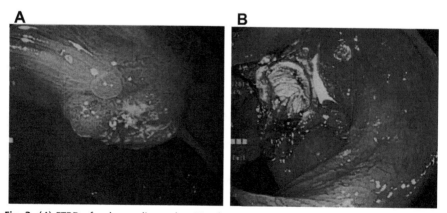

Fig. 3. (*A*) FTRD of a descending colon T1 adenocarcinoma lesion. (*B*) Lesion after EFTR.

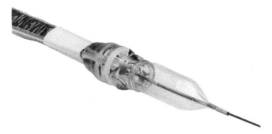

Fig. 4. Gastroduodenal FTRD. (*Courtesy of* Ovesco Endoscopy, Cary, NC.)

The Padlock Clip (Steris, Mentor, OH, USA) is another tool that can be used to perform a nonexposed EFTR. It is a star-shaped ring with 6 inner needles preloaded onto a cap. It offers the potential advantage of having a flat base, which could enhance resection rates.[13] Its tip diameter ranges from the Standard clip (Steris, Mentor, OH, USA) 9.5 to 11 mm to Pro-Select (Steris, Mentor, OH, USA) that is larger at 11.5 to 14 mm[15]. For both clips, the cap diameter is 11 mm. Similar to FTRD, the borders of the lesion are initially typically marked using a snare tip soft coagulation. The endoscope is taken back out to attach the Padlock Clip cap at the tip of the endoscope. The endoscope is reinserted and the cap is positioned over the center of the lesion. This is suctioned into the cap to create a pseudopolyp; if extensive fibrosis is present, a grasping forceps can be used to pull the lesion into the cap. After the lesion is fully captured inside the cap with presumed apposition of the 2 serosal layers, the Padlock Clip is deployed to create a pseudopolyp. The endoscope is withdrawn again to remove the cap. The pseudopolyp is then removed with a snare above the clip; the resection is aimed at about the same length as the diameter of the tube (2.3 mm) above the clip. Hemostasis would have already been achieved by the pressure created by the clip onto the tissue. **Fig. 6** shows a Padlock Clip mounted on an endoscope.

Exposed EFTR (also known as open EFTR) is accomplished by first having a submucosal injection to the lesion then cutting circumferentially around the lesion through the submucosal layer via a standard ESD technique.[11,18] After the ESD is performed, the center of the lesion is suctioned inside the cap and full thickness of the mucosa including the serosal layer is resected, creating an iatrogenic, intentional perforation. This defect is then closed using clips or sutures. Endoloop can also be used as a loop-and-clip technique, for which a double-channel endoscope is used.[14]

OUTCOMES

Schmidt and colleagues published a first experience in using FTRD (nonexposed EFTR) for colorectal EFTRs.[16] They reported R0 resection rate (ie, complete remission

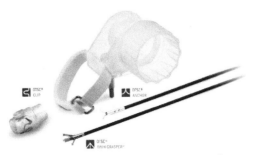

Fig. 5. OTSC, Twin Grasper, and Anchor. (*Courtesy of* Ovesco Endoscopy, Cary, NC.)

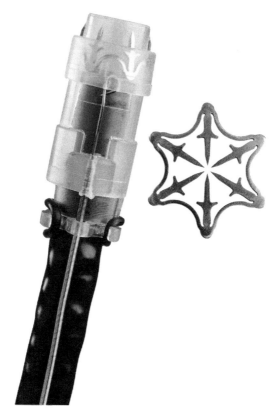

Fig. 6. Padlock Clip mounted on an endoscope. (*Courtesy of* STERIS, Mentor, OH.)

or resection for cure[21]) of 75.0% (18 of 24 lesions) with no perforation or major bleeding and 2 patients with postpolypectomy syndrome that was managed conservatively with antibiotics. Since then, multiple studies on FTRD have been published with comparable and improved safety and success outcomes.[22–25]

A 2022 systematic review and meta-analysis compiled studies using both EFTR with OTSC and snare and FTRD (a total of 14 studies and 1936 patients undergoing EFTRs of lower GI lesions) and showed that overall technical success of EFTR in colorectal lesions was 86.5%, with R0 resection rate of 78.4% and mean procedure time of 45.5 minutes.[6] The median size of the lesions was 15.1 mm, with most lesions being adenomas (57.7%) and 21.2% being T1, carcinoma, or intramucosal cancer. About 75.8% of the lesions were located in the colon and 24.2% in the rectum. This study showed adverse events at 15.4% with GI bleeding of 6.4%, perforation of 4.4%, and postpolypectomy syndrome of 1.7%; and recurrence rate or the rate of having residual lesion was at 8.3%. There were 128 appendiceal lesions included in the study, with 11.5% having appendicitis after EFTR. The overall rate of requiring surgical intervention after EFTR was 5.5%. The use of both FTRD and Padlock Clips has comparable results.[13]

Although there are limited data specifically on neoplasms, emerging data show that EFTR is safe and effective for treatment of T1 colorectal cancers less than 2 cm.[8] One multicenter study evaluated 330 colorectal lesions that were either suspected or diagnosed for adenocarcinoma that underwent EFTR. The median size of the lesions was

15 mm. Of the 330 lesions, 132 were for primary treatment and the rest (198 lesions) for secondary treatment of previous resection (67 were R1, 103 were Rx, and 28 were R0 <1 mm). Technical success was 87.0% (287/330 procedures); out of the failed cases, 10 lesions were could not be reached or retracted inside the cap. In EFTRs that were primary resections, there was 89.4% success rate with 82% R0 resection rate. The overall R0 resection rate was 85.6%, 80.0% for lesions greater than 20 mm and 85.9% for those less or equal to 20 mm, although this difference was not statistically significant (P = .60). Adverse events occurred in 8.1% of the cases including perforation and bleeding. There were 7 severe events (2.2%) that required surgical management. The rest were managed endoscopically or conservatively with antibiotics.

Similarly, when the 2022 meta-analysis performed a subgroup analysis based on type of the colorectal lesions, it demonstrated that technical success rate was 87.2% for adenomatous lesions, whereas technical success rate for subepithelial lesions was 94.6% and 85.2% for T1 carcinomas.[6] R0 resection rate also differed depending on the type of the lesion: About 77.6% for adenomas, 94.5% for subepithelial lesions, and 83.0% for T1 carcinomas. When analyzed based on the average size of the lesion, there was no difference in the technical success or the recurrence rates for lesions less than or greater than 20 mm. Larger lesions (ie, >20 mm) did have higher adverse events (odds ratio 3.5) and lower R0 resection rates (odds ratio 0.3) when compared with the smaller lesions.

These findings are comparable to a previously published study on 156 T1 colorectal cancers (incompletely resected or nonlifting lesions) undergoing EFTR with 92.3% technical success and 71.8% R0 resection rate.[9] Of the 31 lesions that were considered histologically incomplete, the subsequent surgical resection showed no residual tumor in 29% (9 of 31) cases, bringing the adjusted R0 resection rate to 78%. There was a 14% adverse event rate with 3% requiring surgical intervention. This study also showed that although 87 of 156 patients had high-risk lesions requiring surgical resection, only 53 of these patients actually underwent surgical resection; for those who did not undergo surgery, it was primarily due to patient refusal and comorbidities making them unfit for surgery. EFTR may be a reasonable approach in this subset of patients as a first-line management approach; 73% of patients who had high-risk features and no surgical resection had achieved R0 resection with no recurrence at a 12-week follow-up.

Although EFTR is mostly used for lower GI lesions, a multicenter international study in 2020 showed favorable outcomes with EFTR (specifically with FTRDs) in upper GI lesions as well.[20] In this study, 38% of the lesions (n = 21) were in the gastric antrum, technical success with complete endoscopic resection was achieved in 77%; and of those, 88% had R0 resection, yielding an overall rate with 27% in the gastric body, 19% in the gastric cardia and fundus, with 14% in the duodenum, and 2% (n = 1) in the esophagus. The majority were GIST (41%), with 9% adenocarcinoma and another 9% with neuroendocrine tumor. The mean diameter was 15 mm (range 3–35 mm). Technical success was 68% for R0 resection in all FTRD resections for upper GI lesions. When adjusted for size, the R0 resection rate was 73% for lesions less than 15 mm versus 29% for lesions greater than 15 mm (P = .034). Adverse events occurred in 21% of resections, most of them bleeding and no perforations. Of those who received a follow-up endoscopy (55%), 97% showed no recurrent or residual lesions.

Another study evaluating 40 EFTRs for gastric subepithelial tumors (90% GIST, 10% leiomyomas) showed a 100% technical success rate.[26] Similarly, using exposed an EFTR technique for gastric lesions has also been shown to be highly successful in a systematic review with 98.8% rate of complete, R0 resection and 0.8% surgical conversion rate.[18] In this study, the overall adverse events rate was 1.6% including bleeding, perforation, peritonitis, and abdominal abscess formation or infection.

A study evaluating 10 duodenal lesions also showed favorable outcomes with EFTR with 80% technical success rate and 80% R0 resection rate.[27] Five lesions were nonlifting adenomas (see example in **Fig. 7**), 2 were recurrent adenomas, and 3 were subepithelial tumors. Sizes ranged from 12 to 25 mm with mean of 16.7 mm. There were no adverse events including delayed perforation at the time of follow-up. Of note, most of these lesions were performed using a pediatric colonoscope to adequately access the second part of the duodenum, and the EFTRs was performed either with OTSC or FTRD. **Fig. 8** shows an example of a scarred duodenal adenoma resected with FTRD.

COMPARISONS OF DIFFERENT METHODS

When comparing 35 exposed EFTRs with 33 laparoscopic surgical resections of a GIST less than 2 cm, it was shown that the exposed EFTR is performed significantly faster than the laparoscopic approach (91 vs 155 minutes, respectively) and had significantly lower adverse events.[28] Exposed EFTR also had 100% success rate. Of note, of the 33 laparoscopic resections performed, 12 required emergency endoscopic assistance to identify the lesion since lesions smaller than 2 cm in diameter can be difficult to identify from the outside of the serosal layer especially when it is located in the gastroesophageal junction or on the posterior aspect of the stomach.

A recent study published in 2022 compared exposed EFTR with nonexposed (or cap-assisted) EFTR in a retrospective analysis evaluating 113 patients with GIST less than 1.5 cm.[29] In this study, both groups had 100% en-bloc resection rate. The exposed group had significantly longer procedure times compared with the nonexposed group (55.5 vs 41.0 minutes, respectively) even after adjusting for the size and layer of origin. The R0 resection rate for exposed EFTR group was 94.0% and that of the nonexposed EFTR group was 97.8%, which were not statistically significant ($P = .355$). The usage of heat clamp such as coagulation graspers for bleeding control was significantly higher in the exposed EFTR group than the nonexposed EFTR group (65.7% vs 10.9%, respectively) but the incidence of pneumoperitoneum was insignificant between the 2 groups (13.4% vs 6.5%, respectively, $P = .251$). The exposed EFTR group had significantly higher postoperative fever (58.2%) when compared with the nonexposed EFTR group. No lesions needed surgery. There was no recurrence in either group at roughly a 3-year follow-up (38.9 months for exposed EFTR group and 31.3 months for nonexposed EFTR group). This highlights that while both approaches are effective, the nonexposed EFTR is a more preferred EFTR technique for smaller lesions.

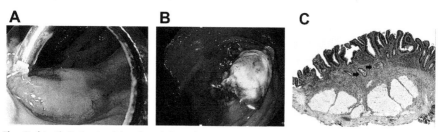

A   **B**   **C**

Fig. 7. (*A, B*) Patient with prior right colon cancer s/p subtotal colectomy and now with a 15 mm distal sigmoid polypoid mass s/p prior incomplete resection showing adenocarcinoma. The patient refused further surgery and lesion was removed using FTRD. (*C*) Final pathologic condition showed 1 mm focus of adenocarcinoma (*arrows*) arising within a tubular adenoma and all margins negative.

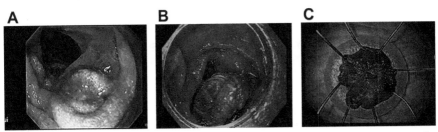

Fig. 8. (*A*) Duodenal adenoma with high-grade dysplasia scarred from prior resection attempt. (*B*) EFTR of the duodenal adenoma using FTRD. (*C*) Resected lesion.

In the lower GI tract, one retrospective study compared transanal endoscopic microsurgery (TEM), ESD, and ESD using FTRD in 76 rectal cancers.[30] The study showed that while the tumor sizes were significantly smaller for patients getting FTRD compared with those getting TEM and ESD, the patients treated with TEM and FTRD had lower perforation rates, shorter hospital stay, and higher en-bloc resection rates when compared with ESD. There was no significant difference in R0 resection rates among these 3 modalities.

Another study compared 50 ESDs to 52 EFTRs in neoplastic lesions less than 30 mm.[31] The mean size was significantly bigger in ESD group (21.7 vs 15.6 mm in EFTR), and although only 10% of lesions treated by ESD were above the splenic flexure, 57% of lesions treated via EFTR were above the splenic flexure. Technical success rate was significantly higher in the EFTR group compared with the ESD group (92% vs 74%, respectively), and R0 resection rate was also significantly higher in the EFTR group (85% vs 62% in ESD group). Of those that had positive margins, there were no positive vertical margins in the EFTR group; the ESD group did have 3 cases of positive vertical margin. Additionally, there were significantly less complication rates in the EFTR group (13% vs 40% in the ESD group), which included perforations (1 EFTR, 4 ESD), bleeding (4 in both groups), postpolypectomy syndrome (20 in ESD only), and appendicitis (2 EFTRs) that were managed conservatively. There was no statistical significance in recurrence rates: 12% in the EFTR group and 5% in the ESD group.

The use of full-thickness resection (FTR; both endoscopic and surgical) as an alternative curative management to the conventional completion surgical approach for a previously resected R1 or Rx T1 colorectal cancers was also studied.[32] R1 refers to having microscopic residual tumor, whereas Rx refers to being unable to assess if there is a residual tumor or not.[21] This study evaluated 334 patients with R1/Rx resected T1 colorectal cancers who underwent completion surgery and 100 who underwent FTRs. Severe complications occurred in 11.1% of completion surgery group including 4 (1.2%) fatal ones. FTR group had a significantly lower serious complication rate at 4.0%, which included bleeding that required reintervention. There were no fatal complications in the FTR group. At a median follow-up of 5 years, those with completion surgery had a 2.2% recurrence rate, whereas those with FTR had 9.0% recurrence rate. Although the 5-year disease-free survival rate was lower in FTR strategy (89.9% vs 96.8% in completion surgery group, $P = .019$), most (63%) were able to get salvage surgery with curative intent, and the overall survival and metastasis-free survival were not significant between the 2 groups. This study did not separate out minimally invasive surgical FTRs from EFTRs; nonetheless, this suggests a new potential role of FTR with surveillance as an alternative option to a completion surgery for patients who do not wish to or are unable to pursue surgical option (see **Fig. 7**).

When compared with various other treatment modalities, EFTR, specifically the nonexposed EFTR, has been consistently shown to have favorable outcomes, although EFTR is limited by the lesion size. Limitations of EFTR will be discussed more in depth in the later section.

COMPLICATIONS

The most common complications of EFTR are bleeding and perforation (sometimes attributed to the malfunctioning of FTRD or misdepolyment of the clips). Others include peritonitis, appendicitis, and postpolypectomy syndrome. Another rare complication for periappendiceal lesions is enterocolonic fistula, only described in 2 case reports to date.[33,34] This may be because the colonic wall in the right colon is very thin and adjacent organs and intestines can easily be suctioned into the cap and resected along with the colonic mucosa. As discussed previously, the rate of additional surgery associated with EFTR remains low.

Appendiceal adenomas can theoretically be at a higher risk for appendicitis because EFTR is associated with a subtotal appendectomy. One study specifically evaluated this with 50 appendiceal lesions undergoing EFTR.[35] The mean size was 18.3 mm, and all patients received antibiotic prophylaxis treatment of a mean of 4 days. Of the 50 patients studied, 7 patients (14%) had postprocedural appendicitis. Of these 7, 4 (57%) were managed conservatively with fluids and antibiotics, and 3 underwent surgical appendectomy. One lesion (2%) had a cecal perforation. It is unclear which patients with an appendiceal lesion are at higher risk for appendicitis, and currently there are no guidelines or a standardized approach on antibiotic regimen (preprocedural or postprocedural) for appendicitis prophylaxis in appendiceal lesions for EFTR.

Although not reported in the literature, anecdotally there have been discussions regarding premature clip passage with the FTRD, which can result in a perforation that requires open surgery because the patient may have a delayed presentation. More data must be gathered to optimize technique before any conclusion regarding technique or device can be made.

Given the risk for perforation if not deployed properly, there is an FDA-mandated training on the use of FTRD that must be completed before using the device in the United States.

LIMITATIONS

There are several limitations to EFTRs. Most of the data using EFTR are derived from retrospective and prospective studies, and there are no randomized controlled trials to compare EFTRs from other treatment modalities. Additionally, in FTRD that uses a cap, the cap diameter is 21 mm and limits the size of lesion being resected. Lesions greater than this have lower rates of R0 resection and higher procedure-related adverse events.[6] The FTRD can also be quite cumbersome to pass through the colon. This is due to multiple factors including a longer cap length that limits endoscopic vision, large size of the clip on the scope tip which makes passage through a tight sigmoid difficult, and the outer setup of the device along the scope shaft can be difficult to obtain a good grip on the scope.

COST ANALYSIS

Although EFTR is more expensive than the standard endoscopic resection with EMR and ESD, EFTR costs are lower than surgical devices. Kuellmer and colleagues analyzed cost effective analysis for EFTR and found that for each R0 resection, EFTR costs €3708.98 (equivalent to US$4106.03) from the care-provider standpoint, whereas surgery would cost €8924.05 (equivalent to US$9879.37), resulting in EFTR having about a third of financial burden when compared with surgery.[9] The cost of EFTR was found to be about 40% higher than the standard endoscopic resection (€2852 vs €1712, respectively).

SUMMARY

Difficult-to-treat lesions in the GI tract result in high complication rates and incomplete resections using the standard endoscopic resection approach via EMR or ESD. T1 carcinoma with submucosal invasion has been traditionally managed surgically due to high rates of Rx or R1 resection rates with EMR or ESD. Although surgical intervention is still standard of care in appropriately fit patients, many patients are poor surgical candidates, and therefore, alternative management strategies such as EFTR can be used. EFTR continues to evolve with more widespread use and gathering of more data but so far for GI tract lesions smaller than 2 cm, it has shown to have high success rates and is a cost-effective approach. Most commonly, FTRD is used for FTRs. Care must be taken for proper training and technique when deploying the device to avoid complications including bleeding and perforation. Furthermore, patients and physicians should also be aware of adverse events associated with appendiceal resections including appendicitis and fistula formation. EFTR can be considered as a viable treatment option in appropriately selected patients that are discussed in a multidisciplinary format.

CLINICS CARE POINTS

- EFTR is a reasonable approach for curative management in locally invasive T1 GI cancers less than 2 cm, especially in patients who are poor surgical candidates.
- If the FTRD clip does not deploy, one can straighten out the scope and reattempt deployment. If this does not work, the scope will need to be removed.
- If the FTRD clip does not deploy but the cut has already been performed, then one may need to convert to an exposed EFTR.
- Rare complications have been associated with FTRD at the appendiceal orifice include fistula and appendicitis.

DISCLOSURE

G.E. Kim has nothing to disclose. S. Kothari is a Consultant for Boston scientific, Olympus. Advisory board castle biosciences. U.D. Siddiqui is a consultant and speaker for Medtronic, Cook, Olympus, and Conmed; and a speaker for Ovesco and Pinnacle Biologic.

REFERENCES

1. Arnold M, Sierra MS, Laversanne M, et al. Global patterns and trends in colorectal cancer incidence and mortality. Gut 2017;66(4):683–91.
2. Benson AB, Venook AP, Al-Hawary MM, et al. Colon Cancer, Version 2.2021, NCCN Clinical Practice Guidelines in Oncology. J Natl Compr Canc Netw 2021;19(3):329–59. https://doi.org/10.6004/jnccn.2021.0012.

3. Fisher DA, Shergill AK, Early DS, et al. Role of endoscopy in the staging and management of colorectal cancer. Gastrointest Endosc 2013;78(1):8–12.

4. Ferlitsch M, Moss A, Hassan C, et al. Colorectal polypectomy and endoscopic mucosal resection (EMR): European Society of Gastrointestinal Endoscopy (ESGE) clinical guideline. Endoscopy 2017;49(03):270–97.

5. Tanaka S, Kashida H, Saito Y, et al. JGES guidelines for colorectal endoscopic submucosal dissection/endoscopic mucosal resection. Dig Endosc 2015;27(4): 417–34.

6. Dolan RD, Bazarbashi AN, McCarty TR, et al. Endoscopic full-thickness resection of colorectal lesions: a systematic review and meta-analysis. Gastrointest Endosc 2022;95(2):216–24. https://doi.org/10.1016/j.gie.2021.09.039, e18.

7. Mizushima T, Kato M, Iwanaga I, et al. Technical difficulty according to location, and risk factors for perforation, in endoscopic submucosal dissection of colorectal tumors. Surg Endosc 2015;29(1):133–9. https://doi.org/10.1007/s00464-014-3665-9.

8. Zwager LW, Bastiaansen BAJ, van der Spek BW, et al. Endoscopic full-thickness resection of T1 colorectal cancers: a retrospective analysis from a multicenter Dutch eFTR registry. Endoscopy 2021. https://doi.org/10.1055/a-1637-9051.

9. Kuellmer A, Behn J, Beyna T, et al. Endoscopic full-thickness resection and its treatment alternatives in difficult-to-treat lesions of the lower gastrointestinal tract: a cost-effectiveness analysis. BMJ Open Gastroenterol 2020;7(1). https://doi.org/10.1136/bmjgast-2020-000449.

10. Guillaumot M-A, Barret M, Jacques J, et al. Endoscopic full-thickness resection of early colorectal neoplasms using an endoscopic submucosal dissection knife: a retrospective multicenter study. Endosc Int Open 2020;8(05):E611–6.

11. Zhou PH, Yao LQ, Qin XY, et al. Endoscopic full-thickness resection without laparoscopic assistance for gastric submucosal tumors originated from the muscularis propria. Surg Endosc 2011;25(9):2926–31. https://doi.org/10.1007/s00464-011-1644-y.

12. Meier B, Stritzke B, Kuellmer A, et al. Efficacy and safety of endoscopic full-thickness resection in the colorectum: results from the German Colonic FTRD Registry. Official J Am Coll Gastroenterol ACG 2020;115(12):1998–2006.

13. Backes Y, Kappelle WF, Berk L, et al. Colorectal endoscopic full-thickness resection using a novel, flat-base over-the-scope clip: a prospective study. Endoscopy 2017;49(11):1092–7.

14. Aslanian HR, Sethi A, Bhutani MS, et al. ASGE guideline for endoscopic full-thickness resection and submucosal tunnel endoscopic resection. VideoGIE 2019;4(8):343–50. https://doi.org/10.1016/j.vgie.2019.03.010.

15. Rajan E, Wong K, Song LM. Endoscopic Full Thickness Resection. Gastroenterology 2018;154(7):1925–37.e2. https://doi.org/10.1053/j.gastro.2018.02.020.

16. Schmidt A, Bauerfeind P, Gubler C, et al. Endoscopic full-thickness resection in the colorectum with a novel over-the-scope device: first experience. Endoscopy 2015;47(8):719–25. https://doi.org/10.1055/s-0034-1391781.

17. von Mehren M, Randall RL, Benjamin RS, et al. Soft Tissue Sarcoma, Version 2.2018, NCCN Clinical Practice Guidelines in Oncology. J Natl Compr Canc Netw 2018;16(5):536–63. https://doi.org/10.6004/jnccn.2018.0025.

18. Antonino G, Alberto M, Michele A, et al. Efficacy and safety of gastric exposed endoscopic full-thickness resection without laparoscopic assistance: a systematic review. Endosc Int Open 2020;8(9):e1173–82. https://doi.org/10.1055/a-1198-4357.

19. Schmidt A, Beyna T, Schumacher B, et al. Colonoscopic full-thickness resection using an over-the-scope device: a prospective multicentre study in various indications. Gut 2018;67(7):1280–9. https://doi.org/10.1136/gutjnl-2016-313677.

20. Hajifathalian K, Ichkhanian Y, Dawod Q, et al. Full-thickness resection device (FTRD) for treatment of upper gastrointestinal tract lesions: the first international experience. Endosc Int Open 2020;8(10):e1291–301. https://doi.org/10.1055/a-1216-1439.

21. Hermanek P, Wittekind C. The pathologist and the residual tumor (R) classification. Pathol Res Pract 1994;190(2):115–23. https://doi.org/10.1016/s0344-0338(11)80700-4.

22. Ichkhanian Y, Vosoughi K, Diehl D, et al. A large multicenter cohort on the use of full-thickness resection device for difficult colonic lesions. Surg Endosc 2021;35(3):1296–306.

23. Zwager LW, Bastiaansen BA, Bronzwaer ME, et al. Endoscopic full-thickness resection (eFTR) of colorectal lesions: results from the Dutch colorectal eFTR registry. Endoscopy 2020;52(11):1014–23.

24. Andrisani G, Soriani P, Manno M, et al. Colo-rectal endoscopic full-thickness resection (EFTR) with the over-the-scope device (FTRD®): A multicenter Italian experience. Dig Liver Dis 2019;51(3):375–81.

25. Bronzwaer ME, Bastiaansen BA, Koens L, et al. Endoscopic full-thickness resection of polyps involving the appendiceal orifice: a prospective observational case study. Endosc Int Open 2018;6(09):E1112–9.

26. Wang W, Liu CX, Niu Q, et al. OTSC assisted EFTR for the treatment of GIST: 40 cases analysis. Minim Invasive Ther Allied Technol 2022;31(2):238–45. https://doi.org/10.1080/13645706.2020.1781190.

27. Andrisani G, Di Matteo FM. Endoscopic full-thickness resection of duodenal lesions (with video). Surg Endosc 2020;34(4):1876–81. https://doi.org/10.1007/s00464-019-07269-w.

28. Wang H, Feng X, Ye S, et al. A comparison of the efficacy and safety of endoscopic full-thickness resection and laparoscopic-assisted surgery for small gastrointestinal stromal tumors. Surg Endosc 2016;30(8):3357–61. https://doi.org/10.1007/s00464-015-4612-0.

29. Yang J, Ni M, Jiang J, et al. Comparison of endoscopic full-thickness resection and cap-assisted endoscopic full-thickness resection in the treatment of small (≤1.5 cm) gastric GI stromal tumors. Gastrointest Endosc 2022;95(4):660–70. https://doi.org/10.1016/j.gie.2021.10.026, e2.

30. Bisogni D, Manetti R, Talamucci L, et al. Comparison among different techniques for en-bloc resection of rectal lesions: transanal endoscopic surgery vs. endoscopic submucosal dissection vs. full-thickness resection device with Over-The-Scope Clip® System. Minerva Chir 2020;75(4):234–43. https://doi.org/10.23736/s0026-4733.20.08298-x.

31. Falt P, Zapletalová J, Urban O. Endoscopic full-thickness resection versus endoscopic submucosal dissection in the treatment of colonic neoplastic lesions ≤ 30 mm-a single-center experience. Surg Endosc 2022;36(3):2062–9. https://doi.org/10.1007/s00464-021-08492-0.

32. Gijsbers KM, Laclé MM, Elias SG, et al. Full-thickness scar resection following R1/Rx excised T1 colorectal cancers as alternative to completion surgery. Am J Gastroenterol 2021. https://doi.org/10.14309/ajg.0000000000001621.

33. Vargas JI, Rowsell C, Mosko JD. Enterocolonic fistula after endoscopic full-thickness resection of a peri-appendiceal orifice adenoma. Gastrointest Endosc 2020;91(6):1405–6. https://doi.org/10.1016/j.gie.2020.01.041.

34. Oliviero G, Gagliardi M, Napoli M, et al. Fatal Outcome Consequent to an Endoscopic Full Thickness Resection of a Colonic Lateral Spreading Tumor: A Case Report. Am J Case Rep 2020;21:e922855. https://doi.org/10.12659/ajcr.922855.

35. Schmidbaur S, Wannhoff A, Walter B, et al. Risk of appendicitis after endoscopic full-thickness resection of lesions involving the appendiceal orifice: a retrospective analysis. Endoscopy 2021;53(4):424–8. https://doi.org/10.1055/a-1227-4555.

Endoscopic Closure
Tools and Techniques

Thomas R. McCarty, MD, MPH[a,b], Pichamol Jirapinyo, MD, MPH[a,b,*]

KEYWORDS

- Endoscopy • Through-the-scope clips • Over-the-scope-clips
- Endoscopic suturing • X-tack endoscopic HeliX tacking system
- Endoscopic submucosal dissection

KEY POINTS

- Proper understanding of endoscopic closure tools is critically important in the field of third space endoscopy.
- Through-the-scope clips are perhaps the most commonly used endoscopic tool to achieve closure of gastrointestinal defects.
- However, over-the-scope-clips and more novel closure techniques including endoscopic suturing and a novel helix tacking system may allow for improved closure rates for larger or irregular-shaped defects.

INTRODUCTION

The field of third space endoscopy has seen a vast expansion in various tools and techniques over the last decade. During these complex procedures such as endoscopic mucosal resection (EMR), endoscopic submucosal dissection (ESD), peroral endoscopic myotomy (POEM), submucosal tunneling endoscopic resection (STER), and endoscopic full-thickness resection (EFTR), mucosal defects are frequently encountered, whether caused by an adverse event (AE) or as a routine part of the procedure. Therefore, as the field of third space endoscopy continues to expand, knowledge of various endoscopic closure tools and techniques remains critically important. This article discusses commonly used endoscopic closure devices, their principles of closure and technique, data on their safety and efficacy, and a description of the authors' own practice patterns. This article focuses on the applications of these devices on mucosal incision and defect closure as part of third space endoscopy. Other applications for these devices are beyond the scope of this review.

Funding: None.
[a] Division of Gastroenterology, Hepatology and Endoscopy, Brigham and Women's Hospital, 75 Francis Street, Boston, MA 02115, USA; [b] Harvard Medical School, Boston, MA, USA
* Corresponding author. Division of Gastroenterology, Hepatology and Endoscopy, Brigham and Women's Hospital, 75 Francis Street, Boston, MA 02115.
E-mail address: pjirapinyo@bwh.harvard.edu

Gastrointest Endoscopy Clin N Am 33 (2023) 169–182
https://doi.org/10.1016/j.giec.2022.08.003
giendo.theclinics.com

THROUGH-THE-SCOPE CLIPS

Through-the-scope clips (TTSCs) are among the most widely adopted tools for the general and advanced endoscopist. Initially used endoscopically by Hayashi and colleagues in 1975, TTSCs consist of 3 main components: a metallic double-pronged clip, a delivery catheter, and a handle used to operate and deploy the clip.[1,2] All TTSCs are designed to be passed through the standard working channel of a gastroscope and are available for all types of endoscopes.[3] To date, there are several TTSCs available commercially, each with unique characteristics including jaw opening width, jaw teeth, and catheter rotatability. A list of currently available TTSCs in the United States is summarized in **Table 1**.

From a technical standpoint, the jaws of the TTSC can be manipulated, rotated (for some clip types), and oriented perpendicular to the mucosal edges of the defect to appropriately appose tissue.[4] Next, suction may be performed to capture additional tissue and aid in securing tissue within the jaws of the TTSC before closure. Once the tissue is apposed and visualized with insufflation, the TTSC may be deployed.

Further technical aspects of the TTSC include considerations of the size and type of the defect. Classically, TTSCs have been demonstrated to be effective at closing a defect up to 2 cm in size, with a decreasing efficacy for larger defects. Closure should be attempted initially at the periphery of the defect, with systematic closure toward the center of the defect. For moderate-to-large defects, serial TTSC application in a line that is perpendicular to the long axis of the lumen (ie, zipper closure technique) may result in a superior defect closure.[4,5] It should be noted that although TTSCs are easy to use, they have limited opening widths and closing strengths, and are usually ineffective in the setting of fibrotic tissue.[6]

It is important to highlight that not all TTSCs are equal, with each type of clip possessing unique physical characteristics and functional profile that should be considered based on the type of gastrointestinal (GI) defect and clinical scenario. In a study by Wang and colleagues, 5 US commercially available TTSCs were evaluated based on multiple features including rotatability, overshoot, open/closure precision, and tensile/closure strength.[7] Additionally, clip performance was examined in 4 different endoscope configurations, including straight, at the duodenal sweep, in full retroflexion, and across the elevator of a duodenoscope. Based on these results, the Resolution 360 clip (Boston Scientific, Marlborough, Massachusetts.) provided the best rotatability in all endoscopic configurations and the least overshoot. Precision opening and closing were best among the SureClip 16 mm (Micro-Tech, Ann Arbor, Michigan) and Dura Clip 11 mm (ConMed, Utica, New York) TTSCs. For tension strength and closure strength, the Quick Clip Pro (Olympus America, Center Valley, Pennsylvania) and Instinct (Cook Medical, Bloomington, Indiana) TTSCs outperformed the others. Ultimately, an understanding of the characteristic of each TTSC should be combined with thorough assessment of the nature of the defect and clinical scenario to assist with clip selection.

With regard to third space endoscopic procedures, TTSCs remain a highly effective and safe option. For GI defect smaller than 2 cm, literature has shown their efficacy to vary from 50% to 90% based on individual lesion characteristic.[3] This, in turn, underscores the need for proper assessment of the defect and understanding of the specific TTSC characteristics to optimize the potential for successful closure. Closure failure may occur because of inability to orient the clip properly (ie, rotatability), inability to grasp or approximate tissue (ie, fibrosis or friable tissue), endoscope position (ie, retroflexion or use of elevator with duodenoscope), and lesion size and location. In the authors' practice, TTSCs are used as a first-line strategy for several third space

Table 1
Currently available through-the-scope-clips and over-the-scope-clips in the US market

Clip Name/Device	Manufacturer	Working Length	Maximal Diameter of Jaw	Advantages or Unique Features
TTSC				
Resolution Clip	Boston Scientific (Marlborough, Massachusetts)	155 and 235 cm	11 mm	Able to be opened/closed up to 5 times before deployment
Resolution 360 Clip	Boston Scientific	155 and 235 cm	11 mm	Rotatable clip for improved orientation
Resolution 360 Ultra Clip	Boston Scientific	155 and 235 cm	17 mm	One of the largest TTSC jaw sizes on the US market
QuickClip Pro	Olympus (Tokyo, Japan)	165 and 230 cm	11 mm	Rotatable clip for improved orientation
QuickClip2 Fixing Device	Olympus	165 and 230 cm	9 and 11 mm	Rotatable clip for improved orientation
Instinct Plus	Cook Medical (Winston-Salem, North Carolina)	230 cm	16 mm	Large jaw with rotatable clip for improved orientation
Dura Clip	ConMed (Utica, New York)	165 and 230 cm	11 and 16 mm	Rotatable clip for improved orientation
SureClip Mini	Micro-Tech Endoscopy (Ann Arbor, Michigan)	235 cm	8 m	One of the smallest jaw sizes on the US market
SureClip	Micro-Tech Endoscopy	235 cm	11 mm	Rotatable clip for improved orientation
SureClip Plus	Micro-Tech Endoscopy	235 cm	16 mm	Rotatable clip for improved orientation
SureClip Max	Micro-Tech Endoscopy	235 cm	17 mm	Rotatable clip for improved orientation
Lockado	Micro-Tech Endoscopy		11, 16, and 22 mm	One of the largest TTSC jaw sizes on the US market
Over-The-Scope Clip (OTSC)				
OTSC Clip	Ovesco Endoscopy (Tübingen, Germany)	165 and 220 cm	8.5–14 mm	Four different sizes of caps, 2 depths of caps, 3 different shapes of teeth
OTSC Mini	Ovesco Endoscopy (Tübingen, Germany)	165 and 220 cm	8.5–10 mm	Compatible with smaller diameter endoscopes and 2 different shapes of teeth

(continued on next page)

Table 1
(continued)

Clip Name/Device	Manufacturer	Working Length	Maximal Diameter of Jaw	Advantages or Unique Features
OTSC StentFix	Ovesco Endoscopy (Tübingen, Germany)	165 and 220 cm	8.5–14 mm	Rounded design to assist with stent fixation/anchoring
Padlock Clip	STERIS (Mentor, Ohio)	165 cm	9.5–11 mm	Circumferential design
Padlock Clip Pro-Select	STERIS	165 cm	11.5–14 mm	Circumferential design with larger diameter

Adapted from Asge Technology Committee, Conway JD, Adler DG, et al. Endoscopic hemostatic devices. Gastrointest Endosc 2009;69(6):987-996.

endoscopic procedures, including closure of EMR defect, incomplete or partial ESD mucosotomy site (for lesions not amenable to complete resection), and mucosotomy site at the end of esophageal POEM (E-POEM) and Zenker POEM (Z-POEM).

Given the efficacy and safety profile of TTSCs, these devices are likely to remain the bedrock of defect and mucosotomy closure. However, it bears repeating that alternative closure devices and techniques may be warranted for defects larger than 2 cm. Additionally, other defect factors such as surface irregularities, defect configuration, and orientation should be taken into consideration when choosing the device and technique.

OVER-THE-SCOPE CLIPS

Over-the-scope-clips (OTSCs) were first described in 2007 by Kirschniak and colleagues.[8] The OTSC device received clearance from the US Food and Drug Administration (FDA) in 2010 for compression of tissue in the gastrointestinal (GI) tract, hemostasis, and treating lesions of the wall of GI organs. Currently, there are 2 OTSC systems available in the United States, including the Padlock Clip (STERIS, Mentor, Ohio) and the Ovesco Clip (GmbH, Tübingen, Germany).[3,8–12] In general, these devices are used to close large defects up to 3 cm and full-thickness defect (such as a perforation) less than 2 cm in size.

Although the Ovesco and Padlock clips are different devices, the mechanisms and principles to achieve defect closure remain the same. The systems include an applicator cap, a specially designed clip (ranging from 8.5 to 14 mm) attached to the outside of the endoscope (different from TTSCs), and an external device to assist in clip deployment.[3] A summary guide of available OTSC devices is highlighted in **Table 1**.[13] To achieve proper closure, the endoscope and OTSC are oriented perpendicular to the defect. The defect is then suctioned into the working channel and inside the applicator with OTSC deployed around the defect, effectively approximating the tissue edges of the defect.

The Ovesco OTSC system consists of a preloaded nitinol clip and applicator cap mounted to the outside of the distal aspect of the endoscope. The Ovesco Clip is deployed in a similar fashion to endoscopic band ligation systems with deployment after the hand-cranked wheel is turned. Notably, the Ovesco system includes a Clip, Mini, and StentFix device with variable applicator sizes and configurations of the clip teeth to optimize grasping and apposition of tissue:

Type a – blunt teeth with a primary compression effect (atraumatic)
Type t – spiked teeth with compression and anchoring effect (traumatic)
Type gc – spiked elongated teeth with anchoring and apposition effect (gastric fistula closure) (**Fig. 1**)

In comparison, the Padlock OTSC system is comprised of a linking cable that runs alongside the endoscope. Additionally, the clip is deployed via a push of the thumb actuation, dissimilar to the hand-crank wheel with the Ovesco device (**Fig. 2**).

Additionally, 2 adjunctive devices including the Ovesco OTSC Twin Grasper and OTSC Anchor are available to assist closure of larger defects and aid in acquiring tissue and improving approximation.[14] These devices are passed down the working channel of the endoscope and then withdrawn within the applicator cap after tissue is grasped to assist in closure of larger defects (typically 2–3 cm in size). The use of the Twin Grasper may also be useful for chronic defects or in situations when suction alone is inadequate to approximate tissue.[14] It should be noted that rat-toothed forceps may also be used to grasp tissue and pull into the working channel and applicator to assist in tissue acquisition and successful defect closure.

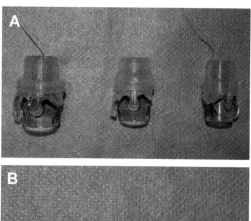

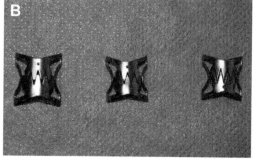

Fig. 1. Ovesco Over-The-Scope Clip (OTSC) system: applicator caps and clip types. (A) Over-the-scope clips: applicator caps; 3 sizes. (B) Over-the-scope clips: type a (left), type t (middle), and type gc (right). (*From* ASGE Technology Committee, Banerjee S, Barth BA, et al. Endoscopic closure devices [published correction appears in Gastrointest Endosc. 2013 May;77(5):833]. Gastrointest Endosc. 2012;76(2):244-251.)

To date, there are no studies comparing characteristics of the 2 OTSCs. One animal study by Dolezel and colleagues compared OTSCs versus an endoloop-plus-TTSC technique, and found both techniques were able to adequately close defects (100% closure in both groups).[15] Another preclinical randomized study in a porcine model compared OTSC versus a traditional surgical approach and found similar results for both groups.[16] One of the largest studies to date has been a multicenter retrospective study by Haito-Chavez and colleagues, which analyzed OTSC closure of GI defects

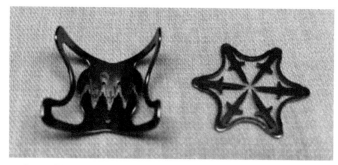

Fig. 2. Comparison of Ovesco versus Padlock Over-The-Scope Clips (OTSCs). Over-the-scope clips: Ovesco (*left*) and Padlock (*right*). (*From* ASGE technology committee, Parsi MA, Schulman AR, et al. Devices for endoscopic hemostasis of nonvariceal GI bleeding (with videos). VideoGIE. 2019;4(7):285-299. Published 2019 Jun 27.)

among 188 patients.[17] This study included 108 patients with fistulas, 48 patients with full-thickness defects, and 32 patients with GI leaks, and found the rates of successful closure for perforations (90%) and leaks (73.3%) were significantly higher than that of fistulas (42.9%, P<.05). On multivariable regression analyses, patients who underwent OTSC placement for perforations and leaks were noted to have significantly greater long-term success compared with those who had fistulas (odds ratio [OR] 51.4 and 8.36, respectively].

OTSCs may also be used to achieve full-thickness resection while simultaneously providing adequate defect closure, a technique that is discussed elsewhere in this collection.[18] Use of OTSCs to aid in stent fixation and treat patients with high-risk stigmata or active peptic ulcer bleeding has also been described.[19] At this time, OTSCs have not been routinely used in the authors' practice for the closure of EMR, ESD, or POEM defect closure, although they remain an important tool for closure of full-thickness defects, leak, and less commonly, fistulas. A previous study by Donatelli and colleagues reported OTSC use for various GI defects among 45 patients (51 OTSCs total). Early or acute defects demonstrated a greater rate of successful closure (clinical success of 100%) compared with chronic defects (37%), suggesting early intervention may improve outcomes with this device.

The most common limitation with OTSC includes the ability to navigate the device to an ideal position and proper deployment. Given that the clip is attached outside of the endoscope, the system may be challenging to pass through the oropharynx or upper esophageal sphincter with deployment issues in a retroflexed position or when the endoscope is acutely angulated.[6] Once deployed, removal may be even more challenging, requiring a specific removal device or direct, high-powered treatment with argon plasma coagulation (APC).[20] Furthermore, OTSCs are more expensive compared with traditional TTSCs, although this cost may be comparable when a multiple TTSCs are required. Another major limitation of the current OTSCs remains the size of the defect able to be closed, that being an upper limit of 2 to 3 cm because of the size of the endoscope, cap, and clip deployment mechanism. Although use of adjunctive tools (ie, Ovesco Twin Grasper) may help approximate tissue for defects between 2 and 3 cm in size, larger or irregular lesions may still be challenging. Given these limitations, OTSCs may be used for moderate-sized rectal defects after EMR or ESD or in simultaneous full-thickness resection techniques for subepithelial lesions.[13]

ENDOSCOPIC SUTURING

The use of endoscopic suturing has become widely adopted to achieve defect closure and overcome the size limitation with current TTSCs and OTSCs. Multiple previous endoscopic suturing devices have been developed over the past 3 decades, including the Bard EndoCinch (C.R. Bard, Murray Hill, New Jersey), the T-Bar (Cook Medical, Bloomington, Indiana.), and the Eagle Claw (Olympus America, Center Valley, Pennsylvania) devices. Currently, there are 3 systems that have FDA clearance for tissue approximation including the OverStitch Endoscopic Suturing System (Apollo Endosurgery, Austin, Texas), the Incisionless Operating Platform (IOP, USGI Medical, San Clemente, California), and the Endomina plication system (Endo Tools Therapeutics, Gosselies, Belgium). Of these, the Overstitch suturing system is the only one that has recently received market authorization from the FDA for the treatment of obesity, specifically for endoscopic sleeve gastroplasty and revision of bariatric surgery, and it is the only system that currently is commercially available in the United States.

The Overstitch system is a disposable single-use endoscopic suturing device with multiple applications for GI defect closure including mucosal resection, POEM, enteral stent fixation, closure of perforations, leaks, and fistulas, and bariatric endoscopy.[21] The original Overstitch device requires a double-channel therapeutic endoscope; however, the Overstitch Sx device can be mounted alongside a single-channel endoscope. Currently, the more commonly used system with more available data is the double channel system, and this will be the focus of this review (**Fig. 3**).

The Apollo Overstitch system was first developed in 2009, and studied by Moran and colleagues, who demonstrated its effectiveness in placing full-thickness sutures for tissue apposition and gastrotomy closure in a porcine model.[22] The device is composed of a needle driver and an anchor exchange catheter.[23] The suture is first mounted onto the anchor exchange catheter and passed through the operating channel. The anchor is then transferred to the needle driver, and suturing is performed by transferring the anchor back and forth between the needle driver and the anchor exchange catheter. Tissue approximation can be facilitated with a tissue helix, which comes with the system, or with any approximator that may be passed down the working double channel gastroscope (often a rat-toothed forceps). When suturing is complete, a release button on the anchor exchange catheter releases the anchor. The suture is threaded onto a cinch device, which is then passed through the operating channel to secure and cut the suture. In this fashion, the Overstitch device allows interrupted or continuous sutures to be placed without needing to remove the device. The device itself can be reloaded multiple times with new needles without removing the endoscope.

With regard to types of suturing patterns for GI defect closure, strategies that may be employed include running suture pattern (1 suture with several stitches) or interrupted suture pattern (several sutures with 2 stitches per suture). In general, a running suture pattern is preferred for defect closure, because it is considered a stronger suture pattern that is associated with a higher leak pressure. When performing a running suture pattern, the authors' group typically closes defects from left to right (for a horizontal defect) or distal to proximal (for a vertical defect). It is also important to pass the

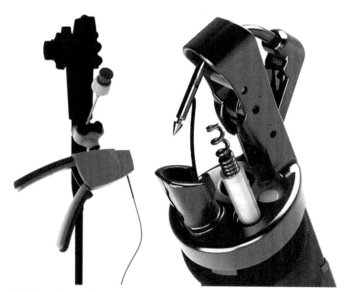

Fig. 3. OverStitch endoscopic suturing system. (*Courtesy* of Apollo Endosurgery, Inc, Austin, Texas, with permission.)

anchor from an outside-inside followed by an inside-outside approach to allow for submucosal-to-submucosal approximation, which leads to better tissue healing that mucosa-to-mucosal approximation. Additionally, when closing a defect, a rotatable rat-toothed forceps is preferred to the tissue helix, as it tends to be less traumatic to the mucosal flap.

One early study by Kantsevoy and colleagues sought to assess the role of endoscopic suturing for defect closure after gastric and colorectal ESD.[24] In this study, ESD was performed and followed by endoscopic suturing of the mucosal defects for 12 patients. Although this study was small, an endoscopic suturing device was technically feasible with a mean closure time of 10.0 plus or minus 5.8 minutes and required only 1 continuous suture for 8 patients and an interrupted suture approach (2–4 stitches per patient) for the remaining 4 patients. Importantly, there were no immediate or delayed adverse events. These results were similar to another small study of 14 patients by Han and colleagues, which demonstrated that endoscopic suturing did not affect endoscopic surveillance and sampling of the resection scar.[25] A recent multicenter registry study of endoscopic suturing by Maselli and colleagues evaluated a total of 137 patients with an overall technical success rate of 99.3%.[26] The overall clinical success was 89% with no adverse events reported. Stratifying these results by type of defect, mucosal defects were associated with 100% clinical success, perforation closure rate of 94.7%, and stent fixation rate of 85%, while leak and fistula closure was lower at 64.7% clinical success rate. Additional analyses revealed no significant correlation between location, suture pattern, or number of sutures; however, a continuous or running suture for smaller fistulas (defined as <10 mm) was more likely to achieve clinical success in the follow-up ($P<.001$).

The most notable advantage of endoscopic suturing is with regard to size of the defect. Given the design, there is no size limitation, with the additional benefit of providing full-thickness closure. Limitations include the inability to access the proximal colon, and a steeper learning curve than TTSCs and OTSCs.

NOVEL HELIX TACKING SYSTEM

One of the newest systems for defect closure is the helix tacking system developed to overcome the limitations of TTSCs, OTSCs and traditional endoscopic suturing devices. The X-Tack Endoscopic HeliX Tacking System (Apollo Endosurgery) has received FDA clearance and is commercially available for GI defect closure. This novel helix tacking system is a TTS, suture-based device that was designed for tissue apposition and closure of large, defects in the upper and lower GI tract (**Fig. 4**). The helix-based suturing system is designed to be passed through the working channel of the gastroscope or colonoscope to achieve defect closure and is not limited by jaw size like traditional TTSCs or OTSCs. The system is designed to be compatible with gastroscopes up to 155 cm and colonoscopes up to 235 cm long with a working channel of 2.8 mm or larger, not requiring a larger double channel gastroscope like a traditional endoscopic suturing system.

To achieve appropriate tissue apposition, independent barbed helical tacks are placed around the periphery of the defect, each tethered together by single polypropylene suture. The first HeliX Tack is preloaded into the system with a total of 3 additional reloadable tacks (a total of 4 tacks around the periphery of the lesion). In the authors' experience, ideal positioning of the barbed tacks is 0.5 to 1 cm from the periphery of the defect and in 4 quadrants to achieve effective closure. Once all tacks have been deployed and fixed, tension is applied to the suture to approximate the margins of the defect and cinching performed, similar to the cinch used with the

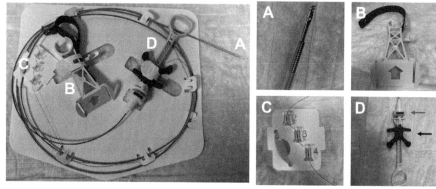

Fig. 4. X-Tack Endoscopic HeliX Tacking System (Apollo Endosurgery, Austin, Texas). (*A*) Push catheter and preloaded helical tack within the protective liner. (*B*) Mounting platform. (*C*) Backing card containing 3 additional helical tacks preloaded on the suture. (*D*) Deployment handle; the tack is advanced by providing forward pressure while pulling back the handle slider (*white arrow*) and additional clockwise rotations, and the tack is then deployed by pushing the blue release button (*black arrow*). (*From* Zhang LY, Ngamruengphong S, Khashab MA. Closing the gap: applications, tips, and tricks for a novel through-the-scope suturing device. Am J Gastroenterol 2022;117(7):1022-1027.)

traditional suturing system. If closure is not adequate, an additional TTSC may be needed to achieve complete closure. Given the design of the system, possible adverse events may include wound dehiscence, delayed perforation, and bleeding if the tacking system is improperly placed.

An early preclinical study in a porcine model sought to compare technical success and closure rates of this novel through-the-scope tissue helix tack and suture device versus TTSCs.[27] In a prehuman study involving mucosal defects in the stomach and colon (ranging in size from 25-50 mm), closure with this helix tacking system outperformed traditional TTSCs (100% vs 81.3%; $P=.0001$), although 1 device-related perforation was noted to occur with the suturing device. To date, this novel helix tacking system has been described for various indications, including closure of a rectal defect after hybrid ESD.[28] In a recent multicenter study by Mahmoud and colleagues, the technical success of the helix tacking system was 89.2% among 93 patients, with a mean defect size of 41.6 plus or minus 19.4 mm.[29] Despite this technical success, adjunctive endoscopic therapy to achieve closure was required in 24.7% of patients. Adverse events occurred in 2 patients (2.2%) over a 34-day follow-up period. The authors concluded that the X-Tack Endoscopic HeliX Tacking System was safe, efficient, and allowed for closure of large and irregularly shaped defects not amenable to traditional endoscopic closure methods (ie, TTSCs or OTSCs).

Potential advantages of this system include the ability to achieve closure for defects greater than 30 mm, irregularly shaped defects, and the ability to perform closure of defects in the proximal colon with no need for endoscopic withdrawal.[29] This last advantage is critical, as the proximal colon is often inaccessible to traditional endoscopic suturing. Yet despite these advances, the exact closure force and ability to close full-thickness defects remain to be determined. Although there remains a lack of truly comparative data to traditional endoscopic closure techniques, this novel helix tacking system may be cost-effective for large defects that require multiple TTSCs or endoscopic suturing. Formal cost-effectiveness analyses are still needed.

ALTERNATIVE CLOSURE METHODS

Although the mainstay of submucosal and third space endoscopy defect closure involves TTSCs, OTSCs, endoscopic suturing, and the more recent helix tacking system, it is important to acknowledge several other adjunctive and primary therapies that may be used. These additional treatments are typically considered outside the scope of traditional submucosal endoscopy and aimed at closing transmural defects including GI perforations, leaks, and fistulas. Perhaps one of the best studied therapies for transmural gastrointestinal defects includes endoscopic vacuum therapy (EVT).[30-32] This technique involves endoscopic placement of a porous sponge or antimicrobial drape connected to a nasogastric tube and wall suction (to create a negative pressure) into the defect cavity or lumen to promote healing through micro/macro-deformation, increase perfusion, exudate control, and bacterial clearance. Tissue adhesives, fibrin glue, and cyanoacrylate glue have also been shown in some studies to aid in mucosal defect closure in combination with other modalities.[33,34] Fistula plugs and cardiac septal defect occluder devices have also been increasingly described for closure of GI defects and fistulas.[33,35-37] Other potential techniques include endoloop and endoclip closure and tissue apposition using T-fasteners or a T-tag system.[33,38-40] Although these alternative closure methods are beyond the scope of this article, proper understanding of adjunctive and alternative endoscopic defect closure tools remains critically important to endoscopists.

SUBMUCOSAL DEFECT CLOSURE IN CLINICAL PRACTICE

This section will describe general patterns for submucosal defect closure and the approach used in the authors' clinical practice. Although variability will certainly exist comparing the authors' practice to other individual endoscopists, the principles of defect closure as discussed previously will remain essential. With regard to the mucosotomy site in esophageal POEM or POEM related to a Zenker diverticulum repair (ie, Z-POEM), the authors' traditional approach is to use TTSCs for defect closure. For gastric POEM, the authors typically use endoscopic suturing for closure of the mucosotomy site, although TTSCs have been described in literature. Similarly, EFTR or STER defect is typically closed via endoscopic suturing, although OTSC may be appropriate for institutions that have limited access or familiarity with endoscopic suturing.

Although defect closure is essential for procedures such as POEM or EFTR, the decision to close EMR or ESD defects remains controversial. Multiple large retrospective studies have demonstrated that prophylactic TTSC closure for lesions larger than 2 cm was beneficial to reduce delayed bleeding after polypectomy or EMR.[41-43] Despite these findings, several randomized trials have demonstrated the opposite, with no reduction in delayed bleeding.[44-46] In their practice, the authors typically do not close ESD defects, but instead perform prophylactic coagulation of visible vessels within the resection bed after resection is complete. For EMR defects, especially those in the right colon, the authors typically are able to achieve closure using TTSCs.

SUMMARY

In summary, as the field of endoscopic surgery continues to evolve, innovative tools and techniques will continue to grow. As this continues, it remains critically important for endoscopists to understand appropriate closure techniques before performing submucosal and third space endoscopy procedures. This article highlighted multiple endoscopic closure devices and techniques including the authors' own practice patterns.

CLINICS CARE POINTS

- TTSCs are used as a first-line strategy for closure of defects of no more than 2 cm.
- OTSCs may achieve adequate closure of larger defects of no more than 3 cm and full-thickness defects less than 2 cm in size.
- Endoscopic suturing may a preferred closure technique for larger defects, as the device is not limited by defect size; however, its use in the right colon may be limited given the device attaches to a gastroscope.
- The novel helix tacking system is ideal for closure for irregularly shaped defects greater than 30 mm and may be used for closure of defects in the proximal colon.

POTENTIAL CONFLICTS OF INTEREST

T.R. McCarty has no conflicts to disclose. P. Jirapinyo has the following disclosures: Apollo Endosurgery – Research Support, Consultant, Advisory Board, Boston Scientific – Research Support, ERBE – Consultant, Fractyl - Research Support, GI Dynamics – Research Support, Endogastric Solutions – Consultant, Endosim – Royalty, Spatz Medical – Consultant, USGI – Research Support.

REFERENCES

1. Asge Technology C, Conway JD, Adlcr DG, et al. Endoscopic hemostatic devices. Gastrointest Endosc 2009;69:987–96.
2. Hayashi I, Yonezawa TM, Kuwabara T, et al. The study on staunch clip for the treatment by endoscopy. Gastrointest Endosc 1975;17:92–101.
3. Abdulfattah Bukhari M, Khashab MA. Optimized training in the use of endoscopic closure devices. Gastrointest Endosc Clin N Am 2020;30:197–208.
4. Sedarat A. Clips for closure of full-thickness defects. Tech Gastrointest Endosc 2015;17(3):129–35.
5. Raju GS, Ahmed I, Shibukawa G, et al. Endoluminal clip closure of a circular full-thickness colon resection in a porcine model (with videos). Gastrointest Endosc 2007;65:503–9.
6. Baron TH, Song LM, Ross A, et al. Use of an over-the-scope clipping device: multicenter retrospective results of the first US experience (with videos). Gastrointest Endosc 2012;76:202–8.
7. Wang TJ, Aihara H, Thompson AC, et al. Choosing the right through-the-scope clip: a rigorous comparison of rotatability, whip, open/close precision, and closure strength (with videos). Gastrointest Endosc 2019;89:77–86 e1.
8. Kirschniak A, Kratt T, Stuker D, et al. A new endoscopic over-the-scope clip system for treatment of lesions and bleeding in the GI tract: first clinical experiences. Gastrointest Endosc 2007;66:162–7.
9. Matthes K, Jung Y, Kato M, et al. Efficacy of full-thickness GI perforation closure with a novel over-the-scope clip application device: an animal study. Gastrointest Endosc 2011;74:1369–75.
10. Rustagi T, McCarty TR, Aslanian HR. Endoscopic treatment of gastrointestinal perforations, leaks, and fistulae. J Clin Gastroenterol 2015;49:804–9.
11. Sandmann M, Heike M, Faehndrich M. Application of the OTSC system for the closure of fistulas, anastomosal leakages and perforations within the gastrointestinal tract. Z Gastroenterol 2011;49:981–5.

12. Disibeyaz S, Koksal AS, Parlak E, et al. Endoscopic closure of gastrointestinal defects with an over-the-scope clip device. A case series and review of the literature. Clin Res Hepatol Gastroenterol 2012;36:614–21.
13. McCarty TR, Ryou M. Endoscopic diagnosis and management of gastric subepithelial lesions. Curr Opin Gastroenterol 2020;36:530–7.
14. committee At, Parsi MA, Schulman AR, et al. Devices for endoscopic hemostasis of nonvariceal GI bleeding (with videos). VideoGIE 2019;4:285–99.
15. Dolezel R, Ryska O, Kollar M, et al. A comparison of two endoscopic closures: over-the-scope clip (OTSC) versus KING closure (endoloop + clips) in a randomized long-term experimental study. Surg Endosc 2016;30:4910–6.
16. von Renteln D, Schmidt A, Vassiliou MC, et al. Endoscopic closure of large colonic perforations using an over-the-scope clip: a randomized controlled porcine study. Endoscopy 2009;41:481–6.
17. Haito-Chavez Y, Law JK, Kratt T, et al. International multicenter experience with an over-the-scope clipping device for endoscopic management of GI defects (with video). Gastrointest Endosc 2014;80:610–22.
18. Dolan RD, Bazarbashi AN, McCarty TR, et al. Endoscopic full-thickness resection of colorectal lesions: a systematic review and meta-analysis. Gastrointest Endosc 2022;95:216–224 e18.
19. Jensen DM, Kovacs T, Ghassemi KA, et al. Randomized controlled trial of over-the-scope clip as initial treatment of severe nonvariceal upper gastrointestinal bleeding. Clin Gastroenterol Hepatol 2021;19:2315–23123.e2.
20. Schmidt A, Riecken B, Damm M, et al. Endoscopic removal of over-the-scope clips using a novel cutting device: a retrospective case series. Endoscopy 2014;46:762–6.
21. Stavropoulos SN, Modayil R, Friedel D. Current applications of endoscopic suturing. World J Gastrointest Endosc 2015;7:777–89.
22. Moran EA, Gostout CJ, Bingener J. Preliminary performance of a flexible cap and catheter-based endoscopic suturing system. Gastrointest Endosc 2009;69:1375–83.
23. Thompson CC, Ge PS. The use of the overstitch to close perforations and fistulas. Gastrointest Endosc Clin N Am 2020 January;30(1):147–61.
24. Kantsevoy SV, Bitner M, Mitrakov AA, et al. Endoscopic suturing closure of large mucosal defects after endoscopic submucosal dissection is technically feasible, fast, and eliminates the need for hospitalization (with videos). Gastrointest Endosc 2014;79:503–7.
25. Han S, Wani S, Kaltenbach T, et al. Endoscopic suturing for closure of endoscopic submucosal dissection defects. VideoGIE 2019;4:310–3.
26. Maselli R, Palma R, Traina M, et al. Endoscopic suturing for gastrointestinal applications: initial results from a prospective multicenter european registry. Gastrointest Endosc 2022. https://doi.org/10.1016/j.gie.2022.06.004.
27. Hernandez A, Marya NB, Sawas T, et al. Gastrointestinal defect closure using a novel through-the-scope helix tack and suture device compared to endoscopic clips in a survival porcine model (with video). Endosc Int Open 2021;9:E572–7.
28. McCarty TR, Aihara H. Hybrid endoscopic submucosal dissection with novel helix tacking system for defect closure. VideoGIE 2021;6:446–9.
29. Mahmoud T, Wong K, Song LM, et al. Initial multicenter experience using a novel endoscopic tack and suture system for challenging GI defect closure and stent fixation (with video). Gastrointest Endosc 2022;95:373–82.
30. de Moura DTH, Hirsch BS, Do Monte Junior ES, et al. Cost-effective modified endoscopic vacuum therapy for the treatment of gastrointestinal transmural

defects: step-by-step process of manufacturing and its advantages. VideoGIE 2021;6:523–8.

31. do Monte Junior ES, de Moura DTH, Ribeiro IB, et al. Endoscopic vacuum therapy versus endoscopic stenting for upper gastrointestinal transmural defects: systematic review and meta-analysis. Dig Endosc 2021;33:892–902.

32. de Moura DTH, de Moura B, Manfredi MA, et al. Role of endoscopic vacuum therapy in the management of gastrointestinal transmural defects. World J Gastrointest Endosc 2019;11:329–44.

33. Yang J, Lee D, Agrawal D. Closure of transmural defects in the gastrointestinal tract by methods other than clips and sutures. Tech Gastrointest Endosc 2015; 17:141–50.

34. Committee AT, Bhat YM, Banerjee S, et al. Tissue adhesives: cyanoacrylate glue and fibrin sealant. Gastrointest Endosc 2013;78:209–15.

35. de Moura DTH, da Ponte-Neto AM, Hathorn KE, et al. Novel endoscopic management of a chronic gastro-gastric fistula using a cardiac septal defect occluder. Obes Surg 2020;30:3253–4.

36. Rabenstein T, Boosfeld C, Henrich R, et al. First use of ventricular septal defect occlusion device for endoscopic closure of an esophagorespiratory fistula using bronchoscopy and esophagoscopy. Chest 2006;130:906–9.

37. Repici A, Presbitero P, Carlino A, et al. First human case of esophagus-tracheal fistula closure by using a cardiac septal occluder (with video). Gastrointest Endosc 2010;71:867–9.

38. Nakagawa Y, Nagai T, Soma W, et al. Endoscopic closure of a large ERCP-related lateral duodenal perforation by using endoloops and endoclips. Gastrointest Endosc 2010;72:216–7.

39. Shi Q, Chen T, Zhong YS, et al. Complete closure of large gastric defects after endoscopic full-thickness resection, using endoloop and metallic clip interrupted suture. Endoscopy 2013;45:329–34.

40. Agrawal D, Chak A, Champagne BJ, et al. Endoscopic mucosal resection with full-thickness closure for difficult polyps: a prospective clinical trial. Gastrointest Endosc 2010;71:1082–8.

41. Dior M, Coriat R, Tarabichi S, et al. Does endoscopic mucosal resection for large colorectal polyps allow ambulatory management? Surg Endosc 2013;27: 2775–81.

42. Liaquat H, Rohn E, Rex DK. Prophylactic clip closure reduced the risk of delayed postpolypectomy hemorrhage: experience in 277 clipped large sessile or flat colorectal lesions and 247 control lesions. Gastrointest Endosc 2013;77:401–7.

43. Omori J, Goto O, Habu T, et al. Prophylactic clip closure for mucosal defects is associated with reduced adverse events after colorectal endoscopic submucosal dissection: a propensity-score matching analysis. BMC Gastroenterol 2022; 22:139.

44. Dokoshi T, Fujiya M, Tanaka K, et al. A randomized study on the effectiveness of prophylactic clipping during endoscopic resection of colon polyps for the prevention of delayed bleeding. Biomed Res Int 2015;2015:490272.

45. Matsumoto M, Kato M, Oba K, et al. Multicenter randomized controlled study to assess the effect of prophylactic clipping on post-polypectomy delayed bleeding. Dig Endosc 2016;28:570–6.

46. Shioji K, Suzuki Y, Kobayashi M, et al. Prophylactic clip application does not decrease delayed bleeding after colonoscopic polypectomy. Gastrointest Endosc 2003;57:691–4.

Management of Adverse Events of Submucosal Endoscopy

Manu Venkat, MD[a], Kavel Visrodia, MD[b],*

KEYWORDS

- ESD • POEM • Submucosal endoscopy • Complications • Dysplasia • Neoplasia

KEY POINTS

- Although generally safe and well tolerated, submucosal endoscopy carries a higher complication risk than most other endoscopic procedures. There are unique considerations in the recognition, management, and prevention of bleeding, perforation, and other complications in the context of submucosal procedures.
- Close monitoring for perforation is necessary during the procedure, especially if the muscularis propria is injured. However, perforations can generally be repaired with clips or endoscopic suturing, after which the procedure can continue.
- Electrocautery with the dissection knife is the first-line tool for small-volume bleeding; larger vessels may require hemostatic forceps.
- Preemptive coagulation of visible vessels in the endoscopic submucosal dissection of ulcer base may reduce the risk of delayed bleeding. Other potential tools being studied to prevent delayed bleeding include hemostatic sprays, over-the-scope clips, snares, and sheets of cultured cells.

INTRODUCTION

The advent of submucosal endoscopic interventions now allows endoscopists to perform procedures that previously necessitated surgical intervention. Despite the relatively recent introduction and evolution of submucosal and third space endoscopy, there is already sufficient evidence to support its efficacy and safety when performed by trained endoscopists in carefully selected patients. However, the learning curve of submucosal endoscopy remains steep, particularly in its initial stages, and the possibility of severe adverse events exists. Fortunately, most acute and delayed

[a] Department of Medicine, Columbia University Irving Medical Center, New York Presbyterian Hospital, 5141 Broadway, New York, NY 10034, USA; [b] Division of Digestive and Liver Diseases, Columbia University Irving Medical Center, New York Presbyterian Hospital, Herbert Irving Pavilion, 161 Fort Washington Avenue, 8th Floor, Street 852A, New York, NY 10032, USA
* Corresponding author.
E-mail address: khv210@cumc.columbia.edu

Gastrointest Endoscopy Clin N Am 33 (2023) 183–196
https://doi.org/10.1016/j.giec.2022.09.005
1052-5157/23/© 2022 Published by Elsevier Inc.

complications can be addressed endoscopically or nonprocedurally with medications and observation. The types of adverse events associated with submucosal endoscopy vary from those typically encountered during less invasive forms of endoscopy, so early recognition and management is paramount in patient and procedure outcomes.

In this article, we will review the spectrum of procedure-related adverse events relevant to submucosal endoscopy. The majority of experience and evidence in this area applies to endoscopic submucosal dissection (ESD), endoscopic mucosal resection, and perioral esophageal myotomy (POEM). Variations of these submucosal endoscopic procedures including G-POEM, Z-POEM, and STER are not specifically discussed but the adverse events herein can similarly occur in those procedures as well.

We categorize adverse events first by their time of presentation relative to the procedure, with certain events likely to occur during the procedure (immediate complications), and others more likely to occur in the following days to weeks (delayed complications; **Table 1**). For each major category of adverse event, we will discuss epidemiology and risk factors, characteristic presentations, immediate treatment recommendations, and recommendations for prevention. There are differences in the types of complications, degree of risk, and presentation of complications depending on the specific procedure being performed and the location within the gastrointestinal (GI) tract being intervened on. We will discuss those differences at a high level but subtle differences remain beyond the scope of this review.

Variability in how adverse events are assessed and categorized has previously hindered the study of the complications of endoscopy. There have been sustained efforts to develop more structured frameworks to categorize complications. In 2010, a working group of the American Society for Gastrointestinal Endoscopy developed a standardized lexicon to categorize endoscopic adverse events as mild, moderate, severe, or fatal.[1] More recently, the Adverse Events in GI Endoscopy (AGREE) classification published in 2022 divides adverse events into 5 grades based on the degree of postprocedural intervention needed to address the event.[2] With regards to POEM, publications have outlined clearer criteria for categories of complications, including insufflation-related adverse events, perforation, bleeding, postprocedural GERD, severe persistent pain, and aspiration pneumonia.[3] Further development and more widespread use of standardized classification systems for complications can aid in the continued study of the adverse events we discuss below and how to better prevent them.

Immediate Complications

Bleeding

Submucosal endoscopic procedures carry among the highest bleeding risk out of any endoscopic procedure.[4] The bleeding risk is greatest in gastric and duodenal submucosal procedures due to the high vascularity of those intestinal regions, with an incidence rate of 2.9% for major bleeding in gastric ESD.[5] Bile exposure in these areas may also increase bleeding risk.[6] Intraprocedural bleeding is less common but still occurs during esophageal and colonic submucosal endoscopy procedures.[7] In POEM, bleeding can happen at multiple stages of the procedure, from the initial mucosal incision through tunneling and myotomy.[3] Although small-volume bleeding is common, bleeding substantial enough to halt the procedure or cause shock is rare.[8,9]

Immediate intraprocedural bleeding should be self-evident, although the rate can vary from oozing to spurting to catastrophic hemorrhage. Nonetheless, even a small amount of bleeding should be addressed to prevent obscuring the field of view or delineation of the submucosal and muscle layers and extending procedure duration and increasing the risk of errors or other complications.

Table 1
Summary of common immediate and delayed complications with submucosal endoscopy

Immediate Complications		
Perforation	**Bleeding**	**Aspiration**
• Perforation risk is higher in esophageal or colonic procedures than in gastric procedures	• In ESD, preprocedural patient positioning should prioritizing placing the dissection site (in ESD) up relative to gravity, helping blood flow away from the work area	• Aspiration and resultant pneumonia can present more commonly on the left side following endoscopy
• CO_2 insufflation should be used for all submucosal endoscopy	• Electrocautery is the first-line tool to address bleeding but should not be overused to avoid causing perforation. Hemostatic forceps or clips can also be helpful in stemming bleeding	• Avoiding excessive insufflation and considering intubation for proximal esophageal procedures can reduce risk of aspiration
• Most perforations identified during the procedure can be closed with clips or endoscopic suturing before continuing with the procedure; postprocedural antibiotic therapy is recommended in case of perforation	• Urgent vascular interventional radiology or surgical consult may be needed in cases of severe hemorrhage but this is very rare	
• Tension pneumothorax or pneumoperitoneum are rare but feared complications of perforation that require emergent decompression	• Low-dose aspirin is likely safe to continue for submucosal procedures, or with only minimal interruption. Other antiplatelet and anticoagulant medications should be held if possible	

Delayed Complications		
Stricture	**Bleeding**	**Delayed Perforation**
• Esophageal ESD, especially with resections involving more than three-fourths of the luminal circumference, has a high risk of postprocedural stricture	• Urgent repeat endoscopy is indicated in case of melena, hematochezia, or other evidence of bleeding following the procedure	• Pneumomediastinum and/or pneumoperitoneum are common postprocedural findings and may not represent complications
• Prophylactic balloon dilations and intraprocedural steroid injections can reduce the risk of stricture	• Preventative hemostasis involving preemptive coagulation of visible vessels at the end of the procedure holds promise but more evidence is needed to definitively recommend it	• Chest/abdominal pain, nausea, and fevers in the postprocedural period should prompt workup for mediastinitis or peritonitis, which in most cases can be treated supportively with antibiotics

Most bleeding can be managed endoscopically and begins with the localization of the bleeding source. Ideally, the patient is already positioned such that the lesion is in an antigravity location, thus promoting contents including blood to pool away from the resection field. Water jet functions available in current generation endoscopes are helpful in rapidly clearing active bleeding to at least momentarily localize the site of bleeding. Underwater visualization can also be used to effectively localize the bleeding (**Fig. 1**). If the resection knife is equipped with an injection channel (manual or automated high-pressure), immediate injection of submucosal agent can provide tamponade effect to stop or reduce small volume bleeding, facilitate treatment, and protect against injury during subsequent electrocautery. If this is ineffective to slow the bleeding, injection of diluted epinephrine may be performed. Gentle tamponade using the side of the cap-fitted endoscope tip can also be helpful while exchanging accessories to administer therapy.

After localization, bleeding can be treated using a variety of electrocautery-based interventions. For example, smaller bleeds can be treated efficiently with coagulation using the knife. More brisk bleeding may require exchanging the knife for hemostatic forceps. These are used by grasping the bleeding vessel/region, gently retracting and then coagulating using "soft-coagulation" mode.[10] The endoscopist should be mindful not to overuse electrocautery because this can increase the risk of deep muscle injury and perforation. Through the scope, clips can also be used for hemostasis but are often considered a secondary measure due to their potential to impair visualization or accessibility and make subsequent dissection more difficult. If severe bleeding cannot be managed endoscopically, IR embolization or urgent surgical intervention may be needed.

Submucosal dissection should be undertaken with great care, with the endoscopist proactively identifying submucosal vessels to be treated prophylactically with electrocoagulation before dissecting (ie, "cutting") through the submucosa. If the identified vessel is large, hemostatic forceps as opposed to the knife can be used instead for the same prophylactic purpose (**Fig. 2**).[11] For smaller vessels, electrocautery using the dissection knife provides the benefit of sparing the endoscopist the time and effort of switching tools frequently. Red dichromatic imaging using a unique light spectrum on equipped endoscopes may be helpful in more easily identifying blood vessels during the procedure.[12]

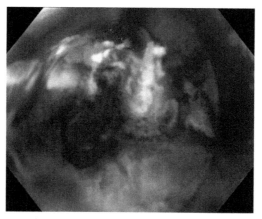

Fig. 1. Bleeding during submucosal dissection. Bleeding during submucosal dissection localized and treated underwater.

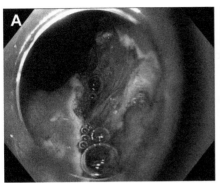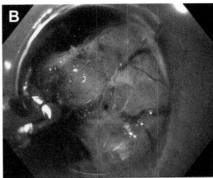

Fig. 2. Prophylactic coagulation of submucosal vessel. A medium-sized submucosal vessel encountered during submucosal dissection (*A*) and prophylactically treated with hemostatic forceps in soft coagulation mode (*B*).

Guidelines from Japan specific to ESD suggest it is acceptable to continue low-dose aspirin monotherapy during ESD, and other guidelines that apply to endoscopic procedures more broadly suggest the same.[13] More recent guidelines provide recommendations on the management of other antiplatelet and anticoagulant medications, depending on the risk of holding those medications. Heparin bridging for patients on warfarin is commonly done, although simply holding warfarin may be noninferior in thrombotic risk based on limited evidence. Overall, making definitive recommendations regarding specific management of nonaspirin antiplatelet agents or anticoagulants is difficult because the designs of past clinical trials in this area are heterogeneous.

Perforation

The incidence of perforation will vary widely depending on endoscopist skill level, difficulty of resection (size, position), intestinal region, procedure technique, and scope maneuverability. Generally, the risk of perforation is lowest in gastric ESD (particularly the distal stomach where the submucosa and muscularis propria is thicker) and thus most suitable for learners. At the opposite end of the spectrum, the duodenum represents the most technically difficult organ due to its thin wall layers and is generally reserved for experts. A recent large German study found perforation rates for ESD to be 2.6% in esophagus, 4.2% in stomach, and 14.1% in colon,[14] whereas meta-analyses have estimated the average perforation risk during ESD at 2.7% for gastric ESD and 4.8% for colonic ESD.[5,15] The risk of perforation into the mediastinum in POEM is low at less than 1%.[9] A small degree of pneumoperitoneum or subcutaneous emphysema during POEM is not uncommon and may not truly need to be considered an adverse event if not associated with tension physiology or other harmful effect.[16]

Large perforations may be directly visualized during the procedure with omentum and/or fat seen, whereas microperforations may only be evident as mediastinal or peritoneal free air palpated or seen on imaging after the procedure. Injury or breech of the muscularis propria should be vigilantly assessed during and at the end of the resection to recognize perforation early. In the esophagus, perforation can result in progressive pneumomediastinum causing compression of intraluminal space. Neck and chest wall crepitus can sometimes be palpated on the patient. Mediastinitis is a feared but an exceedingly rare adverse event. Pneumothorax can also occur, which in exceedingly rare occasions can progress to tension pneumothorax. Perforation in the stomach, duodenum, or colon can cause pneumoperitoneum, which can evolve to tension pneumoperitoneum causing hemodynamic shock that becomes apparent during the procedure.

Endoscopy allows for early recognition of perforation, and provided the range of endoscopic management options, it is also the first-line treatment option. Thus, endoscopists should be trained and comfortable in closure techniques. Endoscopic management of perforation is reviewed in detail elsewhere in the collection. Briefly, closure will depend on the size of the defect and endoscopic accessibility. Through-the-scope clips offer closure of small defects without requiring exchange of the endoscope for setup of alternative closure devices and therefore should be the first consideration. They should be applied carefully without further injury to the muscularis propria or exacerbation of the perforation. Because clips can hinder further dissection, submucosal dissection may be continued in small-to-medium–sized perforations until there is sufficient space around defect to place a clip without entrapping or impairing dissection of the lesion. There are a wide variety of through the scope clips ranging in size (up to 16–17 mm), and selection will typically depend on institutional availability and endoscopist/assistant familiarity. For larger perforations, over-the-scope clips and endoscopic suturing devices are available but require removal of the endoscope. Of note, endoscopic suturing remains limited to a gastroscope length dual-channel therapeutic endoscope, and thus, advancement to the right colon may be challenging. Recently, a through-the-scope suturing device has been released compatible with colonoscope length endoscopes without need for endoscope removal (X-Tack, Apollo).

There exist unique considerations regarding closing perforations in the context of POEM. If a full-thickness perforation is made at the time of the initial mucosal incision (mucosotomy), through the scope clipping may not be sufficient, and suturing or an over-the-scope clip may be preferable.[9]

On recognition of perforation, IV antibiotics should be administered immediately with coverage of enteric organisms (anaerobes and broad gram-negative coverage). If a perforation is small and clipped successfully, the procedure can generally continue safely but the patient will need close postprocedure monitoring for evolving infection. Antibiotics should be continued and the patient should be kept NPO at least until any symptoms subside.

In the event of tension pneumoperitoneum intraprocedurally or postprocedure, emergent needle decompression (pneumoparacentesis) is required. A Veress needle can be used for this purpose.[9] However, pneumomediastinum and/or pneumoperitoneum are common incidental findings on postprocedural imaging, occurring in upward of 50% of cases in some studies of post-POEM patients without any impact on outcomes.[17] If tension pneumothorax were to occur, this requires emergent needle or tube thoracostomy and recruitment of help from pulmonology or anesthesiology colleagues may be necessary.

Endoscopist skill level and appropriate case selection are certainly key variables affecting the risk of perforation but can occur in expert hands as well. From a technical standpoint, endoscopists should avoid injury or breech of the muscularis propria layer by striving to preserve the deepest one-third of submucosa during dissection. Various devices and techniques have also been developed to facilitate safe submucosal dissection including insulated tip knives, scissor knives, and countertraction techniques. There should be a low threshold to consider these when difficult portions of dissection are encountered. Other strategies related to perforation include intubation (owing to positive intrathoracic pressure), which reduces the risk of significant pneumomediastinum, and CO_2 insufflation rather than air because CO_2 can be resorbed relatively rapidly from body cavities. Insufflation CO_2 flow rate should be reduced to the lowest effective setting once perforation is suspected to minimize pneumoperito-neum.[8] Particular care to using minimal CO_2 insufflation flow should be taken when in the submucosal tunnel during POEM.[9] Bleeding should be controlled as discussed earlier to maintain exposure and avoid inadvertence injury. For colonic ESD, poor bowel preparation predisposes patients to poor outcomes in the event of a perforation due to peritoneal contamination, and therefore should only be pursued in the setting of a high-quality preparation.

Although concern is generally for perforation into the space outside of the organ, with POEM, there is also the potential for mucosal perforation from the submucosal tunnel into the gastroesophageal lumen. In a large study reviewing more than 1800 pa-tients who underwent POEM, 2.8% experienced inadvertent mucosectomy.[18] Closure of these defects can be performed with clips or endoscopic suturing. There is not suf-ficient data to advocate for one of these means over the other, with the choice being influenced by the size of the perforation.[8] Generally, in the hands of experienced op-erators, mucosal perforations can be addressed fully during the procedure without long-term sequelae.

Aspiration Pneumonia

Aspiration pneumonia is manifest by hypoxia, sepsis, dyspnea, and or productive cough or sputum. Because GI endoscopy patients are often positioned on their left side, aspiration more often affects the left lung, as opposed to more general contexts when the right lung is at greater risk.[19] Prompt initiation or broadening of antibiotics with enteric (GNR and anaerobe) coverage should occur. To prevent aspiration pneu-monia, patients undergoing procedures of higher aspiration risk (eg, proximal esoph-ageal ESD) may benefit from intubation. Moreover, for upper GI procedures, excessive air insufflation should be avoided. A "flexible overtube" (Sumitomo Bakelite) has also been suggested to lower the risk of aspiration pneumonia.

Delayed Complications

Stricture
Gastrointestinal stricture is of greatest concern in esophageal ESD. However, stricture can occur in other locations especially with large near or fully circumferential resec-tions. Involvement of a greater circumference of the esophagus is a significant predic-tor of stricture risk, with the risk markedly elevated in resections greater than 75% circumference (**Fig. 3**).[20] A case-control study of 134 patients with and without stric-ture after esophageal ESD found that 75% circumferential tumor involvement was associated with refractory stricture with an adjusted odds ratio of 5.49.[21] These man-ifest themselves based on region, such as dysphagia in the esophagus or constipation in the colon (**Fig. 4**). Stricture formation can have a major impact on quality of life and prevention and management is important. As with most benign strictures, balloon di-lations are first-line treatment, with serial dilations usually being required until resolu-tion of symptoms.

There have been significant efforts to prevent stricture formation. Intraprocedural in-jection of steroids (generally triamcinolone injected into the resection or ulcer base) may be effective in reducing stricture and the frequency of postprocedural balloon di-lations.[6] Care must be taken not to inject into the muscularis propria, which can cause abscess formation or perforation. Oral prednisolone moderately reduced stricture rate but the dose of prednisolone trialed was very high.[22] Prophylactic balloon dilations early in the postresection period (theoretically before significant fibrosis has occurred), for example, 3 to 4 days after ESD, can be performed. Other investigational things

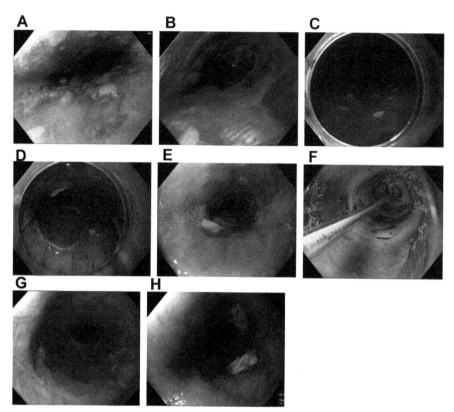

Fig. 3. Esophageal stricture following esophageal ESD. Appearance of esophageal squamous cell carcinoma on NBI (*A*), Lugol's stain (*B*), and white light endoscopy after marking (*C*). ESD was performed of a 7-cm length region that was nearly circumferential (*D*). Three weeks following ESD, an esophageal stricture formed (*E*), and was serially dilated (*F, G*) with eventual intralesional steroid injection resulting in durable stricture improvement and tolerance to solid foods (*H*). (*Courtesy of* Amrita Sethi, MD, MASGE, NYSGEF, New York, NY.)

include dissolving stents, antifibrotic medications, polyglycolic acid sheets, or cultured oral mucosal cells in sheets.[23]

Bleeding

Delayed bleeding occurs much less commonly compared with intraprocedural bleeding. There is significant variability in estimates of delayed bleeding due to lack of consistency in how delayed bleeding is defined, diagnosed, and quantified in the literature, although the AGREE adverse event classification may help standardize the assessment in future studies.[2,24] The rate has been estimated at between 2% and 16% following ESD, with antithrombotic medication therapy and resected specimen size greater than 40 mm being the predominant risk factors for delayed bleeding.[7,25,26] In terms of organ-specific risk, meta-analyses have estimated the risk of delayed major bleeding at 3.6% with gastric ESD and 4.0% for colonic ESD.[5,15] Other factors that may increase the risk of delayed bleeding include prolonged procedure time and chronic hemodialysis.[7] In POEM, delayed bleeding into the submucosal tunnel occurs generally less than 1% of cases, rarely requiring repeat endoscopy for treatment.[9,27,28]

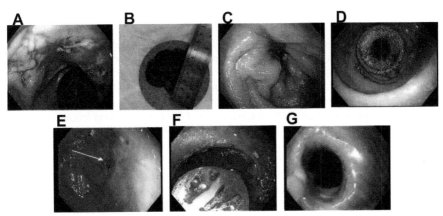

Fig. 4. Rectal stricture following ESD. A 5-cm rectal lesion (*A*) resected by ESD (*B*). The patient returned with constipation 2 months and later and was to have a rectal stricture (*C*). This was treated initially with a fully covered metal stent for 3 months (*D*). However 2 months later the stricture recurred (*E*) and was then treated with aggressive serial balloon dilation (*F*) resulting in durable endoscopic and clinical improvement (*G*). (*Courtesy of* Amrita Sethi, MD, MASGE, NYSGEF, New York, NY.)

Delayed bleeding can present with hematemesis, melena, hematochezia, shock, or a significant hemoglobin drop without another causative explanation depending on the site and severity of bleeding. Vague symptoms including abdominal pain and nausea can sometimes herald the early phase of delayed bleeding. The greatest risk of delayed bleeding is within 24 hours of the procedure.[7] In early Japanese studies, most delayed bleeding occurred while patients were still hospitalized, with only approximately 1 in 5 instances occurring after discharge.[24] However, in the United States, patients typically have a shorter postprocedure length of stay, and so by definition, the risk of delayed bleeding after hospital discharge may be higher.[29,30]

The mainstay of management for delayed bleeding after adequate resuscitation is repeat endoscopy. In most cases, standard tools to treat bleeding ulcer such as epinephrine injection, hemostatic clips, and or electrocautery can be used. To avoid perforation, excessive use of electrocautery on the ESD ulcer base should be avoided but hemostatic forceps may be carefully applied to visible vessels. Generally, delayed bleeding is not catastrophic and responds well to endoscopic interventions, making the need for interventional radiology or surgical intervention is rare.[25] In the event of catastrophic bleeding, or bleeding that cannot be sufficiently addressed by endoscopic means, urgent surgery or embolization should be pursued promptly.

Second-look endoscopy has been proposed as a means to identify patients with bleeding or who may be at high risk of delayed bleeding after ESD. However, data in this area has generally shown no significant benefit of second-look endoscopy.[31,32] Some groups have theorized that second-look endoscopy could offer benefit if performed more selectively in patients with risk factors for increased bleeding risk.[26]

Medical optimization may lower the risk of bleeding. Proton pump inhibitor (PPI) therapy is often used after submucosal procedures in the upper GI tract, although there is insufficient evidence to recommend a specific agent or course.[6] Many centers use between 2 weeks and 2 months of PPI therapy for gastric and distal esophageal submucosal endoscopic procedures. Studies to date are mixed in the degree of benefit PPIs offer, and other more recent studies support the use of lower dose intermittent PPI dosing as noninferior to daily high-dose use.[33] H2 receptor blockers have also been used to reduce the risk of delayed bleeding. However, although there is heterogeneity in results, there is some evidence to suggest PPIs are more effective overall than H2 receptor blockers in reducing bleeding risk.[7] In the authors' view, the risk–benefit profile based on current data favors a course of PPI therapy following gastric and distal esophageal procedures, although more data are needed in this area. Early evidence on the potassium-competitive acid blocking medication vonaprazan, including from phase II clinical trials, suggests that this emerging medication class could be more effective than PPIs in prevention of delayed bleeding following gastric ESD.[34,35] Preprocedural gastric lavage has been theorized as a means to reduce the risk of delayed bleeding, under the hypothesis that bacterial growth in the stomach due to frequent concomitant PPI use may increase the risk of infection and bleeding in the ulcer base.[36] However, there is insufficient evidence to recommend this practice.

Preventative hemostasis is a concept that many experts in the field have suggested as a means to reduce the risk of postprocedural bleeding. It involves the preemptive coagulation of nonbleeding visible vessels in the postdissection ulcer base in ESD. An early retrospective study suggested a benefit of preventative coagulation using forceps.[37] However, the benefits of this preventative coagulation must be weighed against the increased risk of perforation with increased coagulation exposure.[7] Small studies have demonstrated promise in the use of endoscopic Doppler probe ultrasonography to better identify at-risk vessels in the postdissection ulcer base.[7] A suggested alternative to preventative electrocoagulation is the search, coagulation, and clipping (SCC) method. Per the developers of this method, it involves "observing the ulcer floor, identifying blood vessels, and cauterizing and clipping respective blood vessels." A retrospective study of the method compared with standard preventative electrocoagulation suggested a reduced risk of delayed bleeding with the SCC method.[38]

There are ongoing efforts to explore other novel tools and techniques to reduce the risk of delayed bleeding.[6] Most attempt to address the fact that prolonged exposure of the dissection ulcer base to the harsh environment of the gastrointestinal lumen is a major contributing factor to delayed bleeding. A recent pilot study of endoscopic suturing of the mucosal defect in gastric ESD suggested a reduced risk of delayed bleeding after the procedure.[39] However, a single-center retrospective study of a strategy using the endoloop and endoclips for closure after gastric ESD showed no benefit.[40] Some groups have explored the use of polyglycolic acid, a biodegradable material used in surgical settings, in combination with fibrin glue to coat the base of ESD dissection ulcers.[41] A systematic review of the current body of evidence suggested a decreased risk of bleeding, including in patients on antithrombotic agents, although the effect may be attenuated in patients with larger sized mucosal defects after dissection.[42]

Applied hemostatic chemicals are another category of therapies indicated to reduce the risk of delayed bleeding in submucosal procedures. The synthetic hemostatic gel PuraStat can be applied using a dedicated catheter compatible with most endoscopes, and dries transparently to allow the proceduralist to assess the ulcer base or other area to which the compound is applied.[43] A single-center randomized control trial found a reduced need for thermocoagulation and improved wound healing (assessed endoscopically 4 weeks after the primary procedure) in the PuraStat group with equivalent rates of delayed bleeding, as compared with the control group where only thermocoagulation could be used.[44] Other applied chemicals including Hemospray have utility in addressing delayed bleeding during follow-up endoscopy but are less useful as a preventative measure during ESD because they are opaque and would obscure the field of view.[45]

Other potential means to reduce the risk of delayed bleeding include over-the-scope clips, snares, or applied sheets of cultured cells, to treat the ESD ulcer base. There is not yet enough clinical evidence to quantify the benefit or to definitively advocate for one of these possibilities over the others. However, overall these efforts represent one of the most potentially fruitful areas for future clinical studies to target.

Delayed Perforation

Delayed perforation is relatively uncommon as most perforations occur or are apparent during the procedure warranting real-time closure. Meta-analyses have estimated the rate of delayed perforation in gastric ESD at only 0.039%.[15]

Despite its rarity, delayed perforation should be kept in mind as a potential cause of postprocedural decompensation due to the potential for serious downstream complications. Peritonitis can result if the defect was incompletely closed, ineffective (eg, premature clip dislodgment), or unrecognized and left untreated. Delayed perforation can manifest as abdominal pain and/or sepsis. The risk decreases as time from procedure increases but there can be especially delayed presentations if the cause is dehiscence/clips dislodgment. In the esophagus, delayed perforation can manifest as chest pain, sepsis/fever, and XR or computed tomographic (CT) can show free air, with CT having higher sensitivity for mediastinal free air. Rapid surgical evaluation is warranted and multidisciplinary formulation of a plan is critical. Depending on the severity of symptoms, repeat endoscopy may be an option to close the defect. However, in the case of severe clinical deterioration, rapid surgical intervention may be necessary. Methods to prevent delayed perforation are similar to those for preventing and/or addressing acute perforation.

Pneumothorax is a relatively uncommon delayed complication of POEM and, if small, can be managed nonprocedurally because the air will be absorbed over time. Any respiratory compromise or tension physiology necessitates the placement of a thoracostomy tube. The same principles apply for postprocedural pleural effusion, in that small collections can be observed while collections large enough to cause symptoms merit thoracostomy tube placement.

SUMMARY

There is justifiable enthusiasm toward the broader adoption of submucosal endoscopy and familiarizing gastrointestinal proceduralists with its unique spectrum of complications will be essential. As with any procedure, factors such as appropriate case selection, preprocedure preparation, sufficient provider skill/experience, preventative measures are the best means to reduce the risk of complications. Fortunately, most complications can be prevented or managed endoscopically, especially when recognized early. Ongoing efforts are anticipated to further enhance the safety and performance of submucosal endoscopy.

CLINICS CARE POINTS

- Orient the endoscopic submucosal dissection site up relative to gravity to allow fluid and blood to flow away from the work area and improve visualization.
- In cases of intraprocedural bleeding, balance the use of electocautery to neutralize bleeding but avoid excessive perforation risk; hemostatic forceps may be better suited to larger bleeding vessels than knife electrocautery.

- For most submucosal procedures, low-dose aspirin is safe to continue without interruption or with only minimal interruption, although other antiplatelet agents and anticoagulants should be held if possible.
- Use CO_2 rather than air for insufflation to reduce the negative downstream complications of perforation if incurred.
- Maintain a high degree of suspicion for tension pneumothorax, pneumoperitoneum, and/or mediastinitis (depending on location of procedure) because these may require urgent procedural intervention. Similarly, maintain a high degree of suspicion for infections in these compartments following the procedure, especially if a visible perforation occurred during the procedure.
- To reduce the risk of aspiration during esophageal submucosal procedures, avoid excessive insufflation and consider planned intubation.

DISCLOSURE

The authors have nothing to disclose.

REFERENCES

1. Cotton PB, Eisen GM, Aabakken L, et al. A lexicon for endoscopic adverse events: report of an ASGE workshop. Gastrointest Endosc 2010;71(3):446–54.
2. Nass KJ, Zwager LW, van der Vlugt M, et al. Novel classification for adverse events in GI endoscopy: the AGREE classification. Gastrointest Endosc 2022; 95(6):1078–85.e8.
3. Nabi Z, Reddy DN, Ramchandani M. Adverse events during and after per-oral endoscopic myotomy: prevention, diagnosis, and management. Gastrointest Endosc 2018;87(1):4–17.
4. Pal P, Tandan M, Reddy DN. Risk of Gastrointestinal Bleed and Endoscopic Procedures on Antiplatelet and Antithrombotic Agents. J Dig Endosc 2019;10(01): 011–20.
5. Akintoye E, Obaitan I, Muthusamy A, et al. Endoscopic submucosal dissection of gastric tumors: A systematic review and meta-analysis. World J Gastrointest Endosc 2016;8(15):517.
6. Misumi Y, Nonaka K. Prevention and Management of Complications and Education in Endoscopic Submucosal Dissection. J Clin Med 2021;10(11). https://doi. org/10.3390/jcm10112511.
7. Kataoka Y, Tsuji Y, Sakaguchi Y, et al. Bleeding after endoscopic submucosal dissection: Risk factors and preventive methods. World J Gastroenterol 2016; 22(26):5927–35.
8. Bechara R, Ikeda H, Inoue H. Peroral endoscopic myotomy: an evolving treatment for achalasia. Nat Rev Gastroenterol Hepatol 2015;12(7):410–26.
9. Stavropoulos SN, Desilets DJ, Fuchs K-H, et al. Per-oral endoscopic myotomy white paper summary. Gastrointest Endosc 2014;80(1):1–15.
10. Veitch AM, Radaelli F, Alikhan R, et al. Endoscopy in patients on antiplatelet or anticoagulant therapy: British Society of Gastroenterology (BSG) and European Society of Gastrointestinal Endoscopy (ESGE) guideline update. Gut 2021; 70(9):1611–28.
11. Horikawa Y, Fushimi S, Sato S. Hemorrhage control during gastric endoscopic submucosal dissection: Techniques using uncovered knives. JGH Open 2020; 4(1):4–10.

12. Miyamoto S, Sugiura R, Abiko S, et al. Red dichromatic imaging helps in detecting exposed blood vessels in gastric ulcer induced by endoscopic submucosal dissection. Endoscopy 2021;53(11):E403–4.
13. Fujimoto K, Fujishiro M, Kato M, et al. Guidelines for gastroenterological endoscopy in patients undergoing antithrombotic treatment. Dig Endosc 2014;26(1):1–14.
14. Fleischmann C, Probst A, Ebigbo A, et al. Endoscopic Submucosal Dissection in Europe: Results of 1000 Neoplastic Lesions From the German Endoscopic Submucosal Dissection Registry. Gastroenterology 2021;161(4):1168–78.
15. Fuccio L, Hassan C, Ponchon T, et al. Clinical outcomes after endoscopic submucosal dissection for colorectal neoplasia: a systematic review and meta-analysis. Gastrointest Endosc 2017;86(1):74–86.e17.
16. Chavan R, Nabi Z, Reddy DN. Adverse events associated with third space endoscopy: Diagnosis and management. Int J Gastrointest Intervention 2020; 9(2):86–97.
17. Yang S, Zeng M-S, Zhang Z-y, et al. Pneumomediastinum and pneumoperitoneum on computed tomography after peroral endoscopic myotomy (POEM): postoperative changes or complications? Acta Radiol 2015;56(10):1216–21.
18. Haito-Chavez Y, Inoue H, Beard KW, et al. Comprehensive Analysis of Adverse Events Associated With Per Oral Endoscopic Myotomy in 1826 Patients: An International Multicenter Study. Am J Gastroenterol 2017;112(8):1267–76.
19. Saito I, Tsuji Y, Sakaguchi Y, et al. Complications related to gastric endoscopic submucosal dissection and their managements. Clin Endosc 2014;47(5): 398–403.
20. Ono S, Fujishiro M, Niimi K, et al. Predictors of postoperative stricture after esophageal endoscopic submucosal dissection for superficial squamous cell neoplasms. Endoscopy 2009;41(08):661–5.
21. Hanaoka N, Ishihara R, Uedo N, et al. Refractory strictures despite steroid injection after esophageal endoscopic resection. Endosc Int Open 2016;04(03):E354–9.
22. Qiu Y, Shi R. Roles of Steroids in Preventing Esophageal Stricture after Endoscopic Resection. Can J Gastroenterol Hepatol 2019;1–9. https://doi.org/10. 1155/2019/5380815.
23. Hikichi T, Nakamura J, Takasumi M, et al. Prevention of Stricture after Endoscopic Submucosal Dissection for Superficial Esophageal Cancer: A Review of the Literature. J Clin Med 2020;10(1):20.
24. Takizawa K. Prevention, Identification, and Treatment of Hemorrhage. In: Fukami N, editor. Endoscopic submucosal dissection: principles and practicevol. 16. Springer; 2015.
25. Suzuki S, Chino A, Kishihara T, et al. Risk factors for bleeding after endoscopic submucosal dissection of colorectal neoplasms. World J Gastroenterol 2014; 20(7):1839–45.
26. Nam HS, Choi CW, Kim SJ, et al. Risk factors for delayed bleeding by onset time after endoscopic submucosal dissection for gastric neoplasm. Scientific Rep 2019;9(1):2674.
27. Li Q-L, Zhou P-H, Yao L-Q, et al. Early diagnosis and management of delayed bleeding in the submucosal tunnel after peroral endoscopic myotomy for achalasia (with video). Gastrointest Endosc 2013;78(2):370–4.
28. Ren Z, Zhong Y, Zhou P, et al. Perioperative management and treatment for complications during and after peroral endoscopic myotomy (POEM) for esophageal achalasia (EA) (data from 119 cases). Surg Endosc 2012;26(11):3267–72.
29. Antillon MR, Pais WP, Bartalos CR, et al. Endoscopic Submucosal Dissection (ESD) Comes to America: Preliminary Experience with Colorectal ESD At An

American Tertiary Care Academic Medical Center. Gastrointest Endosc 2008; 67(5):AB147.

30. Nakajima Y, Nemoto D, Nemoto T, et al. Short-term outcomes of patients undergoing endoscopic submucosal dissection for colorectal lesions. DEN Open 2022;3(1). https://doi.org/10.1002/deo2.136.

31. Ryu HY, Kim JW, Kim H-S, et al. Second-look endoscopy is not associated with better clinical outcomes after gastric endoscopic submucosal dissection: a prospective, randomized, clinical trial analyzed on an as-treated basis. Gastrointest Endosc 2013;78(2):285–94.

32. Nishizawa T, Suzuki H, Kinoshita S, et al. Second-look endoscopy after endoscopic submucosal dissection for gastric neoplasms. Dig Endosc 2015;27(3): 279–84.

33. Yang L, Qi J, Chen W, et al. Low-dose PPI to prevent bleeding after ESD: A multicenter randomized controlled study. Biomed Pharmacother 2021;136:111251.

34. Hamada K, Uedo N, Tonai Y, et al. Efficacy of vonoprazan in prevention of bleeding from endoscopic submucosal dissection-induced gastric ulcers: a prospective randomized phase II study. J Gastroenterol 2019;54(2):122–30.

35. Hidaka Y, Imai T, Inaba T, et al. Efficacy of vonoprazan against bleeding from endoscopic submucosal dissection-induced gastric ulcers under antithrombotic medication: A cross-design synthesis of randomized and observational studies. PLOS ONE 2021;16(12):e0261703.

36. Yang CH, Qiu Y, Li X, et al. Bleeding after endoscopic submucosal dissection of gastric lesions. J Dig Dis 2020;21(3):139–46.

37. Takizawa K, Oda I, Gotoda T, et al. Routine coagulation of visible vessels may prevent delayed bleeding after endoscopic submucosal dissection–an analysis of risk factors. Endoscopy 2008;40(3):179–83.

38. Azumi M, Takeuchi M, Koseki Y, et al. The search, coagulation, and clipping (SCC) method prevents delayed bleeding after gastric endoscopic submucosal dissection. Gastric Cancer 2019;22(3):567–75.

39. Goto O, Oyama T, Ono H, et al. Endoscopic hand-suturing is feasible, safe, and may reduce bleeding risk after gastric endoscopic submucosal dissection: a multicenter pilot study (with video). Gastrointest Endosc 2020;91(5):1195–202.

40. Ego M, Abe S, Nonaka S, et al. Endoscopic Closure Utilizing Endoloop and Endoclips After Gastric Endoscopic Submucosal Dissection for Patients on Antithrombotic Therapy. Dig Dis Sci 2021;66(7):2336–44.

41. Chen Y, Zhao X, Wang D, et al. Endoscopic Delivery of Polymers Reduces Delayed Bleeding after Gastric Endoscopic Submucosal Dissection: A Systematic Review and Meta-Analysis. Polymers 2022;14(12):2387.

42. Li DF, Xiong F, Xu ZL, et al. Polyglycolic acid sheets decrease post-endoscopic submucosal dissection bleeding in early gastric cancer: A systematic review and meta-analysis. J Dig Dis 2020;21(8):437–44.

43. Branchi F, Klingenberg-Noftz R, Friedrich K, et al. PuraStat in gastrointestinal bleeding: results of a prospective multicentre observational pilot study. Surg Endosc 2022;36(5):2954–61.

44. Subramaniam S, Kandiah K, Chedgy F, et al. A novel self-assembling peptide for hemostasis during endoscopic submucosal dissection: a randomized controlled trial. Endoscopy 2021;53(01):27–35.

45. Hussein M, Alzoubaidi D, Serna A, et al. Outcomes of Hemospray therapy in the treatment of intraprocedural upper gastrointestinal bleeding post-endoscopic therapy. United Eur Gastroenterol J 2020;8(10):1155–62.

A Look into the Future of Endoscopic Submucosal Dissection and Third Space Endoscopy

The Role for Robotics and Other Innovation

Philip Wai-yan Chiu, MD, FRCSEd[a,b,*], Siran Zhou, MMed[a,b], Zhiwei Dong, MSurg[a,b]

KEYWORDS

- Endoscopic submucosal dissection • Third space endoscopy
- Endoluminal robotics • Endoscopic full thickness resection

KEY POINTS

- Third space endoscopy allowed the development of novel endoscopic procedures including POEM, STER, and other related treatments for gastrointestinal diseases.
- Future development in flexible robotics will enhance the performance of ESD and other novel endoscopic devices including suturing.

Video content accompanies this article at http://www.giendo.theclinics.com.

DEVELOPMENT OF ENDOSCOPIC SUBMUCOSAL DISSECTION FOR TREATMENT OF EARLY GASTROINTESTINAL NEOPLASIA

Endoscopic resection for treatment of early gastrointestinal (GI) neoplasia started when the first polypectomy was performed by Dr Shinya using innovative flexible snare in 1969.[1] With advances in diagnostic endoscopy, there was an increasing detection of sessile and lateral spreading early GI neoplasia. This led to the development of endoscopic mucosal resection (EMR), which included preinjection of the submucosa of the lesion before resection.[2] Numerous techniques of EMR had been developed including cap-EMR and strip biopsy.[3] However, the usual size of resected

[a] Division of Upper GI and Metabolic Surgery, Department of Surgery, Institute of Digestive Disease, The Chinese University of Hong Kong, Hong Kong; [b] Multi-Scale Medical Robotics Center
* Corresponding author. Division of Upper GI and Metabolic Surgery, Department of Surgery, Institute of Digestive Disease, The Chinese University of Hong Kong, Hong Kong.
E-mail address: philipchiu@surgery.cuhk.edu.hk

Gastrointest Endoscopy Clin N Am 33 (2023) 197–212
https://doi.org/10.1016/j.giec.2022.09.006
1052-5157/23/© 2022 Elsevier Inc. All rights reserved.

specimen after cap-EMR was 20 mm. Hence, intramucosal early GI neoplasia larger than 20 mm required either surgical treatment or piecemeal resection. Piecemeal EMR led to higher risks of local recurrence because of incomplete resection. The development of endoscopic submucosal dissection (ESD) aimed to achieve en bloc resection for intramucosal early GI neoplasia without size limitation. Ono and colleagues[4] reported first performance of ESD for treatment of early gastric cancer in 278 patients and found the local recurrence rate of only 2%. The apparent advantage of ESD is en bloc resection of any lesion irrespective of size, providing an accurate pathologic review of margin and depth.[5] Currently, more than 60% of patients with early gastric cancer in Japan underwent ESD.[6] Several clinical guidelines and meta-analyses have been stated for ESD's standard process, providing optimal assessment recommendations before clinical application.[7,8] Systematic reviews and meta-analyses confirmed that ESD achieved higher rate of en bloc resection for early gastric and colorectal neoplasia, whereas ESD had higher risks of perforation when compared with EMR.[9,10] Quero and colleagues[11] conducted a propensity score–matched comparison of short- and long-term outcomes between conventional surgery and ESD for early gastric cancer in a European tertiary referral center. Eighty-four patients were matched and found no difference in 5-year disease-free survival rates (70.8% and 75.6%, respectively).

LIMITATIONS OF ENDOSCOPIC SUBMUCOSAL DISSECTION

Although ESD is now the first-line endoscopic treatment of intramucosal early cancer in the GI tract, the practice was limited by the challenge of steep learning curve and high risks of adverse events.[12] ESD can only be safely performed by expert endoscopists. Bleeding, perforation, and stricture are common complications after ESD, whereas most of them can be managed endoscopically.[9] The incidence of bleeding after gastric ESD was reported between 1.8% and 15.6%.[9] Stricture after ESD occurs after near circumferential or circumferential esophageal ESD.[13] Among ESD procedures in GI tract, duodenal ESD carried highest risks of perforation followed by colonic ESD and esophageal ESD. Liu and colleagues[14] compared cap-assisted EMR with ESD in 130 patients with early esophagogastric junction neoplasm from 2008 to 2015. The procedure time and adverse events rate was significantly higher in the ESD groups. The serious complications included bleeding (7.7% vs 3.8%), stenosis (5.1% vs 0%), and perforation (5.1% vs 0%).

One of the major limitations to the current instruments for ESD is the lack of traction. Surgeons usually perform minimally invasive surgical tasks within the human body cavity using two laparoscopic instruments arranged in triangulation with a separate laparoscope, which provide stable vision field and traction. On the contrary, ESD is performed with the dissection instrument passing through the therapeutic channel in the same axis to the endoscope. Hence the dissection device needed to be manipulated using the endoscope without triangulation and induced significant challenges to learning curves for endoscopists (**Fig. 1**).

TRACTION METHODS TO OVERCOME DIFFICULTIES IN ENDOSCOPIC SUBMUCOSAL DISSECTION

At the beginning of ESD, mucosal traction was achieved via a distal attachment using transparent hood, and natural traction by gravitational force. A transparent hood attached to the distal end of the endoscope provides traction by lifting the mucosal flap. However, using this hood would restrict the distance between the dissection knife and the submucosal plane. Gravitational traction is simple and effective, whereas

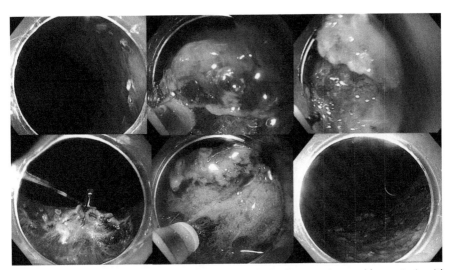

Fig. 1. ESD for treatment of early gastric cancer with clip-line traction and hemostasis with ESD device under red dichromatic imaging.

changing the patients' position may limit the flexibility of the endoscope. The pocket creation method was developed by Dr Yamamoto where a submucosal pocket is created after a small mucosal incision is made and effectively provides a stable dissection plane within the submucosa, followed by the complete circumferential mucosal incision.[15] Kitamura and colleagues[16] analyzed 66 patients from 2006 to 2019 who underwent conventional or pocket creation method ESD. The pocket creation method group had a significantly higher R0 resection rate and dissection speed than the traditional group.

There are different traction methods using a device detached from the endoscope; the clip-with-line method is simple and economical (Video 1). Yoshida and colleagues[17] conducted a randomized multicenter controlled trial comparing conventional and traction-assisted ESD. The clip-with-line traction group showed significantly shorter procedure time for esophageal ESD. However, the direction of traction for clip-with-line was limited to only the pulled side. The pulley method allowed traction force in the desired direction. The pulley method is divided into clip pulley and suture pulley. Ge and colleagues[18] performed a prospective randomized ex vivo study about the suture pulley counteraction method. The ESD procedure time was significantly shorter and there was a reduction in technical demand for new endoscopists with the use of the traction method.

The sheath traction method was designed to combine pull and push force creating a two-way traction during the ESD procedure. The sheath method replaces the line part of the clip-with-line with a hard sheath, and the main types of sheath traction methods include the clip-and-snare method and the Endotrac (Stryker, Kalamazoo, MI).[19] However, the sheath method requires withdrawal and reinsertion before and during the procedure, which means the technique is difficult for colonic ESD. Besides, the friction between endoscope and sheath is unavoidable even with the thinnest sheath currently available.[20]

Unlike the clip-with-line traction method, several methods have been invented to allow traction with various angulations, such as the spring-and-loop with clip (S-O clip) assisted method. The S-O clip allows multiple traction directions, and the traction force is adjusted accordingly because of elasticity of spring. With a high elasticity spring, the S-O clip is suitable for a large lumen, preventing slip-off or breakage of the traction devices.[20] A single-center randomized controlled trial from Japan enrolled 40 patients who underwent the S-O clip–assisted ESD compared with conventional ESD.[21] The results demonstrated that the median ESD procedure time was significantly shorter in the S-O clip–assisted ESD groups (29.1 minutes vs 52.6 minutes; $P = 0.05$). The authors recommended the optimal traction by S-O clip should achieve traction vertical to the gastric wall. However, the S-O clip was only commercialized in Japan and has not been widely used.

Other traction methods including the double scope method and the magnetic anchor method derived similar principles to hasten ESD procedures. Ebigbo and colleagues[22] reported the double scope technique for colorectal ESD, where traction was achieved using a grasping forceps via a small-caliber endoscope while the submucosal dissection was achieved using an ordinary endoscope. Magnetic methods were invented to resist the gravity of the mucosal flap during the ESD procedure. Gotoda and colleagues[23] first reported the use of magnet-assisted gastric ESD where a magnetic controlled anchor was attached to the mucosal flap, and traction was achieved by the external magnetic system. The trial demonstrated clinical safety and efficacy in using magnetic traction in 23 patients without perforation. One of the major disadvantages for the magnetic retraction is the large size of the extracorporeal magnetic system. Recently, Ye and colleagues[24] reported the use of a clip in fixing a magnetic bead with two attached strings to the mucosal flap, exposing the submucosal plane on a change in patient position by gravity and the weight of the bead.

Evidence from studies demonstrated that traction enhances the safety and efficacy in performing ESD in the GI tract. Currently, multiple methods were developed to provide traction during ESD. However, the methods are limited by the unidirectional traction and lack of coordinated submucosal exposure for dissection.

ENDOLUMINAL ROBOTICS FOR ENDOSCOPIC SUBMUCOSAL DISSECTION: CURRENT DEVELOPMENT

Endoluminal multitasking platforms were first developed for more than a decade during the era of natural orifice transluminal endoscopic surgery (NOTES) with a view to achieve more degrees of freedom for endoluminal triangulation and traction.[25] Most of these endoluminal multitasking platforms were mechanically driven using flexible wire and pulley system, hence the degree of freedom and precision was limited.[26] The application of flexible robotics enhanced the precision control and degree of freedom available for endoluminal manipulation from a long distance within the GI tract.[27] Several robotic systems have been tested for performance of ESD through in vitro or in vivo experiments. These included the Master and Slave Transluminal Endoscopic Robot (MASTER; EndoMaster Pte Ltd, Singapore),[28] the Single-access Transluminal Robotic Assistant for Surgeons (STRAS robot; Karl Storz, IRCAD, Tuttlingen, Germany),[29] Flex Robotic System (Medrobotics, Raynham, MA),[30] and the Endoluminal Surgical (ELS) system (Endoquest Robotics; formerly Colubris Mx, Houston, TX).[31]

ENDOLUMINAL ROBOTICS FOR ENDOSCOPIC SUBMUCOSAL DISSECTION: FLEX ROBOTIC SYSTEM

Among all the flexible endoluminal robotic systems, the Flex Robotic System focused on robotizing the endoscope. The Flex Robotic System was originally designed for transoral minimally invasive surgery. The system was later adapted to perform lower GI endoscopic procedures by attaching an additional seal to maintain insufflation.[30]

In a preclinical study, expert supervised colonic ESD was performed in an ex vivo colon model using either the Flex Robotic System or conventional ESD devices.[30] Complete resection was achieved in all 10 procedures using the Flex Robotic System, whereas only 5 of 10 ESD was completed with the conventional approach. Although the Flex Robotic System provided a stable robotized flexible platform, the instruments used for traction and dissection were manually designed, which may hinder the degree of freedom for complex endoluminal procedures.

ENDOLUMINAL ROBOTICS FOR ENDOSCOPIC SUBMUCOSAL DISSECTION: STRAS ROBOT

The flexible Anubiscope (Karl Storz) was a mechanical flexible surgical platform for performance of NOTES.[32] To improve on this mechanical platform, the Isiscope (Isoma, Brügg, Switzerland) was developed as a base to produce the STRAS robot, which is a master-slave system operating through an intuitive control interface. It is a 50-cm-long flexible endoscope with maximal diameter of 18 mm. There were two 4.2-mm working channels for operative instruments and a 2.8-mm working channel for conventional flexible instruments. In a preclinical study, 18 ESDs were attempted in eight live porcine models using STRAS with 12 successfully completed.[32] Six were aborted because of technical failure of the platform or occurrence of perforation. The mean total procedure time was 73 35.5 ± minutes and the mean size of specimen resected was 18.2 ± 9.8 cm².

ENDOLUMINAL ROBOTICS FOR ENDOSCOPIC SUBMUCOSAL DISSECTION: EndoMaster ENDOLUMINAL ACCESS SURGICAL EFFICACY SYSTEM

The EndoMaster Endoluminal Access Surgical Efficacy (EASE) System (Endomaster Pte Ltd) is the second generation of the MASTER, composed of three main components: (1) a master console, (2) a telesurgical workstation, and (3) a slave robotic manipulator.[33] The first prototype endoluminal robotic system, MASTER was successfully applied in performing ESD for treatment of early stage gastric neoplasia in 2011.[34] A total of five patients with early gastric neoplasia were resected completely without complication, and the procedural time ranged between 26 and 68 minutes. After completion of this proof-of-concept study, a clinical ready system was designed to improve on the deficiencies discovered from MASTER. The newly designed Endo-MASTER is built based on a redesigned flexible endoscope with three working channels catering to two robotic arms and one channel for passage of conventional endoscopic instruments. The two arms serve as the grasper and a source of monopolar electrocautery, respectively. The newly designed EndoMaster EASE System is well designed to perform ESD in almost all locations in the GI tract.

The EndoMASTER EASE system was tested in numerous preclinical porcine model studies for performance of esophageal, gastric, and colonic ESD. The system was modified to enable working in a narrow space. Our previous study demonstrated the safety and feasibility in performing esophageal ESD.[35] The use of the EndoMaster EASE System for colorectal ESD was tested in five live porcine models.[36] The average operative time was 73.8 minutes and the mean size of specimens was 1340 mm². There were no cases of perforation; however, there was one episode of sustained profuse bleeding, which was controlled without conversion. The preclinical studies demonstrated the feasibility and safety with EndoMaster EASE system in ESD. A clinical trial is currently being performed and the results will provide insight into the future clinical applications of endoluminal robotics.

FUTURE DEVELOPMENT OF ENDOLUMINAL ROBOTIC SURGICAL SYSTEM

One of the major challenges for endoluminal surgery is the achievement of tissue approximation within the GI tract. Numerous devices had been developed to achieve suturing within the GI tract.[37] A recent multicenter European registry showed that endoscopic suturing had been widely applied for management of GI diseases in 136 patients including closure of mucosal defects, fistula, perforation, postoperative leaks, and stent fixation.[38] The technical success was 99.3% and the overall clinical success was 89%. Endoscopic suturing devices are difficult to use and less intuitive when compared with suturing by robotic surgical system. Moreover, the current endoscopic suturing devices did not achieve a complete loop of surgical knot tying, which may affect the security of tissue approximation especially in full thickness resection.

Flexible endoluminal robotics provide the opportunity to achieve suturing with the GI lumen. In the preclinical study, a figure-of-eight suture was performed using the endoscopic robotic system to close the perforation efficiently.[39] A preclinical animal study confirmed the feasibility of endoscopic full thickness resection (EFTR) using MASTER endoscopic robot, whereas secure closure was achieved using Overstitch endoscopic suturing system (Apollo Endosurgery, Austin, TX).[40] In the future, endoluminal robotic system should be able to achieve tissue resection and approximation.

The current endoluminal flexible robotic systems do not allow exchange of the end-effectors for traction and dissection. In the future, exchange of end-effectors will provide the best solution for performance of complex tasks within the lumen. Moreover, various types of robotic-driven instruments may be designed so as to enhance the performance of specific tasks (eg, a single arm robotic suturing device may improve the ergonomics of suturing within the confined GI lumen). The EndoMaster EASE System required two operators: a surgeon and endoscopist. In the future, partial automation of endoluminal robots will allow a single operator to perform the complex tasks, and the image of the surgical field will be stabilized using artificial intelligence and automation.[41]

INNOVATIVE APPROACH AND CLINICAL APPLICATIONS FOR THIRD SPACE ENDOSCOPY

Third space endoscopy extends the potential of flexible endoscopy for diagnostic and therapeutic purpose beyond the GI lumen. The access to subepithelial space allowed endoscopists to diagnose and treat diseases of the mesenchymal tissue. Inoue and colleagues[42] first reported the performance of per oral endoscopic myotomy (POEM) for treatment of achalasia. POEM was demonstrated in prospective cohort studies to achieve high rates of symptomatic relief for patients with achalasia,[42,43] whereas a prospective multicenter randomized trial showed significantly higher rate of symptomatic response after POEM when compared with pneumatic dilatation.[44] One of the major issues after POEM is the occurrence of gastrointestinal reflux disease (GERD). Although the reported incidence of GERD after POEM varied among varies studies, the typical rate ranged between 20% and 50%.[45,46] Numerous research identified the important factors leading to risks of GERD after POEM, including the transection of sling fibers during myotomy and long myotomy more than 4 cm.[46] Innovative development to tackle GERD after POEM led to the performance of fundoplication after POEM by Inoue and colleagues.[47] In 21 patients with achalasia who received anterior POEM, fundoplication was performed without adverse event. The anterior fundus was fixed to the edge of esophageal myotomy using clips and loop technique. Development of third space endoscopy via POEM opens the potential for endoscopic fundoplication, fulfilling the original concepts of NOTES.[48,49]

The technique of POEM was extended to management of subepithelial tumors with the development of per oral endoscopic tumor resection (POET) and submucosal tunnel endoscopic resection (STER) (**Fig. 2**).[50–52] POET/STER allow resection of subepithelial tumors through a submucosal tunnel without full thickness perforation of the GI tract, avoiding difficulties in secure closure of full thickness defect (**Fig. 3**). These subepithelial tumors included gastrointestinal stromal tumors (GIST), leiomyoma, and schwannoma. A systematic review and meta-analysis confirmed the safety and efficacy of POET/STER in management of upper GI subepithelial tumors with en bloc resection rate of 94.6% and pooled perforation risk of 5.6%.[53]

The family of third space endoscopy had extended quickly to cover the management of numerous GI diseases (see **Fig. 2**).[48] These included diagnostic and therapeutic indications for upper and lower GI tract. In the perspective of therapeutic third space endoscopy in upper GI tract, the procedures covered management of Zenker diverticulum and esophageal diverticulum.[54,55] POET for restoration of the esophagus was described for endoscopic management of a tight esophageal stricture and the restoration of the normal esophageal lumen in the case of a completely occluded esophageal lumen.[56] Recently, our team introduced the performance of cricopharyngeal POEM for management of dysphagia in patients with Parkinson disease.[57] Eight patients with Parkinson disease received cricopharyngeal POEM and had significant improvement in swallowing quality and functional outcomes. Gastric POEM is one of the first extensions of POEM to management of gastroparesis.[58] In a meta-analysis, 10 studies including 482 patients received gastric POEM for management of refractory gastroparesis with at least 1-year follow-up.[59] The results showed that 1-year clinical success in relief of symptoms was 61%, whereas the adverse events rate was 8%.

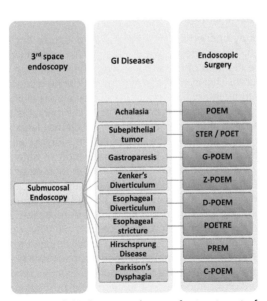

Fig. 2. Current development of third space endoscopy for treatment of various gastrointestinal diseases. C-POEM, cricopharyngeal POEM; D-POEM, diverticulum POEM; G-POEM, gastric peroral endoscopic myotomy; POETRE, peroral endoscopic tunneling for restoration of the esophagus; PREM, per-rectal endoscopic myotomy; Z-POEM, Zenkers POEM

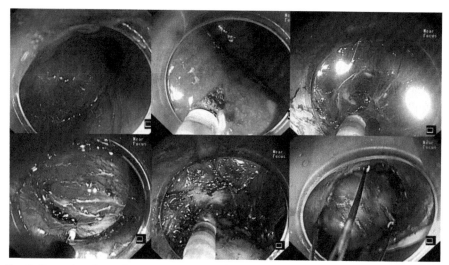

Fig. 3. Peroral endoscopic tumor resection/submucosal tunneling endoscopic resection for treatment of esophageal leiomyoma.

For therapeutic third space endoscopy in lower GI tract, per-rectal endoscopic myotomy was successfully performed for the management of pediatric Hirschsprung disease. In this POEM variant, the aganglionic segment of the muscularis layer in rectum is targeted for the myotomy.[59] Although rectal GIST is uncommon, a recent case report demonstrated the feasibility of rectal STER for treatment of GIST located over the lower rectum.[60]

Limitation of Third Space Endoscopy

Third space endoscopy opened a new horizon in endoscopic access to body space beyond the GI lumen. The concept is safe access with secure closure of the GI window.[49] However, the creation of the submucosal tunnel limits the working space for endoscopic procedures. This is especially important during dissection of GIST when en bloc resection with an intact tumor capsule serves as one of the important oncologic principles in preventing local recurrence.[49,52,61] The manipulation of subepithelial tumors could be difficult within a confined tunnel, which may lead to close dissection plane at the tumor capsule. In a retrospective cohort study comparing endoscopic submucosal excavation, STER, and EFTR for resection of subepithelial tumors in 218 patients, there was no significant difference in en bloc resection and complete resection among these three procedures.[61] However, the en bloc resection and complete resection rate for STER was only 83.7% and 83.7%, respectively, apparently lower than EFTR (en bloc resection 98.4%; complete resection 93.4%) and endoscopic submucosal excavation (en bloc resection 98.2%; complete resection 97.4%).[61] In the management of gastric GIST especially among those with high malignant potential, EFTR may serve as a better procedure to achieve higher en bloc resection without limitation in luminal space for dissection.

Moreover, the creation of submucosal tunnel could be hindered by presence of dense submucosal fibrosis. A retrospective cohort study on 568 patients with achalasia who underwent POEM demonstrated that endoscopic mucosal appearance classified according to Esophageal Mucosa In Achalasia classification correlated significantly with severity of submucosal fibrosis.[62] Among these 568 patients,

POEM procedures were completed in 552 and aborted in 16. The reason for cessation of POEM procedure was severe submucosal fibrosis in 15 of the 16 patients. Submucosal fibrosis could also occur after endoscopic ultrasound–guided fine-needle aspiration/fine-needle biopsy for GI subepithelial tumors, leading to difficulties in creating space for submucosal tunneling during STER/POET.

Although submucosal tunneling allows access to pathologic conditions beyond the GI tract, the access to these pathologic conditions is limited by the tunnel created.[63] A recent retrospective cohort on 1701 cases receiving esophageal STER demonstrated an adverse event rate of 18.8%, whereas 5% of these were categorized as major adverse event.[64] The most common complications included perforation, unintended penetration beyond mucosa, and pneumonitis. The size of the upper GI tract subepithelial tumors retrieved were limited. The largest subepithelial tumors retrieved per orally were less than 6 cm, and most experts would consider the upper limit of the size of resectable tumors to be 4 cm as upper limit to receive STER/POET.[65]

ENDOSCOPIC FULL THICKNESS RESECTION

EFTR was first reported via a transanal endoscopic microsurgery in 1990s.[66] A large operating port was first inserted through the anus and then a laparoscope and other instruments were used for full thickness resection of early rectal neoplasia and suture repair of the luminal defect.[67] Recently, EFTR using the flexible endoscope was developed for the treatment of early GI neoplasia in which dense submucosal fibrosis causes difficulty in ESD and GI subepithelial tumors. EFTR will be able to overcome some of the difficulties of STER/POET in the management of subepithelial tumors, including the challenge of limited space for dissection and the presence of submucosal fibrosis after endoscopic ultrasound–guided fine-needle aspiration.

The American Society for Gastrointestinal Endoscopy Technology committee classified EFTR into "exposed" and "nonexposed," and "exposed" EFTR is subclassified into tunneled and nontunnelled techniques.[67] For exposed EFTR, the techniques originate from ESD where the subepithelial tumor is resected before closure of the luminal defect. The principles of dissection for nontunnelling EFTR are similar to ESD where submucosal dissection should extend beyond the muscularis propria through to the serosa. The resulting luminal full thickness defect results in loss of insufflation during EFTR, and it also requires secure closure without leakage. In our clinical experience on exposed EFTR for gastric GIST, we divided the gastric EFTR into four procedure steps. First, half of mucosa surrounding the gastric GIST is opened after injection to expose the edge of the tumor at the submucosal plane (**Fig. 4**, Video 2). Second, the circumferential edge of tumor further dissects to muscularis propria. After adequate mobilization, we proceed to full thickness incision in the muscularis propria, whereas tumor traction is achieved via transoral clip and line technique. This step is essential to pull the extraluminal component to within the stomach and facilitate endoscopic dissection. Moreover, this exposes the extragastric component at serosa and allows precise dissection to define the serosal tumor border. Third, on further dissection most of the tumor is pulled within the stomach and the dissection is similar to ESD using a combination of a needle-type ESD device and an insulated tip ESD device. After completion of dissection, the tumor is retrieved transorally and avoids dropping of tumor into peritoneal cavity. The fourth step in exposed EFTR is secure closure of the luminal defect. Numerous methods had been reported including multiple clips, clips and loop technique, over-the-scope clip, and endoscopic suturing.[37,67–70] Granata and colleagues[37] reviewed the closure techniques after exposed EFTR. Numerous studies reported the use of pure clip closure techniques after EFTR for gastric lesions.

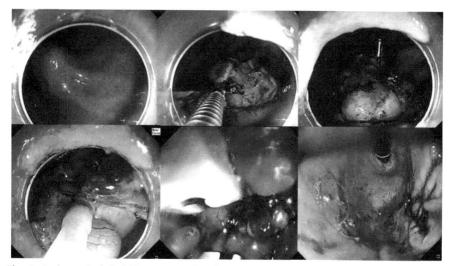

Fig. 4. Endoscopic full thickness resection for treatment of gastric GIST with full thickness closure by single channel overstitch.

The techniques included clips and clips with omental patch with a variation of technical success varied between 80% and 100%.[67] Few patients sustained significant adverse events including peritonitis and abdominal abscess and delayed bleeding. The endoloop-assisted closure method consisted of use of an endoloop with fixation by multiple clips to the edge of the luminal defect before closure. The technical success was 100%, whereas the mean closure time ranged between 9.4 minutes and 22.42 minutes.[67] One patient sustained delayed bleeding after closure. Although there were limited number of cohort studies using OTSC clips for closure, the success of closure was 100% without any adverse events.

Endoscopic suturing provided a secure closure especially after extensive EFTR with luminal defects larger than 20 mm.[68–70] Using the Apollo Overstitch with a double channel or a single channel system allowed continuous full thickness seromucosal suturing.[69] After gastric EFTR, we usually close the full thickness defect via two or three figure-of-eight sutures with overstitch (see **Fig. 3**).

For nonexposed EFTR, the bowel segment containing the target lesion is pulled into the lumen, allowing approximation of the bowel wall before full thickness resection to be performed above the serosal closure.[67] Currently, there are few devices that allow closure of luminal defect before resection including the full thickness resection device (Ovesco Endoscopy, Tubingen, Germany)[71] and endoscopic plicating and suturing devices.[72] In a meta-analysis on the use of full thickness resection device for full thickness resection of colonic lesions not amendable to resection by conventional methods, nine studies including 551 patients showed technical success of 89.25% and complication rates of 10.2%.[73] The pooled rate of major bleeding, postpolypectomy syndrome, and perforation were 0.97%, 2.2%, and 1.2%, respectively. Full thickness resection device seemed to be safe and effective in management of difficult colorectal lesions. However, the size of lesions included in these studies were all less than 20 mm. The Plicator (NDO Surgical, Inc, Mansfield, MA) was used to perform an endoscopic antireflux procedure via full thickness plication. Currently, a similar device named GERDX (G-Surg, Seeon, Germany) was clinically applied for endoscopic antireflux procedure. The use of GERDX for closure of the gastric wall before nonexposed EFTR for resection of gastric subepithelial tumors was reported as one of the methods to overcome the limitation of specimen size obtained using current devices for nonexposure EFTR.[74]

FUTURE OF ROBOTICS AND THIRD SPACE ENDOSCOPY

The current development of third apace endoscopy opens a new horizon for management of GI diseases that are conventionally managed by minimally invasive surgery. We are seeing an extension of third space endoscopy to resection of subepithelial tumors or tumors adjacent to the GI tract.[63] Moreover, third space endoscopy allows secure closure of GI tract, which extends the potential of EFTR to organ resection including purely endoscopic appendicectomy.[75] Recently, endoscopic transgastric cholecystectomy was successfully performed in eight patients without adverse events.[76] Endoscopic transgastric cholecystectomy was performed using instruments for flexible endoscopy, whereas the median operative time was 4 hours. POEM and fundoplication were performed as a transgastric procedure that required manipulation of a flexible endoscope within the peritoneal cavity. The fixation of the fundoplication was achieved either by clip and loop technique or suturing.[47] These procedures demonstrated the potential of endoscopic adjacent organ resection via third space endoscopy, fulfilling the principles and concepts of NOTES. However, it also showed the limitation of current flexible endoscopic devices and instruments especially when laparoscopic cholecystectomy was completed safely in a mean time of 60 minutes.[77]

Flexible robotics provide the potential in enhancing endoscopic devices and instruments for performance of endoscopic adjacent organ resection. With reference to common instruments used for minimally invasive surgery, endoscopic clip applicable to within peritoneal cavity and endoscopic stapling devices should be developed. Palapothu and colleagues[78] reported the use of SurgAssist endoscopic stapler (Power Medical Interventions, Langhorne, PA) for performance of NOTES cystogastrostomy in six patients with 100% technical success. This power-driven endoscopic stapler was also tested in porcine models for the full thickness closure of gastrotomy,[79] and two patients with early gastric cancer and carcinoid tumor received EFTR using this endoscopic stapling device.[80] Unfortunately, there was no further development on this flexible endoscopic power-driven stapling device. Endoscopic stapling provides the optimal approach for nonexposed EFTR especially for management of GISTs, and extends the potential to performing endoscopic sleeve gastrectomy for morbid obesity.[81] The development of an innovative endoscopic suturing device (EndoZip, Nitinotes, Caesarea, Israel) allows full thickness suturing after vacuum wall aspiration to achieve EFTR for endoscopic sleeve gastrectomy. The robotic stapler can also be used to perform endoscopic gastrojejunostomy.[82] The potential of a pure transgastric endoscopic gastrojejunostomy was successfully performed in 11 of 13 porcine models. The mean operative time was 53.6 minutes where the gastrojejunostomy was performed after transgastric retrieval of jejunum through a transgastric introduction of an endostapler. The transgastric endoscopic gastrojejunostomy procedure allows for a pure endoscopic approach with endoscopic stapling and suturing device.

CLINICS CARE POINTS

- POEM and STER are successful procedures based on the concept of third space endoscopy.
- ESD is the standard endoscopic treatment of early gastrointestinal neoplasia. Safe practice of ESD requires intensive training because the skill requires lots of experience.

- Development of flexible robotics aimed to enhance the safe practice of ESD through the use of robotic devices for precise dissection and tissue traction.

DISCLOSURE

Philip Chiu serves as a member of the scientific advisory board of EndoMaster Pte Ltd, Singapore. Siran Zhou and Zhiwei Dong have no conflict of interest to declare.

SUPPLEMENTARY DATA

Supplementary data related to this article can be found online at https://doi.org/10.1016/j.giec.2022.09.006.

REFERENCES

1. Sivak Michael V Jr. Polypectomy: looking back. Gastrointest Endosc 2004;60(6): 977–82.
2. Inoue H. Endoscopic mucosal resection for esophageal and gastric mucosal cancers. Can J Gastroenterol 1998;12(5):355–9.
3. Soetikno R, Kaltenbach T, Yeh R, et al. Endoscopic mucosal resection for early cancers of the upper gastrointestinal tract. J Clin Oncol 2005;23(20):4490–8.
4. Ono H, Kondo H, Gotoda T, et al. Endoscopic mucosal resection for treatment of early gastric cancer. Gut 2001;48(2):225–9.
5. Fujiya M, Tanaka K, Dokoshi T, et al. Efficacy and adverse events of EMR and endoscopic submucosal dissection for the treatment of colon neoplasms: a meta-analysis of studies comparing EMR and endoscopic submucosal dissection. Gastrointest Endosc 2015;81:583–95.
6. Ono H, Yao K, Fujishiro M, et al. Guidelines for endoscopic submucosal dissection and endoscopic mucosal resection for early gastric cancer (second edition). Dig Endosc 2021;33:4–20.
7. Ishihara R, Arima M, Iizuka T, et al. Endoscopic submucosal dissection/endoscopic mucosal resection guidelines for esophageal cancer. Dig Endosc 2020; 32:452–93.
8. Liu Q, Ding L, Qiu X, et al. Updated evaluation of endoscopic submucosal dissection versus surgery for early gastric cancer: a systematic review and meta-analysis. Int J Surg 2020;73:28–41.
9. Facciorusso A, Antonino M, Di Maso M, et al. Endoscopic submucosal dissection vs endoscopic mucosal resection for early gastric cancer: a meta-analysis. World J Gastrointest Endosc 2014;6(11):555–63.
10. Russo P, Barbeiro S, Awadie H, et al. Management of colorectal laterally spreading tumors: a systematic review and meta-analysis. Endosc Int Open 2019;7(2):E239–59.
11. Quero G, Fiorillo C, Longo F, et al. Propensity score-matched comparison of short- and long-term outcomes between surgery and endoscopic submucosal dissection (ESD) for intestinal type early gastric cancer (EGC) of the middle and lower third of the stomach: a European tertiary referral center experience. Surg Endosc 2021;35:2592–600.
12. Tomizawa Y, Friedland S, Hwang JH. Endoscopic submucosal dissection (ESD) for Barrett's esophagus (BE)-related early neoplasia after standard endoscopic management is feasible and safe. Endosc Int Open 2020;8:E498–505.

13. Liu BR, Liu D, Yang W, et al. Mucosal loss as a critical factor in esophageal stricture formation after mucosal resection: a pilot experiment in a porcine model. Surg Endosc 2020;34:551–6.
14. Liu Y, He S, Zhang Y, et al. Comparing long-term outcomes between endoscopic submucosal dissection (ESD) and endoscopic mucosal resection (EMR) for type II esophagogastric junction neoplasm. Ann Transl Med 2021;9:322.
15. Takezawa T, Hayashi Y, Shinozaki S, et al. The pocket-creation method facilitates colonic endoscopic submucosal dissection (with video). Gastrointest Endosc 2019;89(5):1045–53.
16. Kitamura M, Miura Y, Shinozaki S, et al. The pocket-creation method facilitates endoscopic submucosal dissection of gastric neoplasms involving the pyloric ring. Endosc Int Open 2021;9:e1062–6.
17. Yoshida M, Takizawa K, Nonaka S, et al. Conventional versus traction-assisted endoscopic submucosal dissection for large esophageal cancers: a multicenter, randomized controlled trial (with video). Gastrointest Endosc 2020;91:55–65 e2.
18. Ge PS, Thompson CC, Jirapinyo P, et al. Suture pulley countertraction method reduces procedure time and technical demand of endoscopic submucosal dissection among novice endoscopists learning endoscopic submucosal dissection: a prospective randomized ex vivo study. Gastrointest Endosc 2019;89:177–84.
19. Yoshida N, Doyama H, Ota R, et al. Effectiveness of clip-and-snare method using pre-looping technique for gastric endoscopic submucosal dissection. World J Gastrointest Endosc 2016;8:451–7.
20. Nagata M. Advances in traction methods for endoscopic submucosal dissection: what is the best traction method and traction direction? World J Gastroenterol 2022;28:1–22.
21. Nagata M, Fujikawa T, Munakata H. Comparing a conventional and a spring-and-loop with clip traction method of endoscopic submucosal dissection for superficial gastric neoplasms: a randomized controlled trial (with videos). Gastrointest Endosc 2021;93:1097–109.
22. Ebigbo A, Tziatzios G, Gölder SK, et al. Double-endoscope assisted endoscopic submucosal dissection for treating tumors in the rectum and distal colon by expert endoscopists: a feasibility study. Tech Coloproctol 2020;24:1293–9.
23. Gotoda T, Oda I, Tamakawa K, et al. Prospective clinical trial of magnetic-anchor-guided endoscopic submucosal dissection for large early gastric cancer (with videos). Gastrointest Endosc 2009;69:10–5.
24. Ye L, Yuan X, Pang M, et al. Magnetic bead-assisted endoscopic submucosal dissection: a gravity-based traction method for treating large superficial colorectal tumors. Surg Endosc 2019;33:2034–41.
25. Thompson CC, Ryou M, Soper NJ, et al. Evaluation of a manually driven, multitasking platform for complex endoluminal and natural orifice transluminal endoscopic surgery applications (with video). Gastrointest Endosc 2009;70(1):121–5.
26. Ikeda K, Sumiyama K, Tajiri H, et al. Evaluation of a new multitasking platform for endoscopic full-thickness resection. Gastrointest Endosc 2011;73(1):117–22.
27. Yeung BP, Chiu PW. Application of robotics in gastrointestinal endoscopy: a review. World J Gastroenterol 2016;22(5):1811–25.
28. Ho K, Phee SJ, Shabbir A, et al. Endoscopic submucosal dissection of gastric lesions by using a master and slave transluminal endoscopic robot (MASTER). Gastrointest Endosc 2010;72(3):593–9.
29. Zorn L, Nageotte F, Zanne P, et al. A novel telemanipulated robotic assistant for surgical endoscopy: preclinical application to ESD. IEEE Trans Biomed Eng 2018;65(4):797–808.

30. Turiani Hourneaux de Moura D, Aihara H, Jirapinyo P, et al. Robot-assisted endoscopic submucosal dissection versus conventional ESD for colorectal lesions: outcomes of a randomized pilot study in endoscopists without prior ESD experience (with video). Gastrointest Endosc 2019;90(2):290–8.
31. Atallah S, Sanchez A, Bianchi E, et al. Envisioning the future of colorectal surgery: preclinical assessment and detailed description of an endoluminal robotic system (ColubrisMX ELS). Tech Coloproctol 2021;25(11):1199–207.
32. Légner A, Diana M, Halvax P, et al. Endoluminal surgical triangulation 2.0: a new flexible surgical robot. Preliminary pre-clinical results with colonic submucosal dissection. Int J Med Robot 2017;13(3).
33. Sun Z, Ang RY, Lim EW, et al. Enhancement of a master-slave robotic system for natural orifice transluminal endoscopic surgery. Ann Acad Med Singap 2011; 40(5):223–30.
34. Phee SJ, Reddy N, Chiu PW, et al. Robot-assisted endoscopic submucosal dissection is effective in treating patients with early-stage gastric neoplasia. Clin Gastroenterol Hepatol 2012;10(10):1117–21.
35. Takeshita N, Ho KY, Phee SJ, et al. Feasibility of performing esophageal endoscopic submucosal dissection using master and slave transluminal endoscopic robot. Endoscopy 2017;49(S 01):E27–8.
36. Chiu PWY, Ho KY, Phee SJ. Colonic endoscopic submucosal dissection using a novel robotic system (with video). Gastrointest Endosc 2021;93(5):1172–7.
37. Granata A, Martino A, Ligresti D, et al. Closure techniques in exposed endoscopic full-thickness resection: overview and future perspectives in the endoscopic suturing era. World J Gastrointest Surg 2021;13(7):645–54.
38. Maselli R, Palma R, Traina M, et al. Endoscopic suturing for gastrointestinal applications: initial results from a prospective multicenter European registry. Gastrointest Endosc 2022. S0016-5107(22)01740-0.
39. Kaan HL, Ho KY. Endoscopic robotic suturing: the way forward. Saudi J Gastroenterol 2019;25(5):272–6.
40. Chiu PW, Phee SJ, Wang Z, et al. Feasibility of full-thickness gastric resection using master and slave transluminal endoscopic robot and closure by Overstitch: a preclinical study. Surg Endosc 2014;28:319–24.
41. Kaan HL, Ho KY. Robot-assisted endoscopic resection: current status and future directions. Gut Liver 2020;14(2):150–2.
42. Inoue H, Minami H, Kobayashi Y, et al. Peroral endoscopic myotomy (POEM) for esophageal achalasia. Endoscopy 2010;42(4):265–71.
43. Chiu PW, Wu JC, Teoh AY, et al. Peroral endoscopic myotomy for treatment of achalasia: from bench to bedside (with video). Gastrointest Endosc 2013;77(1): 29–38.
44. Ponds FA, Fockens P, Lei A, et al. Effect of peroral endoscopic myotomy vs pneumatic dilation on symptom severity and treatment outcomes among treatment-naive patients with achalasia: a randomized clinical trial. JAMA 2019;322(2): 134–44.
45. Inoue H, Shiwaku H, Kobayashi Y, et al. Statement for gastroesophageal reflux disease after peroral endoscopic myotomy from an international multicenter experience. Esophagus 2020;17(1):3–10.
46. Mota RCL, de Moura EGH, de Moura DTH, et al. Risk factors for gastroesophageal reflux after POEM for achalasia: a systematic review and meta-analysis. Surg Endosc 2021;35(1):383–97.
47. Inoue H, Ueno A, Shimamura Y, et al. Peroral endoscopic myotomy and fundoplication: a novel NOTES procedure. Endoscopy 2019;51(2):161–4.

48. Manolakis AC, Inoue H, Ueno A, et al. 2007-2019: a "third"-space odyssey in the endoscopic management of gastrointestinal tract diseases. Curr Treat Options Gastroenterol 2019;17(2):202–20.
49. Chiu PW, Inoue H, Rösch T. From POEM to POET: applications and perspectives for submucosal tunnel endoscopy. Endoscopy 2016;48(12):1134–42.
50. Onimaru M, Inoue H, Bechara R, et al. Clinical outcomes of per-oral endoscopic tumor resection for submucosal tumors in the esophagus and gastric cardia. Dig Endosc 2020;32(3):328–36.
51. Xu MD, Cai MY, Zhou PH, et al. Submucosal tunneling endoscopic resection: a new technique for treating upper GI submucosal tumors originating from the muscularis propria layer (with videos). Gastrointest Endosc 2012;75(1):195–9.
52. Chiu PWY, Yip HC, Teoh AYB, et al. Per oral endoscopic tumor (POET) resection for treatment of upper gastrointestinal subepithelial tumors. Surg Endosc 2019;33(4):1326–33.
53. Lv XH, Wang CH, Xie Y. Efficacy and safety of submucosal tunneling endoscopic resection for upper gastrointestinal submucosal tumors: a systematic review and meta-analysis. Surg Endosc 2017;31(1):49–63.
54. Zhang H, Huang S, Xia H, et al. The role of peroral endoscopic myotomy for Zenker's diverticulum: a systematic review and meta-analysis. Surg Endosc 2022;36(5):2749–59.
55. Maydeo A, Patil GK, Dalal A. Operative technical tricks and 12-month outcomes of diverticular peroral endoscopic myotomy (D-POEM) in patients with symptomatic esophageal diverticula. Endoscopy 2019;51(12):1136–40.
56. Wagh MS, Draganov PV. Per-oral endoscopic tunneling for restoration of the esophagus: a novel endoscopic submucosal dissection technique for therapy of complete esophageal obstruction. Gastrointest Endosc 2017;85(4):722–7.
57. Wu PI, Szczesniak MM, Omari T, et al. Cricopharyngeal peroral endoscopic myotomy improves oropharyngeal dysphagia in patients with Parkinson's disease. Endosc Int Open 2021;9(11):E1811–9.
58. Khashab MA, Stein E, Clarke JO, et al. Gastric peroral endoscopic myotomy for refractory gastroparesis: first human endoscopic pyloromyotomy (with video). Gastrointest Endosc 2013;78(5):764–8.
59. Kamal F, Khan MA, Lee-Smith W, et al. Systematic review with meta-analysis: one-year outcomes of gastric peroral endoscopic myotomy for refractory gastroparesis. Aliment Pharmacol Ther 2022;55(2):168–77.
60. Wallenhorst T, Jacques J, Lièvre A, et al. Endoscopic resection of a rectal gastrointestinal stromal tumor using the submucosal tunneling endoscopic resection (STER) technique. Endoscopy 2022;54(6):E273–7.
61. Xiu H, Zhao CY, Liu FG, et al. Comparing about three types of endoscopic therapy methods for upper gastrointestinal submucosal tumors originating from the muscularis propria layer. Scand J Gastroenterol 2019;54(12):1481–6.
62. Zhang WG, Linghu EQ, Chai NL, et al. Ling classification describes endoscopic progressive process of achalasia and successful peroral endoscopy myotomy prevents endoscopic progression of achalasia. World J Gastroenterol 2017;23(18):3309–31.
63. Cai MY, Zhu BQ, Xu MD, et al. Submucosal tunnel endoscopic resection for extraluminal tumors: a novel endoscopic method for en bloc resection of predominant extraluminal growing subepithelial tumors or extra-gastrointestinal tumors (with videos). Gastrointest Endosc 2018;88(1):160–7.
64. Xu JQ, Xu JX, Xu XY, et al. Landscape of esophageal submucosal tunneling endoscopic resection-related adverse events in a standardized lexicon: a large

volume of 1701 cases. Surg Endosc 2022. https://doi.org/10.1007/s00464-022-09241-7.

65. Du C, Chai N, Linghu E, et al. Clinical outcomes of endoscopic resection for the treatment of gastric gastrointestinal stromal tumors originating from the muscularis propria: a 7-year experience from a large tertiary center in China. Surg Endosc 2022;36(2):1544–53.

66. Middleton PF, Sutherland LM, Maddern GJ. Transanal endoscopic microsurgery: a systematic review. Dis Colon Rectum 2005;48(2):270–84.

67. ASGE Technology Committee, Aslanian HR, Sethi A, Bhutani MS, et al. ASGE guideline for endoscopic full-thickness resection and submucosal tunnel endoscopic resection. VideoGIE 2019;4(8):343–50.

68. Mori H, Kobara H, Nishiyama N, et al. Current status and future perspectives of endoscopic full-thickness resection. Dig Endosc 2018;30(Suppl 1):25–31.

69. Pawlak KM, Raiter A, Kozłowska-Petriczko K, et al. Optimal endoscopic resection technique for selected gastric GISTs. the endoscopic suturing system combined with ESD-a new alternative? J Clin Med 2020;9(6):1776.

70. Chiba H, Ohata K, Mori H, et al. A novel endoscopic suturing device after endoscopic full-thickness resection of gastric submucosal tumor. Endoscopy 2021. https://doi.org/10.1055/a-1581-7679.

71. Schmidt A, Bauerfeind P, Gubler C, et al. Endoscopic full-thickness resection in the colorectum with a novel over-the-scope device: first experience. Endoscopy 2015;47(8):719–25.

72. Rothstein R, Filipi C, Caca K. Endoscopic full-thickness plication for the treatment of GERD: a randomized, sham-controlled trial. Gastroenterology 2006;131:704–12.

73. Fahmawi Y, Hanjar A, Ahmed Y, et al. Efficacy and safety of full-thickness resection device (FTRD) for colorectal lesions endoscopic full-thickness resection: a systematic review and meta-analysis. J Clin Gastroenterol 2021;55(4):e27–36.

74. Bauder M, Schmidt A, Caca K. Non-exposure device assisted endoscopic full-thickness resection. Gastrointest Endosc Clin N Am 2016;26:297–312.

75. Kantsevoy SV, Robbins G, Raina A, et al. Purely endoscopic appendectomy. VideoGIE 2022;7(7):265–7.

76. Liu XY, Li QL, Xu XY, et al. Endoscopic transgastric cholecystectomy: a novel approach for minimally invasive cholecystectomy. Endoscopy 2021;53(2):E50–1.

77. Pucher PH, Brunt LM, Davies N, et al, SAGES Safe Cholecystectomy Task Force. Outcome trends and safety measures after 30 years of laparoscopic cholecystectomy: a systematic review and pooled data analysis. Surg Endosc 2018;32(5):2175–83.

78. Pallapothu R, Earle DB, Desilets DJ, et al. NOTES(®) stapled cystgastrostomy: a novel approach for surgical management of pancreatic pseudocysts. Surg Endosc 2011;25(3):883–9.

79. Meireles OR, Kantsevoy SV, Assumpcao LR, et al. Reliable gastric closure after natural orifice translumenal endoscopic surgery (NOTES) using a novel automated flexible stapling device. Surg Endosc 2008;22(7):1609–13.

80. Kaehler G, Grobholz R, Langner C. A new technique of endoscopic full-thickness resection using a flexible stapler. Endoscopy 2006;38:86–9.

81. Bove V, Matteo MV, Pontecorvi V, et al. Robotic endoscopic sleeve gastroplasty. Gut 2022;2022:327548. Epub ahead of print. PMID: 35820781.

82. Chiu PW, Wai Ng EK, Teoh AY, et al. Transgastric endoluminal gastrojejunostomy: technical development from bench to animal study (with video). Gastrointest Endosc 2010;71(2):390–3.

Moving?

Make sure your subscription moves with you!

To notify us of your new address, find your **Clinics Account Number** (located on your mailing label above your name), and contact customer service at:

Email: journalscustomerservice-usa@elsevier.com

800-654-2452 (subscribers in the U.S. & Canada)
314-447-8871 (subscribers outside of the U.S. & Canada)

Fax number: 314-447-8029

Elsevier Health Sciences Division
Subscription Customer Service
3251 Riverport Lane
Maryland Heights, MO 63043

*To ensure uninterrupted delivery of your subscription, please notify us at least 4 weeks in advance of move.

Printed and bound by CPI Group (UK) Ltd, Croydon, CR0 4YY

08/05/2025

01864719-0002